Autoimmune Disorders: Diagnosis, Prognosis and Therapeutics

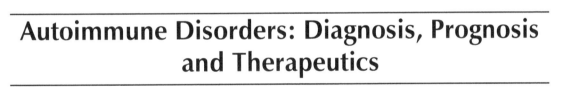

Autoimmune Disorders: Diagnosis, Prognosis and Therapeutics

Editor: Chloe Weber

AMERICAN
MEDICAL PUBLISHERS
www.americanmedicalpublishers.com

AMERICAN
MEDICAL PUBLISHERS
www.americanmedicalpublishers.com

Cataloging-in-publication Data

Autoimmune disorders : diagnosis, prognosis and therapeutics / edited by Chloe Weber.
p. cm.
Includes bibliographical references and index.
ISBN 978-1-63927-906-7
1. Autoimmune diseases. 2. Autoimmune diseases--Diagnosis.
3. Autoimmune diseases--Prognosis. 4. Autoimmune diseases--Treatment.
5. Immunologic diseases. 6. Autoimmunity. I. Weber, Chloe.
RC600 .A88 2023
616.978--dc23

American Medical Publishers,
41 Flatbush Avenue,
1st Floor, New York,
NY 11217, USA

ISBN 978-1-63927-906-7 (Hardback)

Contents

Preface

This book has been a concerted effort by a group of academicians, researchers and scientists, who have contributed their research works for the realization of the book. This book has materialized in the wake of emerging advancements and innovations in this field. Therefore, the need of the hour was to compile all the required researches and disseminate the knowledge to a broad spectrum of people comprising of students, researchers and specialists of the field.

Autoimmune disorders are those health conditions in which the body's immune system attacks and damages the healthy tissues of the body. Some common types of autoimmune disorders are type 1 diabetes, rheumatoid arthritis, psoriatic arthritis, multiple sclerosis, systemic lupus erythematosus, inflammatory bowel disease, Addison's disease, etc. The initial signs and symptoms of many autoimmune disorders share common similarity that includes fatigue, achy muscles, swelling and redness, low-grade fever, trouble concentrating, numbness and tingling in the hands and feet, etc. These disorders are diagnosed by performing antinuclear antibody test (ANA). There are no treatments available to cure autoimmune disorders, but some can help relieve the symptoms. Nonsteroidal anti-inflammatory drugs (NSAIDs), such as ibuprofen and naproxen, and immune-suppressing drugs are used to control the overactive immune response. This book is compiled in such a manner, that it will provide in-depth knowledge about the diagnosis, prognosis and therapeutics of autoimmune disorders. It presents researches and studies performed by experts across the globe. This book will prove to be immensely beneficial to students and researchers in the study of these disorders.

At the end of the preface, I would like to thank the authors for their brilliant chapters and the publisher for guiding us all-through the making of the book till its final stage. Also, I would like to thank my family for providing the support and encouragement throughout my academic career and research projects.

Editor

1

Treatment of Pediatric-Onset Lupus Nephritis: A New Option of Less Cytotoxic Immunosuppressive Therapy

Hiroshi Tanaka[1,2] and Tadaatsu Imaizumi[3]
Department of School Health Science, Faculty of Education Hirosaki University,
[2]Department of Pediatrics, Hirosaki University Hospital and
[3]Department of Vascular Biology, Hirosaki University Graduate School of Medicine
Japan

1. Introduction

Optimal treatment for lupus nephritis in adolescents is still a great challenge. Systemic lupus erythematosus (SLE) is a chronic disease characterized by frequent disease flares for which effective and safe maintenance therapy is required (Chan et al., 2005; Lai et al., 2005). Since diffuse proliferative lupus nephritis (DPLN) is a major concern regarding treatment of young patients with SLE, the optimal immunosuppressive therapy for controlling the activity of DPLN in this population remains controversial (Niaudet, 2000; Tanaka et al., 2004, 2009). Intermittent monthly pulses of intravenous cyclophosphamide (CPA) have been reported to be effective even for patients with pediatric-onset SLE (Lehman & Onel, 2000); however, CPA is a potent immunosuppressive agent associated with myelotoxicity, gonadal toxicity, and an increased risk of secondary malignancy (Chan et al., 2000; Lai et al., 2005). Since therapy related-adverse events are a major therapeutic risk of the immunosuppressive treatment in patients with SLE, selecting a safe and effective treatment protocol poses a big dilemma for physicians treating young patients. Thus, optimal maintenance treatment for controlling the clinical activity of SLE, particularly in young patients with pediatric-onset SLE, remains to be established (Yang et al., 1994; Niaudet, 2000; Tanaka et al., 2001).

Mycofenolate mofetil (MMF) has recently been reported to be as effective as and less toxic than oral CPA or monthly intermittent pulse therapy with intravenous CPA (iv-CPA) for SLE patients (Chan et al., 2000; Lai et al., 2005; Sinclair et al., 2007). However, clinical use of MMF, in patients other than those undergoing solid organ transplantation, has not been approved by the Japanese Ministry of Health and Welfare yet. On the other hand, mizoribine (MZR), a selective inhibitor of inosine monophosphate dehydrogenase in the *de novo* pathway of purine nucleotides, which acts very similar to MMF (Burkhardt & Kalden, 1997; Yokota, 2002), has been successfully used without any serious adverse effects for the long-term treatment of young patients with lupus nephritis (Tanaka et al., 2004; Yumura et al., 2005). We hypothesized that calcineurin inhibitors, other than MZR, might be a feasible alternative treatment for patients with pediatric-onset lupus nephritis (Tanaka et al., 2007a, 2009). Tacrolimus (Tac) is a T-cell-specific calcineurin inhibitor that prevents the activation of helper T cells, thereby inhibiting the transcription of the early activation genes of interleukin (IL)-2

and suppressing the T cell-induced activation of tumor necrosis factor (TNF)-α, IL-1β and IL-6 (Kawai & Yamamoto, 2006). Therefore, Tac is an attractive therapeutic option for young patients with lupus nephritis. We believe that both MZR and Tac may be new options of less cytotoxic immunosuppressive therapy for pediatric patients with lupus nephritis. Recently, a multidrug regimen comprising prednisolone (PDN), Tac, and MMF has been reported to be safe and effective for the treatment of adult lupus (Lanta et al., 2010). We also propose that as an alternative to CPA, a multidrug therapy consisting the immunosuppressive agents, MZR and Tac, which have different modes of action, combined with PDN would be an effective and safe treatment for pediatric-onset SLE (Watanabe et al., 2011).
From our recent clinical experiences, we would like to introduce this new less cytotoxic immunosuppressive therapy for the treatment of pediatric-onset lupus nephritis. Furthermore, we would like to discuss the novel signaling pathways in mesangial cells, which may be involved in the pathogenesis of lupus nephritis.

2. A new option of less cytotoxic immunosuppressive therapy for pediatric-onset lupus nephritis

Recent advances in the management of lupus nephritis, together with earlier renal biopsy and selective use of aggressive immunosuppressive therapy, have contributed to a favorable outcome in children and adolescents with SLE (Yang et al., 1994; Niaudet, 2000; Tanaka et al., 2001). Nevertheless, for optimal control of the activity of lupus nephritis, we believe that more effective and less toxic treatment strategies need to be developed. Although it has been reported that iv-CPA is effective for preserving renal function in adult patients (Austin & Balow, 1999), CPA is a potent immunosuppressive agent that induces severe toxicity, including myelotoxicity, gonadal toxicity, and an increased risk of secondary malignancy (Chan et al, 2000). Thus, the optimal treatment strategy for controlling the activity of lupus nephritis, especially in children and adolescents, is still controversial (Niaudet, 2000; Tanaka et al., 2004).

2.1 Mizoribine, a selective inhibitor of inosine monophosphate dehydrogenase in the *de novo* pathway

The mode of action of mizoribine (MZR) is, very similar to that of MMF, owing to the selective inhibition of inosine monophosphate dehydrogenease (IMPD) in the *de novo* pathway of purine nucleotide synthesis. MZR inhibits T cell and B cell proliferation (Burkhardt & Kalden, 1997; Yokota, 2002). MZR inhibition of IMPD is competitive and different from that induced by MMF (Sonda et al., 1996). Indeed, it has been reported that the concentrations of MZR required to effectively inhibit human mixed-lymphocyte reaction, must reach peak blood levels ranging approximately from 3.0 to 6.0 μg/mL, while beyond the 6.0 μg/mL level, it may lead to myelotoxicity (Sonda et al., 1996). It has also been reported that following MZR administration, 14-3-3 proteins, that is, MZR-binding proteins in *vivo*, interact with glucocorticoid receptors to enhance the transcriptional activity of these receptors (Takahashi et al., 2000). In *vitro*, the MZR concentration required to effectively enhance steroid receptor activity has been reported to be more than 10 μM, which corresponds to a blood MZR level of approximately 2.6 μg/mL. Clinically, MZR has been successfully used without any serious adverse effects for the long-term treatment of young patients with lupus nephritis (Tanaka et al., 2004; Yumura et al., 2005). Based on previous clinical observations, the efficacy of MZR may depend on the peak serum level of the drug

(Tanaka et al., 2003; Nozu et al., 2006; Kuroda et al., 2007). In addition, it has been reported that a peak serum MZR level of at least 2.5-3.0 μg/mL may be needed to effectively suppress of serum anti-dsDNA antibody titers and attain satisfactory clinical efficacy in lupus nephritis patients (Tanaka et al., 2005). However, when using MZR with the conventional protocol of low-dose (3-4 mg/kg) daily MZR (MZR-C) in young patients with lupus nephritis, the peak blood level of the drug usually remains at around 1.0 μg/mL (Tanaka et al., 2003), which may explain the relatively mild efficacy of MZR observed in clinical practice (Kuroda et al., 2007).

In this context, we conducted a trial of relatively long-term (at least 12 months or longer) intermittent pulse therapy with oral MZR (up to 10 mg/kg as a single dose before breakfast on 2 days of the week, MZR-P), to attain increased peak blood levels of MZR, in young patients with flares of lupus nephritis (Tanaka et al., 2008a). Our results suggested that this new treatment protocol was beneficial and resulted in higher efficacy and lower toxicity, in terms of reduction of proteinuria, decrease in the serum anti-dsDNA antibody titer, recovery of hypocomplementemia, preservation serum creatinine level, and decrease in the European Consensus Lupus Activity Measurement index (ECLAM) (Masca et al., 2000) than the MZR-C (Tanaka et al., 2008a and b). The rationale for using MZR-P was as follows: 1) MZR is rapidly excreted into the urine: about 90% of the drug is completely eliminated from the circulation within about 12 hours after oral intake; thus, the accumulation of the drug is not considered to be a problem, at least under the condition of normal renal function (Yokota, 2002). Considering this point, the intermittent use of high-dose MZR may be relatively safe. 2) Higher doses of MZR increase the area under the serum concentration-time curve (AUC) in lupus patients (Yumura et al., 2005); thus, the efficacy of MZR may depend on the peak serum level of the drug, which, in turn, may be closely correlated with the AUC of the drug (Tanaka et al., 2003). 3) In an SLE mouse model, the intermittent administration (every other day) of MZR effectively reduced anti-DNA antibody production (Kamata et al., 1984). In our recent multicenter study, we confirmed that the MZR-P protocol was more effective than the MZR-C protocol, with no serious adverse events occurring during the long-term treatment of young patients with DPLN (Tanaka et al., 2008a). Also, MZR-P showed the potential usefulness of MZR-P as induction therapy in young patients even in those with DPLN (Tanaka et al., 2008a and b). Follow-up renal biopsy specimens obtained after the initiation of MZR-P revealed an apparent improvement in the 2003 classification of lupus nephritis by the International Society of Nephrology/Renal Pathology Society (ISN/RPS), with a decrease in the activity indices without a significant progression in the chronicity indices described by Austin et al. (1984). It is noteworthy that no clinical toxicity, not even amenorrhea- a serious problem in female patients, occurred in any of the study patients. This low clinical toxicity is an important advantage of MZR-P treatment, especially for long-term treatment of young patients.

Besides its immunosuppressive effects, MZR has recently been reported to suppress the progression of histologic chronicity in selected patients with lupus nephritis and IgA nephropathy (Kawasaki et al., 2004; Tanaka et al., 2007b and c; Ikezumi et al., 2008). Moreover, MZR has been reported to attenuate tubulointerstitial fibrosis in a dose-dependent manner in rat models of unilateral ureteral obstruction, non-insulin-dependent diabetes and peritoneal fibrosis via suppression of macrophage infiltration of the interstitium (Sato et al., 2001; Kikuchi et al., 2005; Takahashi et al., 2009). Interestingly, MZR has been reported to bind specifically to heat shock protein (HSP) 60, which results in interference of the chaperone activity of HSP60 *in vitro* (Itoh et al., 1999). This may, in turn, lead to suppression of the activity of α3β1-integrin, which is known to play a role in the

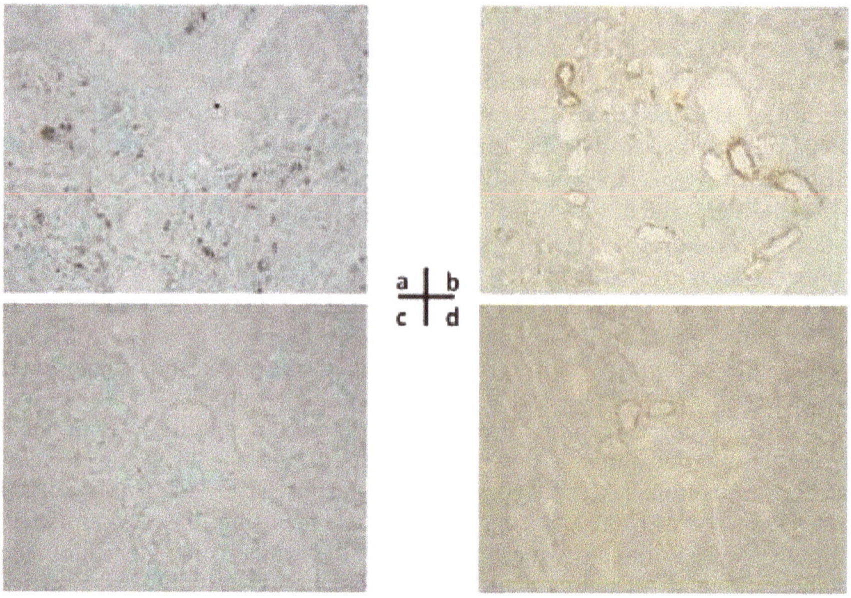

Pre-treatment renal biopsy specimen of a patient with diffuse proliferative lupus nephritis (DPLN) showing numerous CD68-positive cells (a), and the area expressing osteopontin (b) Post-MZR treatment renal biopsy specimen of a patient with DPLN who received MZR treatment showing a significant decrease in the infiltration by CD68-positive cells (c) associated with markedly decrease in the area expressing osteopontin (d)

Fig. 1. (Tanaka H, et al. Clin Rheumatol 2010)

development of interstitial fibrosis. Indeed, in a clinical setting, it has also been reported that posttreatment renal biopsy specimen from patients with severe IgA nephropathy treated with MZR, showed marked attenuation of glomerular and interstitial lesions, and significantly reduced the number of activated macropharges, associated with the expression of 14-3-3 proteins and HSP60, which are known to be MZR-binding proteins, in the inflamed glomerular cells (Ikezumi et al., 2008). Thus, it is speculated that MZR may bind directly to inflamed glomerular cells and prevent progressive damage by suppressing activated macrophages and intrinsic renal cells. Therefore, MZR itself may have a favorable effect against the progression of interstitial fibrosis in the diseased kidney. These laboratory and clinical observations suggest another beneficial mechanism of action of MZR in the treatment of renal diseases. From our recent study, we confirmed the reported beneficial histologic effects of MZR, that is, we found a significant suppression of intraglomerular macrophage infiltration accompanied with significant suppression of the chronicity indices following MZR treatment (Tanaka et al., 2010). MZR treatment also resulted in a decreasing tendency of interstitial macrophage infiltration and the expression of osteopontin, known to be a chemoattractant protein for macrophages (Fig. 1). Since the inflamed glomeruli express 14-3-3 proteins and HSP60 (Ikezumi et al., 2008), MZR may directly interact with inflamed glomerular cells, because MZR is directly excreted into the urine. Moreover, Takeuchi et al. (2010) reported that MZR directly prevented podocyte injury in experimental puromycin aminonucleoside-induced nephropathy, suggesting an anti-proteinuic effect of MZR besides its immunosuppressive effects. These beneficial mechanisms of action of MZR would warrant its use in the treatment of patients with lupus nephritis, although this theory remains speculative. We suspect that this mechanism may represent a mode of action different from that of MMF, although we could not demonstrate whether MZR was superior to MMF treatment for DPLN patients.

Further detailed studies involving a larger number of patients are needed to draw a conclusion. We believe that MZR is an attractive treatment for young patients with lupus nephritis because of attenuated histologic progression resulting from a suppressed accumulation of activated macrophages in the glomeruli. From the view point of the balance between suppression of disease activity and the adverse effects of treatment, we believe that long-term MZR treatment, including use of our MZR-P protocol, may become the new treatment of choice for young patients with lupus nephritis.

2.2 Tacrolimus, a calcineurin inhibitor

Some studies have recently suggested that cyclosporine A (CsA), a calcineurin inhibitor similar to Tac, might replace cytotoxic agents and reduce the dosage of concomitantly administered PDN for maintenance therapy in selected patients with lupus nephritis (Rihova et al., 2007; Moroni et al., 2008). It has been reported CsA treatment has beneficial effects in some pediatric patient with SLE resistant to conventional immunosuppressive therapy, including iv-CPA (Sakano et al., 2004; Suzuki et al., 2006). However, CsA-related nephrotoxicity, posterior reversible encephalopathy syndrome, as well as unfavorable cosmetic effects, such as hypertrichosis and gingival hypertrophy, remain major concerns for young patients with SLE, especially female adolescents.

Tacrolimus (Tac) is a T cell-specific calcineurin inhibitor that prevents activation of helper T cells, thereby inhibiting transcription of the early activation genes of IL-2 and suppressing the production of TNF-α, IL-1β, and IL-6. Considering its effects, Tac is expected to have clinical benefits in the treatment of patients with active SLE. Indeed, to date several papers have described the efficacy and safety of Tac in patients with active SLE (Duddridge & Powell, 1997). Recently, Tac combined with PDN has been successfully administered without serious adverse effects, as induction and maintenance treatment for patients with proliferative and membranous lupus nephritis (Politt et al., 2004; Maruyama et al., 2005; Mok et al., 2005; Tse et al., 2007; Szeto et al., 2008). However, there is little information regarding the efficacy and safety of Tac in young patients with lupus nephritis (Tanaka et al., 2007a, 2009). The safety of Tac treatment is important because of its potent nephrotoxicity. Although these patients did not necessarily have permanently high blood levels of Tac (Duddridge & Powell, 1997; Tse et al., 2007), the development of an optimal Tac treatment strategy for lupus nephritis, with a dose as low as possible, is sought to minimize treatment toxicity while maintaining treatment efficacy. In this context, in Japan, Tac is usually administered once daily for patients with rheumatoid arthritis (RA) or lupus nephritis since once-daily administration of Tac is the governmental approved protocol (Kawai & Yamamoto, 2006; Tanaka et al., 2007a, 2009; Asamiya et al., 2009). Kawai and Yamamoto (2006) reported the safety of Tac administered at a dose of 1.5-3.0 mg once daily for the treatment of RA even in the elderly. Although further studies, including a histologic evaluation following Tac treatment, are needed, we consider that a once-daily regimen could shorten the exposure to Tac, would be more cost-beneficial than the conventional twice-daily protocol, and might result in better treatment compliance. Interestingly, Tac has been reported to stimulate glucocorticoid receptor (GR) transactivity through its ligands (Davies et al., 2005), which may explain the tendency to exacerbate glucose intolerance in selected patients (Mok et al., 2005). However, some patients who had experienced new flares of SLE while receiving CsA were successfully treated with Tac (Tanaka et al., 2007a, 2009). Differential control of the GR hormone-binding function by immunosuppressive ligands, such as Tac, reportedly stimulates GR transactivity beyond the effect of the ligand on hormone retention although this is not the case with CsA (Davies et al., 2005). These laboratory observations may explain the superior effect of Tac to that of CsA in selected patients with lupus, although this hypothesis remains speculative.

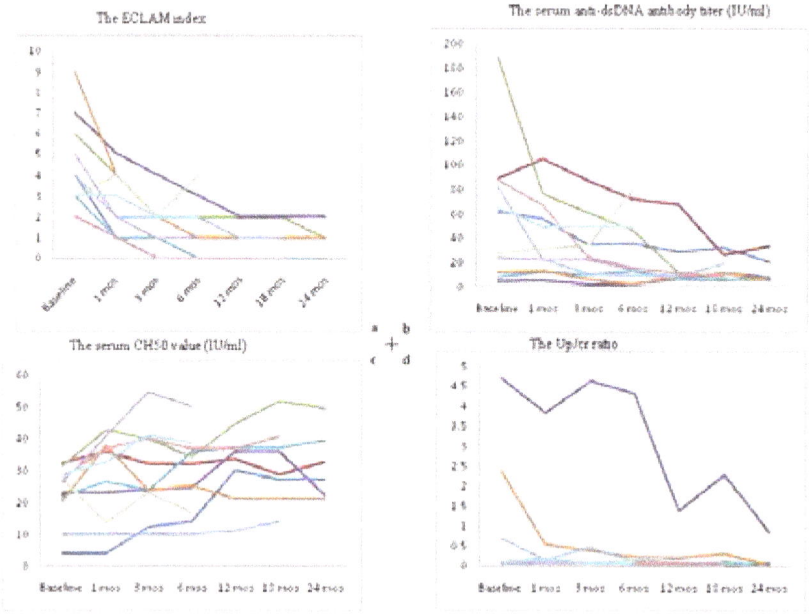

Individual changes in the ECLAM index (a), the serum anti-dsDNA antibody titer (b), the serum complement hemolytic activity (CH50) value (c) and the urinay protein/creatinone (Up/cr) ratio (d) in patients with lupus nephritis (LN) treated with tacrolimus administered once daily. A significant decrease in the ECLAM index was noted after 1 month treatment (a). A significant decrease was also noted in the serum anti-dsDNA antibody titer and the serum CH50 value after 3 months treatment (b, c). One patient with class V LN associated with massive proteinuria showed a significantly decrease in the Up/cr ratio after 12 months treatment (d).

Fig. 2. (Tanaka H, et al. Clin Nephrol 2009)

In our recent study, 11 consecutive patients with long-standing biopsy-proven lupus nephritis were recruited for at least 6 months or longer (6-24 months) as part of an open-label trial of single-daily-dose administration of Tac (3 mg/day, 0.04-0.075 mg/kg). As a result, despite the gradual tapering of the PDN dose, a marked improvement of the ECLAM index, compared with the baseline values, was observed even at 1 month after the start of treatment and in the serological parameters at 3 months. These favorable results persisted until the end of the study. Proteinuria gradually decreased and had dropped significantly by 24 months after the start of treatment (Fig. 2). After a mean of 18 months, a complete response was achieved in 8 patients (73%) and a partial response was achieved in two patients (Tanaka et al., 2009). Adverse reactions to Tac treatment were not severe and were well tolerated. Although the blood levels of Tac in the participants ranged from 1.5 ng/mL to 7.5 ng/mL, no definite relationship between the efficacy of the drug and its blood level was noted. Even though the absorption profile of Tac showed some variations among the study patients, the appropriate blood levels and doses of Tac for the treatment of young patients with lupus nephritis remains to be determined. Measuring the AUC in the pharmacokinetic profile of Tac obtained from each patient is also needed to confirm whether its efficacy depends on its blood levels. From our recent studies, although further studies involving a larger number of patients, including a histologic evaluation following Tac treatment, are needed, we believe that low-dose Tac treatment, administered once daily, may be an effective and safe method for managing selected young patients with pediatric-onset, long-standing lupus nephritis (Tanaka et al., 2007, 2009).

Tac has been reported to reduce proteinuria and mesangial alterations due to its suppressive effects on glomerular expression of IFN-γ mRNA in rat models (Ikezumi et al., 2002) In addition, it has recently been reported that Tac may overcome treatment unresponsiveness through the blockade of the drug exclusion effect of P-glycoprotein, leading to restoration of the intracellular therapeutic levels of corticosteroids and clinical improvement (Suzuki et al., 2010). These laboratory and clinical observations suggest that Tac might have other useful mechanisms of action besides its immunosuppressive effects, which would warrant its use in the treatment of patients with active and steroid-resistant SLE with lupus nephritis.

2.3 New multidrug therapy using tacrolimus and mizoribine

Combination therapy consisting of two immunosuppressive agents with different modes of action is useful and frequently used for immunosuppression in solid organ transplantation.The efficacy of multidrug therapy using MMF and Tac as induction therapy in patients with class V+IV lupus nephritis (DPLN with membranous lesions; Bao et al., 2008), has recently been reported. This multidrug therapy resulted in less cytotoxicity than iv-CPA therapy; the authors concluded that multidrug therapy MMF and Tac was superior to iv-CPA for inducing remission of class V+IV lupus nephritis and was well tolerated. Also, Lanta et al. (2010) reported the efficacy of adding Tac to the MMF plus PDN treatment regimen in some patients with DPLN resistant to MMF and PDN, although clinical toxicity, such as ketoacidosis, infections and muscle pain, limited the use of this combination therapy. Since the mechanisms of action of MMF and Tac are probably complementary, these clinical observations suggested the potential usefulness of multidrug therapy for the treatment of lupus nephritis. However, therapy related-adverse events remain a major therapeutic risk of the immunosuppressive treatment for patients with lupus patients.

The inhibitor of purine synthesis, MZR has reportedly exhibits relatively low clinical toxicity in patients with lupus nephritis (Tanaka et al., 2004; Yumura et al., 2005). Interestingly, aside from its immunosuppressive effect, MZR also appears to have a beneficial effect against the adverse effects of calcineurin inhibitors, such as CsA-induced intimal hyperplasia and perivascular inflammatory cell infiltration observed in rat models (Shimizu et al., 2003; Hara et al., 2009). We recently documented significant suppression of intraglomerular and interstitial macrophage infiltration accompanied by significant suppression of chronicity indices following MZR treatment in patients with lupus nephritis (Tanaka et al., 2010). Thus, we speculate that these histological observations may further support the use of MZR to treat selected patients with glomerular diseases, especially those treated with calcineurin inhibitors, such as CsA or Tac. Moreover, we hypothesized that combination therapy using low-dose Tac administered once-daily and MZR, instead of MMF, might be a beneficial alternative for the treatment of pediatric-onset refractory renal diseases including lupus nephritis (Aizawa-Yashiro et al., 2011; Watanabe et al., 2011).

We present here typical cases of pediatric-onset lupus nephritis in which the efficacy and safety of our novel multidrug therapy were observed. Patient 1 was an 11-year-old Japanese girl with a 2-year history of SLE with ISN/RPS classification class V lupus nephritis. She suddenly developed refractory epistaxis due to severe thrombocytopenia (7,000/μL) associated with serum C4 depression. The patient had been successfully managed with PDN combined with Tac. Consequently, the patient was given an emergency intravenous infusion of high-dose immunoglobulin, which transiently raised her platelet count to 36,000/μL. Because the patient was in a near-pubertal state, we avoided the use of iv-CPA. Thus, we used MZR in addition to Tac. After this combination therapy, her platelet count remained normal at 200,000/μL. The dose of concomitantly administered PDN was tapered without recurrence of thrombocytopenia. At present, 18 months after administration of this therapy, she is free of SLE signs and symptoms without therapy-related clinical toxicity (Watanabe et al., 2011). Patient 2 was a 14-year-old Japanese girl. She was treated with PDN because of hemophagocytic syndrome that she had developed 6 months earlier. When PDN was tapered, she developed malar rash, significant proteinuria/hematuria, hypocomplemententemia and elevation of serum anti-dsDNA antibody titers. Percutaneous renal biopsy revealed ISN/RPS class IIIa lupus nephritis (activity index, 8; chronicity index, 2). She was administered 2 courses of methyprednisolone pulse therapy followed by multidrug therapy consisting of Tac, MZR and PDN. Because she was of pubertal age, the PDN dose was reduced to a minimum at a relative early stage. Her clinical and laboratory signs improved, and the second renal biopsy, performed 12 months after the initial biopsy, revealed marked improvement to ISN/RPS class II lupus nephritis (activity index, 4; chronicity index, 1) without any significant increase in the number of chronic lesions. At present, 36 months after the start of the administration of this therapy, she is free of SLE signs and symptoms without therapy-related clinical toxicity. In lupus nephritis patients, it is well known that flares may occur during long-term immunosuppressive treatment, even after at least a 12 month-long successful treatment with MMF or MZR (Tanaka et al., 2006; Posalski et al., 2009). Although the optimal treatment strategy for managing long-standing SLE, especially in pediatric patients, remains controversial, we believe that our treatment protocol is both effective and safe, and also easy to comply with for patients with pediatric-onset lupus. However, the long-term efficacy and safety of this regimen remains unclear. Further studies in a larger number of young patients with lupus nephritis are necessary to confirm the long-term efficacy and safety of our current protocol.

3. A potential new therapeutic strategy for pediatric-onset lupus nephritis: targeting the IFN regulatory factor signaling pathways

Recently, the importance of innate immunity in the pathogenesis of glomerulonephritis has been reported (Robson, 2009; Coppo et al., 2010). Toll-like receptors (TLRs), which are cell surface and intracelluar receptors for pathogen-associated molecules, play a central role in the response of both the innate and adaptive immune systems to microbial ligands (Robson, 2009). Once presumptive antigenic ligands bind to TLRs, the activation of transcriptional factors, such as interferon regulatory factors (IRF) and nuclear factor kappa B (NF-κB) is induced through intracellular signaling cascade activation. The activation results in the release of adhesion molecules, cytokines and chemokines, which play a pivotal role in the innate and adaptive immune responses (Coppo et al., 2010). Interestingly, recent studies revealed the expressions of TLRs in resident renal cells, suggesting the involvement of the TLR signaling pathway in the pathogenesis of glomerular diseases (Patole et al., 2006).

3.1 The retinoic acid-inducible gene-I (RIG-I) and lupus nephritis

Retinoic acid-inducible gene-I (RIG-I) encodes a DExH box protein, which is a RNA helicase. The DExH box family of proteins regulates RNA metabolism and has various biological functions. Like toll-like receptor (TLR)-3, RIG-I may detect viral RNAs and mediate immune reactions against RNA viruses (Yoneyama et al., 2004). RIG-I has also been suggested to be involved in immune and inflammatory responses in various physiological and morbid conditions (Imaizumi et al., 2009)

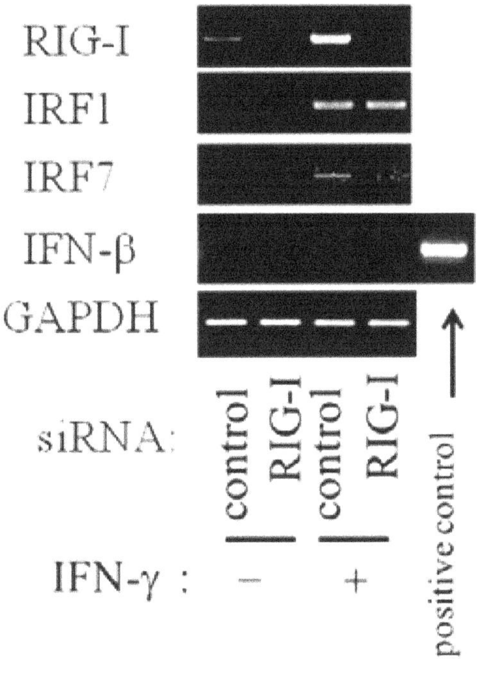

The cells were transfected with siRNA against RIG-I or a negative control non-silencing siRNA. At 24 h after the transfection, the cells were treated with 5 ng/ml IFN-γ for 24 h. RNA was extracted from the cells and RT-PCR analyses for RIG-I, IRF1, IRF7, IFN-β and GAPDH were performed.

Fig. 3. (Imaizumi et al., Lupus 2010)

In a recent study, we showed that RIG-I controlled the immune and inflammatory responses by regulating the expression of various downstream genes, including IFNs regulatory factor (IRF) genes, in mesangial cells (Imaizumi et al., 2010). We previously found RIG-I was highly expressed in the glomeruli examined in biopsy specimens from patients with lupus nephritis, and the level of expression correlated with the severity of acute inflammatory lesions (Suzuki et al., 2007). In addition, we found that the levels of RIG-I mRNA in the urinary sediment of patients with lupus nephritis were higher than those in patients with IgA nephropathy and controls (Tsugawa et al. 2008). Interestingly, repeated measurements of RIG-I mRNA in the urinary sediment of lupus patients revealed a reduction of the expression following immunosuppressive treatment (Tsugawa et al., 2008). These findings suggest that RIG-I may be involved in the acute inflammatory process in human lupus nephritis. In order to examine the involvement of RIG-I in lupus nephritis, we conducted experimental studies using human mesangial cells. Because Th1-derived cytokines are known to be key mediators in the

progression of lupus-associated renal injury, and IFN-γ is one of the major Th1 type cytokines with potent proinflammatory effects that exerts its effects through the upregulation of IFN-inducible genes (Patole et al., 2006), we examined the effects of IFN-γ on the expression of RIG-I in human mesangial cells. As a result, IFN-γ treatment resulted in a concentration-dependent upregulation of the expression of RIG-I mRNA and protein in human mesangial cells. Treatment of cells with IFN-γ also induced the expression of mRNA of both IRF 1 and IRF7, which are important IFN-inducible transcriptional factors. Furthermore, knockdown of RIG-I expression by RNA interference inhibited the IFN-γ-induced expression of IRF7, but not that of IRF1. In contrast, IFN-γ did not induce the expression of IFN-β, which is known to be a target gene of IRF-7, in mesangial cells (Fig. 3) (Imaizumi et al., 2010)
Interestingly, pretreatment of cells with dexamethasone inhibited the IFN-γ-induced expression of monocyte chemoattractant protein (MCP)-1 mRNA but did not affect the induction of RIG-I or IRF7 mRNA in mesangial cells. The induction of MCP-1 mRNA by IFN-γ was not inhibited by the knockdown of NF-κB p65, indicating that the NF-κB signaling pathway was not involved. Our results suggest selective regulation of the expression of IRFs by RIG-I in human mesangial cells. The function of IRF7 has been well studied, mainly in dendritic cells and in mouse embryonic fibroblasts, and IRF7 is thought to be an important transcriptional factor that affects anti-viral responses by inducing the production of type I IFN (Honda et al., 2005).

3.2 Treatment of pediatric-onset lupus nephritis by direct targeting the IFN-γ/RIG-I/IRF7 pathway

Although the functional significance of IRF7 expression in mesangial cells remains to be elucidated, our recent observations suggest that the IFN-γ/RIG-I/IRF7 signaling pathways may be involved in the pathogenesis of lupus nephritis. We believe that the involvement of the newly observed IFN-γ/RIG-I/IRF7 pathway in mesangial cells may contribute to mesangial inflammation, and the intervention of this signaling pathway may lead to the development of optimal future therapeutic strategies for patients with lupus nephritis. However, further clinical and experimental issues remain to be examined in future studies.

4. Acknowledgements

Part of these studies was supported by a Grant from the Japan Society for the Promotion of Science (#21591259 and #22591175) and a grant from The Mother and Child Health Foundation, Osaka, Japan.

5. Conflict of interest statement

None declared.

6. References

Aizawa-Yashiro T, Tsuruga K, Watanabe S, Oki E, Ito E, Tanaka H (2011). Novel multidrug therapy for children with cyclosporine-resistant or -intolerant nephrotic syndrome. *Pediatr Nephrol* DOI: 10.1007/s00467-011-1876-z

Asamiya Y, Uchida K, Otsubo S, Takei T, Nitta K (2009). Clinical assessment of tacrolimus therapy in lupus nephritis: One-year follow-up study in a single center. *Nephron Clin Pract* 113: c330-c336.

Austin HA & Balow JE (1999) Natural history and treatment of lupus nephritis. *Semin Nephrol* 19: 2-11.

Austin HA, Muenz LR, Joyce KM, Antonnovych TT & Balow JE (1984) Diffuse proliferative lupus nephritis: Identification of specific pathologic features affecting renal outcome. *Kidney Int* 25: 689-695.

Bao H, Liu ZH, Xie HL, Hu WX, Zhang HT & Li LS (2008) Successful treatment of class V+IV lupus nephritis with multitarget therapy. *J Am Soc Nephrol* 19: 2001-2010.

Burkhardt H & Kalden JR (1997) Xenobiotic immunosuppressive agents: therapeutic effects in animal models of autoimmune diseases. *Rheumatol Int* 17: 85-90.

Chan TM, Li FK, Tang CSO, Wong RWS, Fang GX, Ji YL, Lau CS, Wong AKM, Tong MKL, Chan KW & Lai KN (2000) Efficacy of mycophenolate mofetil in patients with diffuse proliferative lupus nephritis. *N Engl J Med* 343:1156-1162

Chan TM, Tse KC, Tang CSO, Lai KN & Li FK (2005) Long-term outcome of patients with diffuse proliferative lupus nephritis treated with prednisolone and oral cyclophosphamide followed by azathioprine. *Lupus* 14: 265-272.

Coppo R, Amore A, Peruzzi L, Vergano L & Camilla R (2010). Innate immunity and IgA nephropathy. *J Nephrol* 23: 626-632.

Davies TH, Ning YM, Sanchez ER (2005) Differential control of glucocorticoid receptor hormone-binding function by tetratricopeptide repeat (TPR) proteins and immunosuppressive ligand FK506. *Biochemistry* 44: 2030-2038.

Duddridge M & Powell RJ (1997) Treatment of severe and difficult cases of systemic lupus erythematosus with tacrolimus. A report of three cases. *Ann Rheum Dis* 56: 690-692.

Hara S, Umino D, Someya T, Fujinaga S, Ohtomo Y, Murakami H & Shimizu T (2009) Protective effects of mizoribine on cyclosporine A nephropathy in rats. *Pediatr Res* 66: 524-527

Honda K, Yanai H, Negishi H, Asagiri M, Sato M, Mizutani T, Shimada N, Oba Y, Takaoka A, Yoshida N & Taniguchi T (2005). IRF-7 is the master regulator of type-I interferon-dependent immune responses. *Nature* 434: 772-777.

Ikezumi Y, Kanno K, Koike H, Tomita M, Uchiyama M, Shimizu F, Kawachi H (2002) FK506 ameliorate proteinuria and glomerular lesions induced by anti-Thy 1.1 monoclonal antibody 1-22-3. *Kidney Int* 61: 1339-1350.

Ikezumi Y, Suzuki T, Karasawa T, Kawachi H, Nikolic-Paterson DJ & Uchiyama M (2008) Use of mizoribine as a rescue drug for steroid-resistant pediatric IgA nephropathy. *Pediatr Nephrol* 23: 645-650.

Imaizumi T, Matsumiya T, Yoshida H, Naraoka T, Uesato R, Ishibashi Y, Ota K, Toh S, Fukuda S & Satoh K (2009). Tumor-necrosis factor-α induces retinoic acid-inducible gene-I in rheumatoid fibroblast-like synoviocytes. *Immunol Lett* 122: 89-93.

Imaizumi T, Tanaka H, Tajima A, Tsuruga K, Oki E, Sashinami H, Matsumiya T, Yoshida H, Inoue I & Ito E (2010) Retinoic acid-inducible gene-I (RIG-I) is induced by IFN-γ in human mesangial cells in culture: possible involvement of RIG-I in the inflammation in lupus nephritis. *Lupus* 19: 830-836.

Itoh H, Komatsuda A, Wakui H, Miura AB & Tashima Y (1999) Mammalian HSP60 is a major target for an immunosuppressant mizoribine. *J Biol Chem* 274: 35147- 35151.

Kamata K, Okubo M, Uchiyama T, Masaki Y, Kobayashi Y & Tanaka T (1984) Effect of mizoribine on lupus nephropathy of New Zealand black/white F1 hybrid mice. *Clin Immunol Immunopathol* 33: 31-38.

Kawai S & Yamamoto K (2006) Safety of tacrolimus, an immunosuppressive agent, in the treatment of rheumatoid arthritis in elderly patients. *Rheumatology* (Oxford) 45: 441-444.

Kawasaki Y, Hosoya M, Suzuki J, Onishi N, Takahashi A, Isome M, Nozawa R & Suzuki H (2004) Efficacy of multidrug therapy combined with mizoribine in children with diffuse IgA nephropathy in comparison with multidrug therapy without mizoribine and with methyprednisolone pulse therapy. *Am J Nephrol* 24: 576-581.

Kikuchi Y, Imakiire T, Yamada M, Saigusa T, Hyodo T, Hyodo N, Suzuki S & Miura S (2005) Mizoribine reduces renal injury and macropharge infiltration in non-insulin-dependent diabetic rats. *Nephrol Dial Transplant* 20: 1573-1581.

Kuroda T, Hirose S, Tanabe N, Sato H, Nakatsue T, Ajiro J, Wada Y, Murakami S, Hasegawa H, Ito S, Sakatsume M, Nakano M & Gejyo F (2007) Mizoribine therapy for patients with lupus nephritis: the association between peak mizoribine concentration and clinical efficacy. *Mod Rheumatol* 17: 206-212.

Lai KN, Tang SCW & Mok CC (2005) Treatment for lupus nephritis: a revisit. *Nephrology* (Carlton) 10: 180-188.

Lanata CM, Mahmood T, Fine DM & Petri M (2010) Combination therapy of mycophenolate mofetil and tacrolimus in lupus nephritis. *Lupus* 19: 935-940.

Lehman TJ & Onel K (2000) Intermittent intravenous cyclophosphamide arrests progression of the renal chronicity index in childhood systemic lupus erythematosus. *J Pediatr* 136: 243-247.

Maruyama M, Yamasaki Y, Sada K, Sarai A, Ujike K, Maeshima Y, Nakamura Y, Sugiyama H & Makino H (2006) Good response of membranous lupus nephritis to tacrolimus. *Clin Nephrol* 65: 276-279.

Mok CC, Tong KH, To CH, Siu YP, & Au TC (2005) Tacrolimus for induction therapy of diffuse proliferative lupus nephritis: an open-labeled pilot study. *Kidney Int* 68: 813-817.

Moroni G, Doria A & Ponticelli C. Cyclosporine (CsA) in lupus nephritis: assessing the evidence. Nephrol Dial Transplant 2009; 24: 15-20.

Mosca M, Bencivelli W, Vitali C, Carrai P, Neri R & Bombardieri S (2000) The validity of the ECLAM index for the retrospective evaluation of disease activity in systemic lupus erythematosus. *Lupus* 9: 445-450.

Niaudet P (2000) Treatment of lupus nephritis in children. *Pediatr Nephrol* 14: 158-166.

Nozu K, Iijima K, Kamioka I, Fujita T, Yoshiya K, Tanaka R, Nakanishi K, Yoshikawa N & Matsuo M (2006) High-dose mizoribine treatment for adolescents with systemic lupus erythematosus. *Pediatr Int* 48: 152-157.

Patole PS, Pawar RD, Lech M, Zecher D, Schmidt H, Segerer S, Ellwart A, Henger A, Kretzler M & Anders HJ (2006). Expression and regulation of Toll-like receptors in lupus-like immune complex glomerulomephritis of MRL-Fas (lpr) mice. *Nephrol Dial Transplant* 21: 3062-3073.

Politt D, Heintz B, Floege J & Mertens PR (2004). Tacrolimus- (FK506) based immunosuppression in severe systemic lupus erythematosus. *Clin Nephrol* 62: 49-53.

Posalski JD, Ishimori ML, Wallace DJ & Weisman MH (2009) Does mycophenolate mofetile prevent extra-renal flares in systemic lupus eruthematosus? Results from an observational study of patients in a single practice treated for up to 5 years. *Lupus* 18: 516-521.

Rihova Z, Vankova Z, Maixnerova D, Dostal C, Jancova E, Honsova E, Merta M, Rysava R & Tesar V (2007) Treatment of lupus nephritis with cyclosporine- An outcome analysis. *Kidney Blood Press Res* 30: 124-128.

Robson MG (2009). Toll-like receptors and renal disease. *Nephron Exp Nephrol* 113: e1-e7.

Sakano T, Ohta T, Kinoshita Y. Fujiwara M & Wakai M (2004) Treatment of steroid-resistant systemic lupus erythematosus with extremely low dose of cyclosporine A. *Pediatr Int* 46: 468-470.

Sato N, Shiraiwa K, Kai K, Watanabe A, Ogawa S, Kobayashi Y, Yamagishi-Imai H, Utsunomiya Y & Mitarai T (2001) Mizoribine ameliorates the tubulointerstitial fibrosis of obstructive nephropathy. *Nephron* 89: 177-185.

Shimizu H, Takahashi M, Takeda S, Tahara K, Inoue S, Nakamata Y, Kaneko T, Takeyoshi I, Morishita Y & Kobayashi E (2003) Effect of conversion from cyclosporine A to mizoribine on transplant arteriosclerosis in rat aortic allograft models. *Microsurgery* 23: 454-457

Sinclair A, Appel G, Dooley MA, Ginzler E, Isenberg D, Jayne D, Wofsy D & Solomons N (2007) Mycophenolate mofetil as induction and maintenance therapy for lupus nephritis: rationale and protocol for the randomized, controlled Aspreva Lupus Management Study (ALMS). *Lupus* 16: 972-980.

Sonda K, Takahashi K, Tanabe K, Fuchinoue S, Hayasaka Y, Kawaguchi H, Teraoka S, Toma H & Ota K (1996) Clinical pharmacokinetic study of mizoribine in renal transplantation patients. *Transplant Proc* 28: 3643-3648.

Suzuki K, Imaizumi T, Oki E, Tsugawa K, Ito E & Tanaka H (2007) Expression of retinoic acid-inducible gene-I in lupus nephritis. *Nephrol Dial Transplant* 22: 2407-2409.

Suzuki K, Saito K, Tsujimura S, Nakayamada S, Yamaoka K, Sawamukai N, Ieata S, Nawata M, Nakano K & Tanaka Y (2010) Tacrolimus, a calcineurin inhibitor, overcomes treatment unresponsiveness mediated by p-glycoprotein on lymphocytes in refractory rheumatoid arthritis. *J Rheumatol* 37: 512-520.

Suzuki K, Tanaka H, Tsugawa K & Ito E (2006) Effective treatment with cyclosporine A of a child with systemic lupus erythematosus resistant to cyclophosphamide pulse therapy. *Tohoku J Exp Med* 208: 355-359.

Szeto CC, Kwan BCH, Lai FMM, Tam LS, Li EKM, Chow KM, Gang W & Li PKT (2008) Tacrolimus for the treatment of systemic lupus erythematosus with pure class V nephritis. *Rheumatology* (Oxford) 47: 1678-1681.

Takahashi S, Taniguchi Y, Nakashima A, Arakawa T, Kawai T, Doi S, Ito T, Masaki T, Kohno N & Yorioka N (2009) Mizoribine suppresses the progression of experimental peritoneal fibrosis in a rat model. *Nephron Exp Nephrol* 112: e59-e69.

Takahashi S, Wakui H, Gustafsson JA, Zilliacus J & Itoh H (2000) Functional interaction of the immunosuppressant mizoribine with the 14-3-3 protein. *Biochem Biophys Res Commun* 274: 87-92.

Takeuchi S, Hiromura K, Tomioka M, Takahashi S, Sakairi T, Maeshima A, Kaneko Y, Kuroiwa T & Nojima Y (2010) The immunosuppressive drug mizoribine directory prevents podocyte injury in puromycin aminosucleoside nephrosis. *Nephron Exp Nephrol* 116: e3-e10

Tanaka H, Oki E, Tsuruga K, Aizawa-Yashiro T, Ito Y, Sato N, Kawasaki Y & Suzuki J (2010) Mizoribine attenuates renal injury and macrophage infiltration in patients with severe lupus nephritis. *Clin Rheumatol* 29: 1049-1054.

Tanaka H, Oki E, Tsugawa K, Nonaka K, Suzuki K & Ito E (2007a). Effective treatment of young patients with pediatric-onset, long-standing lupus nephritis with tacrolimus given as a single daily dose: An open-label pilot study. *Lupus* 16: 896-900.

Tanaka H, Oki E, Tsuruga K, Sato N, Matsukura H, Matsunaga A, Kondo Y, Suzuki J (2008a) Mizoribine treatment of young patients with severe lupus nephritis: A clinicopathologic study by the Tohoku Pediatric Study Group. *Nephron Clin Pract* 110: c73-c79.

Tanaka H, Oki Es, Tsugawa K, Suzuki K, Tsuruga K & Ito E (2007b) Long-term intermittent pulse therapy with mizoribine attenuates histologic progression in young patients with severe lupus nephritis: Report of two patients. *Nephrology* (Carlton) 12: 376-379.

Tanaka H, Oki E, Tsuruga K, Yashiro T, Hanada I & Ito E (2009) Management of young patients with lupus nephritis using tacrolimus administered as a single daily dose. *Clin Nephrol* 72: 430-436.

Tanaka H, Suzuki K, Nakahata T, Tsugawa K, Ito E & Waga S (2003) Mizoribine oral pulse therapy for patients with disease flare of lupus nephritis. *Clin Nephrol* 60: 390-394.

Tanaka H, Tateyama T & Waga S (2001) Methylprednisolone pulse therapy in Japanese children with severe lupus nephritis. *Pediatr Nephrol* 16: 817-819.

Tanaka H, Tsugawa K, Nakahata T, Kudo M, Suzuki K & Ito E (2005) Implication of peak serum level of mizoribine for control the serum anti-dsDNA antibody titer in patients with lupus nephritis. *Clin Nephrol* 63: 417-422.

Tanaka H, Tsugawa K, Oki E, Suzuki K & Ito E (2008b) Mizoribine intermittent pulse therapy for induction therapy for systemic lupus erythematosus in children: an open-label pilot study with five newly diagnosed patients. *Clin Rheumatol* 27: 85-89.

Tanaka H, Tsugawa K, Oki E, Suzuki K, Waga S & Ito E (2007c) Long-term mizoribine intermittent pulse therapy, but not azathioprine therapy, attenuated histologic progression in a patient with severe lupus nephritis. *Clin Nephrol* 68: 198-200.

Tanaka H, Tsugawa K, Suzuki K, Nakahata T & Ito E (2006) Long-term mizoribine intermittent pulse therapy for young patients with flare of lupus nephritis. *Pediatr Nephrol* 21: 962-966.

Tanaka H, Tsugawa K, Tsuruga K, Nakahata T, Suzuki K, Ito E &Waga S (2004) Mizoribine for the treatment of lupus nephritis in children and adolescents. *Clin Nephrol* 62: 412-417.

Tse KC, Lam MF, Tang SCW, Tang CSO & Chan TM (2007) A pilot study on tacrolimus treatment in membranous or quiescent lupus nephritis with proteinuria resistant to angiotensin inhibitor or blockade. *Lupus* 16: 46-51.

Tsugawa K, Oki E, Suzuki K, Imaizumi T, Ito E & Tanaka H (2008) Expression of mRNA for functional molecules in urinary sediment in glomerulonephritis. Pediatr Nephrol 23: 395-401.

Watanabe S, Tsuruga K, Aizawa-Yashiro T, Oki E, Ito E & Tanaka H (2011) Addition of mizoribine to the prednisolone plus tacrolimus treatment regimen in a patient with lupus flare. *Rheumatol Int* DOI: 10.1007/s00296-011-1858-2.

Yang LY, Chen WP & Lin CY (1994) Lupus nephritis in children. A review of 167 patients. *Pediatrics* 94:335-340

Yokota S (2002) Mizoribine: Mode of action and effects in clinical use. *Pediatr Int* 44: 196-198.

Yoneyama M, Kikuchi M, Natsukawa T, Shinobu N, Imaizumi T, Miyagishi M, Taira K, Akira S & Fujita T (2004). The RNA helicase RIG-I has an essential function in double-stranded RNA-induced innate antiviral responses. *Nat Immunol* 5: 730-737.

Yumura W, Suganuma K, Uchida K, Moriyama T, Otsubo S, Takei T, Naito M, Koike M, Nitta K & Nihei H (2005) Effects of long-term treatment with mizoribine in patients with proliferative lupus nephritis. *Clin Nephrol* 64: 28-34.

2

Intravenous Immunoglobulins in Neurological Diseases: Established and Novel Clinical Applications

Konstantina G. Yiannopoulou
Neurological Department, Laiko General Hospital of Athens
Greece

1. Introduction

Over the last decade, high-dose polyclonal intravenous immunoglobulin (IVIg) is used increasingly in the management of autoimmune conditions of the central and peripheral nervous system. Despite the expanded use of IVIg, the consensus on its optimal use is insufficient. Currently chronic idiopathic demyelinating polyneuropathy (CIDP), Guillain - Barre syndrome (GBS) and multifocal motor neuropathy (MMN) are the three major immune neuropathies, in which the latest evidence strongly supports the use of IVIg as a first-line therapy. In addition to these disorders, there is a rising number of other neurological indications in which IVIg has been used as a therapy, even though the available evidence-based data are relatively sparse and less convincing. Due to increasing costs of this treatment and relative shortage of products, careful selection of patients who will benefit from IVIg is extremely important (Elovaara & Hietaharju, 2010).
In this paper the current literature on the use of IVIG in treatment of neurological diseases has been reviewed and evidence-based recommendations, as well as less convincing data and future possibilities for its use in these disorders are presented.

2. IVIg in therapy of autoimmune neuropathies

Currently CIDP, GBS and MMN are the three major immune neuropathies, in which the latest evidence strongly supports the use of IVIg as a first-line therapy (level A recommendation). However, questions remain regarding the dose, timing and duration of IVIg treatment in these disorders. The efficacy of IVIg has been also proven in some paraneoplastic neuropathies (level B) (European Federation of Neurology Society [EFNS] task force, 2008; Elovaara & Hietaharju, 2010). There are other peripheral neuropathies in which there are reports of the efficacy of IVIg. These include diabetic amyotrophy, vasculitic peripheral neuropathy and painful sensory neuropathy associated with Sjogren's syndrome. The evidence for these conditions has been insufficient to earn a recommendation for the use of IVIg from national or international guidelines (Hughes et al, 2009).

2.1 Guillan-barre syndrome (GBS)

GBS is an autoimmune disorder of the peripheral nervous system. The incidence of GBS is approximately two per 100 000/year in adults. It may lead to respiratory failure requiring artificial ventilation in up to 30% of patients and about 5% die in this disease (Hughes et al, 2006).

GBS consists of four major subtypes: acute inflammatory demyelinating polyneuropathy (AIDP); acute motor axonal neuropathy (AMAN); acute motor and sensory axonal neuropathy (AMSAN); and Fisher syndrome. The subtypes can be differentiated by clinical, electrophysiological and pathological findings. Diagnosis of GBS is made in the setting of the classic clinical scenario of a monophasic illness reaching a nadir within 4 weeks with symmetric weakness and sensory loss, areflexia and elevated cerebrospinal fluid (CSF) protein without pleocytosis. Presumed antecedent inciting events, such as infections, occur in up to 80% (van Doorn P.A. et al, 2008).

Molecular mimicry probably plays an important role in the pathogenesis. Infection with a pathological agent such as *Campylobacter jejuni* leads to the formation of cross-reacting antibodies. In AIDP, such cross-reacting anti-myelin or anti-ganglioside antibodies attack Schwann cell surface epitopes of motor and sensory fibres. Subsequent complement activation and macrophage infiltration leads to multi-focal inflammatory demyelination with conduction failure and secondary axonal degeneration. AMAN and AMSAN are characterized by axonal/nodal antibody binding, complement activation, macrophage attachment at nodes, opening of the periaxonal space and macrophage infiltration in motor axons in AMAN, or in motor and sensory axons in AMSAN (van Doorn P.A. et al, 2008).

The proposed autoimmune aetiology led to the introduction of immunotherapy. Before its introduction, 10% of patients died and 20% were left seriously disabled (EFNS task force, 2008). Plasma exchange (PE) was the first treatment of GBS that was shown to offer a significant benefit in randomized controlled trials (RCT) and became. The first RCT on the use of IVIg was published in 1992, followed later by other trials.

Even though both IVIG and PE are considered as first-line therapy for GBS, IVIG is usually favored over PE due to its simplicity and better availability. Standard therapy of IVIG is 0.4 g / kg given for 5 days, but there is only limited evidence concerning the optimal dosage. There are also other unanswered questions. Additional primary treatments are needed, as up to 20% of patients with GBS die or are unable to walk after 1 year. Treatments to enhance nerve regeneration and to improve function in existing but partially repaired nerves are also required. The Inflammatory Neuropathy Consortium of the Peripheral Nerve Society defined a need for trials of IVIg treatment in mild GBS and Fisher syndrome, an IVIg dose-finding study in GBS and studies on the use of complement inhibitors and sodium channel blockers (Hughes et al, 2009).The most urgent question is whether patients who continue to deteriorate after a standard course of IVIG should receive a second course or receive some other additional treatment An international study concerning this last issue is about to be launched in the near future (Elovaara & Hietaharju, 2010).

Recommendations:

- IVIg 0.4 g/kg/day for 5 days or PE can be used as first line treatment and are considered to be equally effective (level A).
- IVIg has lesser side effects than PE and this would favour IVIg over PE treatment (level B). --IVIg treatment after PE, as standard combination, does not produce significant extra benefit and can not be recommended (level B).
- Combining high-dose intravenous methylprednisolone with IVIg may have a minor shortterm benefit (level C).
- Children, who generally have a better prognosis, should be treated with IVIg as firstline treatment (level C).

- Patients who improve after IVIg and then relapse should preferentially be retreated with a second course of IVIg (good practice point).
- In patients who seem to be unresponsive to the first course of IVIg a second course may be tried, but evidence supporting such a strategy is lacking (good practice point).
- No recommendations can be given whether mildly affected GBS patients or patients with Miller Fisher syndrome should be treated with IVIG. (EFNS task force, 2008).

2.2 Chronic Inflammatory Demyelinating Polyneuropathy (CIDP)

CIDP is a progressive or relapsing autoimmune disease that targets the myelin sheaths of the peripheral nerves, leading to weakness, sensory loss and impairment of gait and coordination. It has a variable clinical course causing both temporary and permanent disability. There is no definitive test for CIDP, and in most patients diagnosis is based on the clinical presentation and demonstration of demyelinating abnormalities in electrodiagnostic studies (Hughes et al, 2009).

It has been shown to respond to several therapies, including corticosteroids, PE and IVIg. The efficacy of IVIg has been assessed in five RCTs including 235 participants. In addition, there is one RCT, which has compared IVIg with PE, and one study, which has compared IVIg with prednisolone. A recently published Cochrane review summarizes the results of these studies and concludes that IVIg therapy improves disability for at least 2-6 weeks compared with placebo (Eftimov et al., 2009). During this induction period IVIg has an efficacy similar to PE and corticosteroids.

The ICE study (Hughes et al, 2008) that is included in this review is not only the largest but also the longest reported RCT ever performed in CIDP patients. Furthermore, it was the first trial aimed to assess the long-term efficacy of IVIg. The results of ICE study unequivocally demonstrated a beneficial effect on disability that is sustained up to 48 weeks.

The initial dose used in the ICE study (2 g/kg) was similar to that used in practice. This dose was shown to be more effective than 1 g/kg or 0·25 g/kg, although higher doses were not examined. The initial dose is usually given over one or several days, depending on tolerability or convenience. Patients who do not respond to an initial dose may respond to subsequent doses. In the ICE study, 44% of responders improved by 3weeks after the initial treatment, and an additional 50% of patients responded only after a second dose of 1 g/kg at week 3, as measured at week 6 of the study. However, it is not known whether even more patients would have improved if additional treatments had been given, as patients who did not show improvement, including those who were stable, were crossed-over at week 6. In clinical practice, initial responses have been seen up to 3 months into the treatment, and stabilization of previously progressive disease is considered to be a positive response (Hughes et al, 2009).

IVIg responsive patients in the ICE trial were treated with 1 g/kg every 3 weeks for up to 24 weeks, with the responsive patients re-randomized to continue treatment or placebo in phase 2 of the study for an additional 24 weeks. Continued improvement was observed in some patients at up to 32 weeks into the study. Approximately 50% of the responders in the first phase of the study suffered a relapse during phase 2 when switched to placebo. Given the goal of achieving maximal improvement, a reasonable strategy would be to continue treatment until the improvement plateaus, before stopping to see whether additional treatments are still needed. Discontinuing the treatments prior to that point would risk leaving the patient with less than optimal function.

CIDP patients with very mild symptoms may not need any treatment at all. Approximately 20% of the CIDP patients seem to improve spontaneously. Treatment should be considered for patients with moderate or severe disability. IVIg (2 g / kg in 2-5 days) or corticosteroids (1 mg / kg or 60 mg daily) are recommended as first-line treatment in sensory and motor CIDP (EFNS task force, 2008). For pure motor CIDP, IVIg treatment should be the first choice and if corticosteroids are used, patients should be monitored closely for deterioration. In patients with relapsing-remitting CIDP responding to IVIg, attempts should be made to reduce the dose in order to find out if the patient still needs IVIg and what is the adequate dose. In addition to IVIg, PE can be considered as a treatment of choice in long-term therapy of relapsing-remitting CIDP. A number of immunosuppressant and chemotherapeutic agents have been reported to be effective in open studies, but only azathioprine and interferon beta have been investigated in RCT, with negative results (Hughes et al, 2004).
CIDP is a treatable disease whose manifestations can be prevented by early diagnosis and treatment with IVIg. Additional efforts are needed, however, to develop more reliable diagnostic tests, establish optimal treatment regimens and increase awareness of this condition.
Recommendations:

- Patients with very mild symptoms which do not or only slightly interfere with activities of daily living may be monitored without treatment (good practice point).
- Treatment should be considered for patients with moderate or severe disability.
- IVIg (2 g/kg in 2-5 days) (level A) or corticosteroids (1 mg/kg or 60 mg daily) (level B) can be used as first-line treatment in sensorimotor CIDP. The presence of relative contraindications to either treatment should influence the choice (good practice point). - For pure motor CIDP IVIg treatment should be first choice and if corticosteroids are used, patients should be monitored closely for deterioration (good practice point).
- If a patient responds to IVIg, attempts should be made at intervals to reduce the dose to discover whether the patient still needs IVIg and what dose is needed (good practice point).
- It is important to avoid deterioration sometimes seen just before the next IVIg course. The treatment intervals should be such that this deterioration does not happen.
- If a patient becomes stable on intermittent IVIg the dose should be reduced before the frequency of administration is lowered (good practice point) (EFNS task force, 2008).

2.3 Multifocal motor neuropathy (MMN)

MMN is a rare autoimmune disorder which may cause prolonged periods of disability due to progressive weakness of one or more limbs.
There are four RCTs, which have examined the effects of IVIg vs placebo in patients with MMN. The total number of participants in these trials was only 34. A Cochrane review, however, showed that muscle strength improved in 78% of patients treated with IVIg and only in 4% of those who received placebo (van Schaik et al, 2005).
Because both prednisolone and PE have proved to be ineffective and even harmful, and cyclophosphamide, even though moderately effective, has significant side effects in long-term use, IVIg remains the only beneficial treatment for MMN.
Approximately one third of patients with MMN have a sustained remission (>12 months) with IVIg alone and approximately half of the patients need repeated IVIg infusions (Leger et al, 2008). The effect of IVIg declines during prolonged treatment, even if the dosage is increased, probably due to ongoing axonal degeneration (Terenghi et al, 2004).

There is only one RCT on the use of an immunosuppressive agent as an additional therapy (Piepers et al, 2007). This study with 28 patients showed that mycophenolate mofetil neither produced significant benefit nor reduced the need for IVIg.
Elevated anti-ganglioside GM1 antibodies and definite conduction block have been shown to be correlated with a favourable response to IVIg (class IV evidence) (EFNS task force, 2008). However, in one retrospective study, treatment with higher than normal maintenance doses of IVIg (1.6–2.0 g/kg given over 4–5 days) promoted re-innervation, decreased the number of conduction blocks and prevented axonal degeneration in 10 MMN patients for up to 12 years (Vucic et al, 2004).
Recommendations:

- As there is no other treatment of proven benefit, the recommendation is to use IVIg (2 g/kg in 2–5 days) as a first-line treatment (level A).
- If the initial IVIg treatment is effective, repeated infusions should be considered (level C).
- A considerable number of patients need prolonged treatment, but attempts should be made to decrease the dose to discover whether a patient still needs IVIg (good practice point).
- Furthermore, the frequency of maintenance therapy should be guided by the individual response, whereby typical treatment regimens are 1 g/kg every 2–4 weeks or 2 g/kg every 4–8 weeks (good practice point) (EFNS task force, 2008).

2.4 Paraproteinaemic demyelinating neuropathy

Paraproteinaemia, also known as monoclonal gammopathy, is characterized by the presence of abnormal immunoglobulin (M protein) produced by bone marrow cells in blood. The different types of immunoglobulin are classified according to the heavy chain class as IgG, IgA or IgM. The non-malignant paraproteinaemias are generally referred to as monoclonal gammopathy of undetermined significance (MGUS).
Paraproteins are found in up to 10% of patients with peripheral neuropathy which is not secondary to another primary illness. In about 60% of patients with MGUS-related neuropathy the paraprotein belongs to the IgM subclass. In almost 50% of patients who have IgM MGUS and a peripheral neuropathy, the M protein reacts against myelin-associated glycoprotein. The most common type of IgM MGUS related peripheral nerve involvement is a distal, symmetrical demyelinating neuropathy. Patients with IgG or IgA paraproteinaemic neuropathy usually have both proximal and distal weakness and sensory impairment that is indistinguishable from CIDP.
Two RCTs with IVIg have been performed, encompassing 33 patients with IgM paraproteinaemic demyelinating neuropathy (class II). A third randomized study was an open parallel group trial with 20 patients which compared IVIg and recombinant interferon-a (class II). The results of these three trials have been summarized in a Cochrane review, which concluded that IVIg is relatively safe and may produce some short-term benefit (Lunn & Nobile-Orazio, 2006).
No RCTs are available on the effects of IVIg in IgG or IgA paraproteinaemic neuropathy. There is one retrospective review of 20 patients with IgG MGUS neuropathy treated with IVIg; beneficial response was found in eight of them (class IV). An open prospective trial of IVIg reported clinical improvement in two of four patients with IgG MGUS (class IV). In a review which included 124 patients with IgG MGUS neuropathy, 81% of the 67 patients with a predominantly demyelinating neuropathy responded to the same immunotherapies

used for CIDP (including IVIg) as compared with 20% of those with axonal neuropathy (class IV). A Cochrane review states that observational or open trial data provides limited support for the use of immunotherapy, including IVIg, in patients with IgG and IgA paraproteinaemic neuropathy (Allen et al, 2007).

Recommendations:

- IVIg should be considered as initial treatment of demyelinating IgM MGUS-related neuropathy (level B recommendation).
- As long as long-term effects and cost-benefit aspects are not known, routine use of IVIg cannot be recommended in patients without significant disability (good practice point).
- However, in patients with significant disability or rapid worsening, IVIg may be tried, although its efficacy is not proven (good practice point).
- In patients with CIDP-like neuropathy, the detection of paraproteinaemia does not justify a different therapeutic approach from CIDP without a paraprotein. (EFNS task force, 2008).

2.5 Diabetic amyotrophy

Lumbosacral radiculoplexus neuropathy (LRPN) originally described in diabetic patients as diabetic amyotrophy is a distinct clinical condition characterized by debilitating pain, weakness and atrophy most commonly affecting the proximal thigh muscles asymmetrically. The syndrome is usually monophasic and preceded by significant weight loss (at least more than 10 lbs). Though a self-limited condition, recovery is gradual with some residual weakness (Bhanushai & Muley, 2008).

- There are reports and small open studies of the efficacy of IVIg in diabetic amyotrophy (Hughes et al, 2009).

Recommendations:

- The evidence for this condition has been insufficient to earn a recommendation for the use of IVIg.

2.6 Vasculitic peripheral neuropathy

Vasculitic neuropathy is routinely considered as a vasculitis associated with neuropathy. The consensus definition of pathologically definite vasculitic neuropathy requires that vessel wall inflammation is accompanied by vascular damage. A case definition of clinically probable vasculitic neuropathy in patients lacking biopsy proof incorporates clinical features typical of vasculitic neuropathy: sensory or sensory-motor involvement, asymmetric/multifocal pattern, lower-limb predominance, distal-predominance, pain, acute relapsing course, and non-demyelinating electrodiagnostic features (Good Practice Points from class II/III evidence). (Collins et al, 2010). There are reports of the efficacy of IVIg in vasculitic peripheral neuropathy (Hughes et al, 2009).

Recommendations:

- The evidence for this condition has been insufficient to earn a recommendation for the use of IVIg.

2.7 Painful sensory neuropathy of Sjogren's syndrome

Primary Sjogren's syndrome is associated with seven forms of neuropathy: sensory ataxic neuropathy, painful sensory neuropathy without sensory ataxia, multiple mononeuropathy, multiple cranial neuropathy, trigeminal neuropathy, autonomic neuropathy and radiculoneuropathy, based on the predominant neuropathic symptoms. The majority of patients are diagnosed with Sjogren's syndrome after neuropathic symptoms appearance. Painful sensory neuropathy without sensory ataxia is the second more frequent form of neuropathy associated with Sjogren's syndrome. It is characterised by chronic progression of sensory symptoms without substantial motor involvement, although the affected sensory modalities and distribution pattern vary. Autonomic symptoms, like abnormal pupils and orthostatic hypotension are often seen. Unelicited somatosensory evoked potentials and spinal cord posterior column abnormalities in MRI are observed. Sural nerve biopsy specimens reveal variable degrees of axon loss, predominantly small fibre loss (Mori et al, 2005). Patients usually suffer from severe neuropathic pain, with small-fiber neuropathy causing lancinating or burning pain which can disproportionately affect the proximal torso or extremities, and the face (ie, in a "non-length-dependent distribution") (Birnbaum, 2010).

There are reports and small open studies of the efficacy of IVIg in painful sensory neuropathy associated with Sjogren's syndrome (Hughes et al, 2009).

Recommendations:

- The evidence for this condition has been insufficient to earn a recommendation for the use of IVIg.

3. IVIg in therapy of myasthenia gravis (MG)

Myasthenia gravis (MG) is caused by autoantibodies against antigen in the post-synaptic neuromuscular membrane; in most patients against the acetylcholine receptor (AChR), in 5% against muscle-specific tyrosin kinase (MuSK), and in 5% against undefined antigen. A direct induction of muscle weakness by the autoantibodies has been shown.

The efficacy of IVIg in the treatment of MG has been confirmed by five controlled, prospective studies that are summarized in a Cochrane review. In acute exacerbations of MG, IVIG and PE have roughly the same efficacy, but when using IVIg the effect is slightly slower and there are less side effects (Gajdos et al, 2006).

The optimal dose of IVIG in MG has also been debated. So far no marked superiority of IVIg 2 g/kg over 2 days compared to 1 g/kg in a single day has been detected. The dose used has mostly been 2 g / kg resulting in the improvement after 3-6 days. Although IVIg is an effective treatment for acute exacerbations of MG, it is not recommended as maintenance therapy. Importantly, IVIg is often used in preparing MG patients for thymectomy or other types of surgery in case they have severe weakness, bulbar symptoms, poor pulmonary function, or a thymoma, even though there are no controlled studies justifying this practice. IVIg therapy has also been considered as rescue therapy in worsening MG, exacerbations of the disease during pregnancy and before giving birth, and neonatal MG. IVIg is considered safe in children and in elderly patients (EFNS task force, 2008).

Recommendations

- Intravenous immunoglobulin is an effective treatment for acute exacerbations of MG and for short-term treatment of severe MG (level A).
- IVIG is similar to PE regarding effect.
- This treatment is safe also for children, during pregnancy and for elderly patients with complicating disorders.
- There is not sufficient evidence to recommend IVIG for chronic maintenance therapy in MG alone or in combination with other immunoactive drugs (EFNS task force, 2008).

4. IVIg in therapy of inflammatory myopathies

The inflammatory myopathies are rare autoimmune diseases characterized by muscle weakness, which is usually proximal, painless and of insidious onset. The three groups of autoimmune myopathies are dermatomyositis (DM), polymyositis (PM) and inclusion body myositis (IBM). There are some controlled trials on the use of IVIg in patients with dermatomyositis (DM) and inclusion body myositis (IBM), and only one with polymyositis (PM) (EFNS task force, 2008; Hughes et al, 2008).

4.1 DM

DM is an inflammatory disease, affecting skin and muscle and causing varying degrees of muscle weakness, ranging from mild to severe. Prominent inflammation is observed usually at the periphery of the fascicle, leading to atrophy of the fibres around the fascicle (Hughes et al, 2008).

In a majority of DM patients a favourable response has been reported and therefore IVIg is recommended as a second line treatment in combination with prednisone for those who have not improved with corticosteroids alone. A total dose of 2 g / kg given over 2–5 days for adults and over 2 days for children is a safe initial treatment option. In severe, life-threatening DM, IVIg can be considered as the first line treatment together with other immunosuppressive therapy (Elovaara et al, 2010; EFNS task force, 2008).

Recommendations:

- IVIg is recommended as a second-line treatment in combination with prednisone for patients with DM who have not adequately responded to corticosteroids (level B).
- IVIg is recommended, in combination with immunosuppressive medication, as a measure to lower the dose of steroids in patients with DM (level C).
- IVIg is not recommended as monotherapy for DM (good practice point).
- In severe, life-threatening DM IVIg can be considered as the first-line treatment together with other immunosuppressive therapy (good practice point) (EFNS task force, 2008).

4.2 IBM

IBM is a progressive inflammatory skeletal muscle disease that presents with a distinctive pattern of weakness in the wrist and finger flexors and quadriceps muscles. It is characterized by inflammatory cells surrounding myofibres and rimmed vacuoles.

In IBM, the available evidence based on trials with small to moderate numbers of patients suggests an overall negative outcome even if a small number of patients reported improvement in swallowing difficulties. Therefore, IVIg cannot be recommended for the treatment of sporadic IBM (Hughes et al, 2008).

Recommendation:

- IVIg can not be recommended for the treatment of sporadic IBM (level A) (EFNS task force, 2008).

4.3 PM

Polymyositis is an inflammatory myopathy with no rash. It is defined by symmetric proximal muscle weakness, elevated serum muscle enzymes, myopathic changes on electromyography, characteristic muscle biopsy abnormalities and the absence of histopathologic signs of other myopathies. Muscle weakness is indeed the most common

presenting feature of polymyositis. The onset is usually insidious and the distribution of weakness is typically symmetric and proximal. Myalgias occur in less than 30% of the patiens (Dalakas & Hohlfeld, 2003).
Only one non-RCT (evidence class III) and two case series (evidence class IV) on IVIg therapy for polymyositis have been published. Only the first one used IVIg exclusively in patients with polymyositis. This study reported clinical improvement in 71% of patients with significant improvement in muscle power, muscle disability scores, and creatinine kinase levels ($P < 0.01$). Steroid doses could be reduced after IVIg ($P < 0.05$) (Hughes et al, 2008).
Recommendation:

- IVIg may be considered amongst the treatment options for patients with polymyositis not responding to first line immunosuppressive treatment (level C).

5. IVIg in therapy of demyelinating diseases of central nervous system

5.1 Multiple sclerosis (MS)

Multiple sclerosis (MS) is a central nervous system chronic inflammatory disease that is characterized by an extensive and complex immune response. It is the most common demyelinating disease of the central nervous system in young adults. MS can cause a variety of symptoms, including changes in sensation, visual problems, muscle weakness, depression, difficulties with coordination and speech, severe fatigue, cognitive impairment, problems with balance, overheating, and pain. MS will cause impaired mobility and disability in more severe cases. Multiple sclerosis may take several different forms, with new symptoms occurring either in discrete attacks or slowly accruing over time. Between attacks, symptoms may resolve completely, but permanent neurologic problems often persist, especially as the disease advances. MS currently does not have a cure, though several treatments are available that may slow the appearance of new symptoms (Baumstarck-Barrau et al, 2011)
Although earlier trials on the efficacy of IVIg in Relapsing Remitting MS (RRMS) have demonstrated a reduction in relapses, a recent study investigating the prevention of relapses with IVIg (PRIVIG trial) failed to confirm these earlier observations (Fazekas et al, 2008). In this study 127 patients with RRMS participated in a double blind, placebo-controlled trial, in which 44 and 42 patients received treatment with 0.2 or 0.4 g / kg of IVIg and 42 patients received placebo every 4 weeks for 48 weeks. After 1 year, the proportion of relapse-free patients did not differ between the groups, and there was no difference in MRI activity assessed 6-weekly. The authors of the study suggested that the obtained results may be related to short disease duration and overall disease activity of the study population that was more like that observed in a population with a clinically isolated syndrome.
The efficacy of IVIg in the treatment of MS exacerbations has been addressed in small add-on type studies that could not demonstrate any additional benefits due to addition of IVIg to conventional treatment of acute exacerbations with high-dose IV methylprednisolone. However, a recent study reported that IVIg might have a beneficial effect in patients with insufficient recovery from optic neuritis, if treatment with high-dose IV methylprednisolone fails (Achiron, 2008). No clinically significant effects were seen in progressive forms of MS, and consequently IVIg is not recommended in these conditions (Elovaara et al, 2010).
Currently the main indication for the use of IVIg in MS is to reduce relapses during pregnancy or breastfeeding when other therapies may not be used safely (Haas & Homes, 2007).
Recommendations:

- IVIG could still be considered as a second or third-line therapy in RRMS if conventional immunomodulatory therapies are not tolerated because of side effects or concomitant diseases (level B), and in particular in pregnancy where other therapies may not be used (good clinical practice point).
- IVIG cannot be recommended for treatment in secondary progressive MS (level A).
- IVIg does not seem to have any valuable effect as add-on therapy to methylprednisolone for acute exacerbations (level B)
- IVIg cannot be recommended as treatment for chronic symptoms in MS (level A).
- In clinically isolated syndromes and in primary progressive MS there is not sufficient evidence to make any recommendations.

5.2 Neuromyelitis optica (NMO)

Neuromyelitis optica (NMO) termed also Devic's disease, is a demyelinating disease of the spinal cord and optic nerves that may manifest by recurrent attacks and tends to have a poor prognosis.

There is only one case type study suggesting that monthly IVIg was associated with cessation of relapses (class IV evidence) (Bakker & Metz, 2004).

5.3 Balo's concentric sclerosis

Balo's concentric sclerosis is a severe demyelinating disease with poor prognosis. There is a case report suggesting that IVIg (0.4 g/kg/daily for 5 days) and interferon-beta-1a given post-partum may result partial neurological improvement (class IV evidence) (Airas et al, 2005).

5.4 Acute disseminated encephalomyelitis (ADEM)

Acute-disseminated encephalomyelitis (ADEM) is a monophasic immune-mediated demyelinating disease of the central nervous system that is associated with significant morbidity and mortality. Controlled studies on therapy in ADEM are not available. Standard treatment is high-dose steroids. The use of IVIg (0.4 g/kg/day for 5 days or 1 g/kg/2 days) has been reported in case reports and small series suggesting that IVIg may have favourable effects when used as an initial therapy in both adults and children (class IV evidence). IVIg may have beneficial effects also as second line therapy (class IV evidence) [149–152] especially in patients who could not receive or failed to respond to steroids (class IV evidence) or in patients with peripheral nervous system involvement and steroid failure (class IV evidence). Alternatively combination therapy by steroids and IVIG (class IV evidence) or steroids, IVIg and PE were suggested to have favourable effects especially if given early in the course of disease (class IV evidence) (EFNS task force 2008).

Recommendations:

- IVIg may have a favourable effect in the treatment of ADEM and therefore it should be tried (0.4 g/kg/day for 4–5 consecutive days) in patients with lack of response to high-dose steroids (good practice point). The cycles may be repeated. PE could also be considered in patients with a lack of response to high-dose steroids.

6. IVIg in therapy of paraneoplastic syndromes

Due to the rarity of immunologically mediated paraneoplastic diseases, there are very few prospective, randomized, double-blind and placebo-controlled studies.

6.1 Lambert – eaton myasthenic syndrome (LEMS)

Lambert-Eaton myasthenic syndrome (LEMS) is an immune-mediated disorder of the presynaptic neuromuscular transmission, which more frequently occurs as the remote effect of a neoplasm. The clinical features described are proximal weakness, especially in the lower limbs, with diminished tendon reflexes and post-tetanic potentiation. Autonomic symptoms are often reported, including pupil abnormalities, dry eyes and mouth, and erectile dysfunction (Maddison & Newsom-Davis, 2005).

LEMS is considered to respond best to immunosupressive treatment. However, there is only one report showing the beneficial but short-term effect of IVIg on the muscle strength in LEMS (class II evidence) and there is also a recent Cochrane review that has concluded that limited data from one placebo-controlled study show improvement in muscle strength after IVIg (Maddison & Newsom-Davis, 2005).

The IVIg response regarding improvement of muscle strength does probably not differ in paraneoplastic and non-paraneoplastic LEMS.

Recommendations:

- IVIg therapy may be tried in paraneoplastic LEMS (good practice point).

6.2 Neuromyotonia

Acquired neuromyotonia is a condition associated with muscle hyperactivity that includes muscle stiffness, cramps, myokymia, pseudomyotonia and weakness, most common in the limbs and trunk. The typical finding on electromyography is spontaneous motor unit discharges occurring in distinctive doublets, triplets, or longer runs with high intraburst frequency (Hart et al, 2002).

Only one case report describes the beneficial effect of IVIg in patient with neuromyotonia, whilst another case report demonstrated worsening after IVIG therapy (EFNS task force, 2008).

6.3 Paraneoplastic opsoclonus ataxia syndrome (OMS)

Opsoclonus refers to involuntary, conjugate, multivectorial, saccadic eye movements. It can occur as an isolated neurologic anomaly but, when it occurs with involuntary multifocal jerking movements of the skeletal musculature, the phenomenon is known as opsoclonus-myoclonus syndrome (OMS). The syndrome often includes features of ataxia, or incoordination with voluntary movements. In the setting of malignancy, opsoclonus is linked most clearly to neuroblastoma, occurring in 3% of childhood cases. Anti-neuronal antibodies, usually to nuclear antigens, are considered markers of immune system activation in this disorder, detected in 81% of pediatric patients (Pittock et al, 2003).

Symptoms in paraneoplastic opsoclonus - ataxia syndrome in paediatric neuroblastoma patients are stated to improve, although data concerning the long-term benefits of the treatment is lacking (class IV evidence). In adult patients the response is less immunosuppressive, although IVIg is suggested to accelerate recovery (class IV evidence) (EFNS task force, 2008).

Recommedation:

- -IVIg therapy may be tried in opsoclonus-ataxia especially in paediatric neuroblastoma patients (good practice point).

6.4 Paraneoplastic cerebellar degeneration

Cerebellar dysfunction is one of the most common paraneoplastic presentations of cancer. The tumours more commonly involved are small-cell lung cancer, gynaecological and breast tumours, and Hodgkin's lymphoma. Neurological deficits are sometimes preceded by prodromal symptoms, such as a viral-like illness, dizziness, nausea, or vomiting that might be attributed to a peripheral vestibular process. These symptoms are followed by gait unsteadiness that rapidly develops into ataxia, diplopia, dysarthria, and dysphagia. Some patients have blurry vision, oscillopsia, and transient opsoclonus.Initial MRI is normal in most patients, although over time, MRI shows cerebellar atrophy and PET demonstrates hypometabolism (Dalmau & Rosenfeld, 2008).

6.5 Limbic encephalitis

Autoimmune limbic encephalitis (LE) can arise both by paraneoplastic and non-paraneoplastic mechanisms. Patients with LE usually have a subacute onset of memory impairment, disorientation and agitation, but can also develop seizures, hallucinations and sleep disturbance. The following investigations may aid the diagnosis: analysis of cerebrospinal fluid (CSF), electroencephalography, magnetic resonance imaging, fluorodeoxyglucose positron emission tomography and neuronal antibodies in the serum and CSF. Neuronal antibodies are sometimes, but not always, pathogenic. Autoimmune LE may respond to corticosteroids, intravenous IgG (IVIG) or plasma exchange. The cornerstone of paraneoplastic LE therapy is resection of the tumour and/or oncological treatment. Several differential diagnoses must be excluded, among them herpes simplex encephalitis (Vedeler & Storstein, 2009)

6.6 Paraneoplastic sensory neuronopathy (SSN)

Paraneoplastic sensory neuronopathy (SSN) is characterized by primary damage of the sensory nerve cell body of the dorsal root ganglia. A paraneoplastic origin is only one of the causes of SSN The most common low associated tumor is small cell lung carcinoma. The main clinical complains at onset are pain and paresthesias with asymmetric distribution that involves the arms rather than the legs. Later, pain is replaced by numbness, limb ataxia, and pseudoathetotic movements of the hands. The neurologic examination shows abolition of the deep tendon reflexes and involvement of all modalities of sensation with clear predominance of the joint position. Electrophysiologic studies show marked, but not restricted, involvement of the sensory fibres (Dalmau & Rosenfeld, 2008).

Evidence for the effect of IVIg in paraneoplastic cerebellar degeneration, limbic encephalitis and sensory neuropathy is scarce. In previously published reports, patients were treated with a combination of immunosupressive or immunomodulatory drugs, including IVIG, with a poor response (class IV evidence) (EFNS task force, 2008).

Recommendations:

- No clear recommendations of the effect of IVIG in paraneoplastic neuromyotonia, cerebellar degeneration, limbic encephalitis or sensory neuronopathy can be made due to lack of data (EFNS task force, 2008).

7. IVIg in therapy of Stiff-Person Syndrome (SPS)

Stiff-person syndrome (SPS) is characterized by muscle stiffness and episodic spasms. A significant decline of the stiffness scores was found in a randomized trial of 16 SPS patients treated with IVIg . Based on this study IVIg may be considered as a safe and effective second-line therapy for patients with SP incompletely responding to diazepam and / or baclofen and who have significant disability requiring a cane or a walker due to truncal stiffness and frequent falls. The recommendation is to use IVIg (2 g / kg in 2-5 days) (EFNS task force, 2008).

Recommendations:

- In patients with SPS incompletely responding to diazepam and/or baclofen and with significant disability requiring a cane or a walker due to truncal stiffness and frequent falls, the recommendation is to use IVIg (2 g/kg in 2-5 days) (level A based on class I evidence).

8. IVIg in therapy of post-polio syndrome (PPS)

Post-polio syndrome (PPS) is characterized by new muscle weakness, muscle atrophy, fatigue and pain developing several years after acute polio. The prevalence of PPS in patients with previous polio is 20-60%.

Post-polio syndrome is caused by an increased degeneration of enlarged motor units, and some motor neurones cannot maintain all their nerve terminals. Muscle overuse may contribute. Immunological and inflammatory signs have been reported in the cerebrospinal fluid and central nervous tissue (EFNS task force, 2008).

There are two RCTs of treatment with IVIg in PPS (class I evidence) including 155 patients. In the study with highest power, a significant increase of mean muscle strength of 8.3% was reported after two IVIg treatment cycles during 3 months. Physical activity and subjective vitality also differed significantly in favour of the IVIG group (Farbu et al., 2007).

Post-polio syndrome is a chronic condition. Although a modest IVIG effect has been described short term, nothing is known about long-term effects. Responders and non-responders have not been defined.

Any relationship between the clinical response to IVIG treatment and PPS severity, cerebrospinal fluid inflammatory changes and cerebrospinal fluid changes after IVIg is unknown. Optimal dose and IVIG cycle frequency has not been examined. Cost-benefit evaluation has not been performed.

Recommendations:

- IVIG has a minor to moderate positive effect on muscle strength and some aspects of quality of life in PPS (class I evidence).
- As long as responding subgroups, long term effects, dosing schedules and cost-benefit aspects are not known, routine use of IVIG for PPS cannot be recommended (good practice point).
- However, in the very few patients with especially rapid progression of muscle weakness and atrophy, especially if there are indications of ongoing low-grade inflammation in the spinal cord, IVIg may be tried if a rigorous follow-up of muscle strength and quality of life can be undertaken (good practice point) (EFNS task force, 2008).

9. IVIg in therapy of drug resistant epilepsy (DRIE)

Drug-resistant infantile epilepsy (DRIE) syndromes include a number of diseases such as Landau-Kleffner syndrome (LKS), West syndrome, Lennox-Gastaut syndrome, severe myoclonic epilepsy or RE that typically manifest in childhood or adolescence and are characterized by epilepsy and progressive neurological dysfunction.

Standard treatment of RE consists of anti-epileptic drugs, high-dose steroids or PE. Surgical treatment also may be considered.

Case studies and small series have reported that some patients with RE respond in some measure to treatment with IVIG (class IV).

Approximately a hundred patients with West or Lennox-Gastaut syndromes have been treated with IVIg with widely varying results. The treatment has resulted in reduction in the number of seizures with improvement in the EEG in about half of the cases. The positive effects were noted few days to several weeks to months after treatment. Relapses have been common.

Successful use of IVIg as initial monotherapy in LKS has been reported in case studies and after initial therapy by steroids or antiepileptic drugs and steroids in only few patients. Case studies on the use of IVIg in RE have suggested that monthly IVIg therapy (0.4 g/kg for 5 days at 4-week interval followed by monthly maintenance IVIg) may ameliorate disease in patients who are refractory to antiepileptic drugs or steroids and PE (EFNS task force, 2008).

Recommendation:

- IVIg seems to have a favourable effect in RE and may be tried in selected patients that are refractory to other therapies (good practice point).
- IVIg has been administered at doses of 0.4 g/kg/day for 4–5 consecutive days, the cycles may be repeated after 2–6 weeks.

10. IVIg in therapy of narcolepsy with cataplexy (NC)

Narcolepsy with cataplexy (NC) is caused by substantial loss of hypocretin neurons. NC patients carry the HLA-DQB1*0602 allele suggesting that hypocretin neuron loss is due to an autoimmune attack.

There are some case studies that report that IVIg treatment initiated before 9 months disease duration has some clinical efficiency. The unaffected CSF hypocretin-1 levels and lack of autoantibodies suggest that any autoimmune process occurs very early in NC. The final IVIg effect needs to be investigated in RCTs (Knudsen et al, 2010).

11. IVIg in therapy of Alzheimer's disease (AD)

Alzheimer's Disease (AD) is the most common neurodegenerative disorder leading to dementia. The pathological hallmarks of AD are extracellular accumulation of Ab peptides, as senile plaques and intracellular neurofibrillary tangles composed of tau proteins.

Clinical studies of active immunization in humans with AD were complicated by the development of meningoencephalitis in 6% of the patients treated with vaccine AN1792 in a phase II clinical trial. Furthermore, only 20% of the patients immunized with AN1792 developed a twofold increase in anti-Ab antibodies.

However, progress was made with the discovery that peripheral administration of antibodies against Ab peptide could reduce amyloid burden to a similar extent as active immunization. Passive immunization had the advantage that the potentially harmful activation of host T cells could be avoided.

Based on the finding that externally administered antibodies were able to protect mice from AD, it was hypothesized that high titres of natural anti-Ab antibodies may protect humans from AD, while low levels may predispose certain individuals to the development of AD. Studies have found reduced levels of anti-Ab antibodies both in the serum and CSF of patients with AD. Autoantibody-decorated plaques were found frequently in patients with AD and patients with low antibody-levels were shown to harbour more diffuse plaques than patients with high levels. Autoantibodies against Ab may therefore be important for maintaining plaque homeostasis.

IVIg has been shown to contain autoantibodies against many states of Ab peptide aggregation including monomers, oligomers and fibrils and may therefore have a distinct advantage over monoclonal anti-Ab until the precise pathogenic state(s) of the Ab peptide is known (Hughes et al, 2008).

Recently, commercially available IVIg have been used in small pilot trials for the treatment of patients with AD, based on the hypothesis that IVIG contains naturally occurring autoantibodies (nAbs-Abeta) that specifically recognize and block the toxic effects of Abeta. Furthermore, these nAbs-Abeta are reduced in AD patients compared with healthy controls, supporting the notion of replacement with IVIg. Beyond the occurrence of nAbs-Abeta, evidence for several other mechanisms associated with IVIg in AD has been reported in preclinical experiments and clinical studies. In 2009, a phase III clinical trial involving more than 360 AD patients was initiated and may provide conclusive evidence for the effect of IVIg as a treatment option for AD in 2011(Dodel et al, 2010).

12. Conclusion

IVIg is used increasingly in neurological diseases.

Its efficacy has been proved in GBS, CIDP and MMN, where it is considered as the first-line treatment. However, questions remain regarding the dose, timing and duration of IVIg treatment in these disorders.

It is also successfully used in acute exacerbations of MG and as a short-term treatment of severe MG. It is recommended in SPS, in some paraneoplastic syndromes and as a second-line treatment in combination with prednisone in dermatomyositis and a treatment option in polymyositis.

In MS, IVIg is indicated mainly in reducing disease activity during pregnancy and breastfeeding.

In addition to these major indications, IVIg is increasingly used even in such conditions where the strong evidence is currently lacking, like refractory epilepsy, narcolepsy, post polio syndrome.

According to preliminary data, IVIg might be a promising candidate for the treatment of (AD). Large-scale randomized trials are under way, and the results of these studies are awaited eagerly worldwide.

When considering treatment options, it is important to notify that uncontrolled use may lead to high costs and limited availability of IVIg. Careful selection of patients who will benefit from IVIg is extremely important.

ABBREVIATIONS:

AChR: acetylcholine receptor

AD: Alzheimer's Disease

ADEM: Acute-disseminated encephalomyelitis

AIDP: acute inflammatory demyelinating polyneuropathy

AMAN: acute motor axonal neuropathy

AMSAN: acute motor and sensory axonal neuropathy

CIDP: chronic idiopathic demyelinating polyneuropathy

CSF: cerebrospinal fluid
DM: dermatomyositis
DRIE: Drug-resistant infantile epilepsy
GBS: Guillain - Barre syndrome
IBM: inclusion body myositis
IVIg: intravenous immunoglobulin
LEMS: Lambert-Eaton myasthenic syndrome
LRPN: Lumbosacral radiculoplexus neuropathy
MGUS: monoclonal gammopathy of undetermined significance
MMN: multifocal motor neuropathy
MG: Myasthenia gravis
MS: Multiple Sclerosis
MuSK: muscle-specific tyrosin kinase
NC: Narcolepsy with cataplexy
NMO: Neuromyelitis optica
OMS : opsoclonus–myoclonus syndrome
PE: Plasma exchange
PM: polymyositis
PPS: Post-polio syndrome
RCT: randomized controlled trials
RRMS: Relapsing Remitting Multiple Sclerosis
SPS: Stiff-person syndrome
SSN: Paraneoplastic sensory neuronopathy

13. References

Achiron, A. (2008). Winning combination: the additive / synergistic benefits of IVIg in corticosteroid refractory optic neuritis. *Eur J Neurol*, Vol.15, pp.1145.

Airas, L., Kurki, T., Erjanti, H. & Marttila RJ. (2005). Successful pregnancy of a patient with Balo's concentric sclerosis. *Multiple Sclerosis,* Vol.11, pp. 346–348.

Allen, D., Lunn, M.P.T., Niermeijer, J. & Nobile-Orazio, E. (2007). Treatment for IgG and IgA paraproteinaemic neuropathy. *Cochrane Database of Systematic Reviews,* CD005376.

Bakker, J. & Metz, L. (2004). Devic's neuromyelitis optica treated with intravenous gamma globulin (IVIG). *Canadian Journal of Neurological Sciences,* Vol. 31, pp. 265–267.

Baumstarck-Barrau, K., Simeoni, M-C., Reuter, F., Klemina, I., Aghababian, V., Pelletier, J. & Auquier, P. (2011).Cognitive function and quality of life in multiple sclerosis patients: a cross-sectional study *BMC Neurology*,Vol.11, No.17, doi:10.1186/1471-2377

Bhanushali, M.J., Muley, S.A. (2008). Diabetic and non-diabetic lumbosacral radiculoplexus neuropathy. *Neurology India,* Vol. 56 No.4, pp.420-5.

Birnbaum, J. (2010). Peripheral nervous system manifestations of Sjφgren syndrome: clinical patterns, diagnostic paradigms, etiopathogenesis, and therapeutic strategies. *Neurologist,* Vol.16, No. 5, pp. 287-297.

Collins, M.P., Dyck, P.J., Gronseth, G.S., Guillevin, L., Hadden, R.D., Heuss, D., Lıger, J.M., Notermans, N.C., Pollard, J.D., Said, G., Sobue, G., Vrancken, A.F.& Kissel, J.T.; Peripheral Nerve Society (2010). Peripheral Nerve Society Guideline on the classification, diagnosis, investigation, and immunosuppressive therapy of non-systemic vasculitic neuropathy: executive summary. *J Peripher Nerv Syst.*, Vol.15, No.3, pp.176-84.

Dalakas, M.C., Hohlfeld, R. (2003). Polymyositis and dermatomyositis. *Lancet*, Vol.362, pp.971-982.

Dalmau, J.& Rosenfeld, M.R.(2008). Paraneoplastic syndromes of the CNS. *Lancet Neurology*, Vol. 7, No. 4, pp. 327-340.

Dodel, R., Neff, F., Noelker, C., Pul, R., Du Y, Bacher, M., Oertel, W. (2010). Intravenous immunoglobulins as a treatment for Alzheimer's disease: rationale and current evidence. *Drugs,* Vol., 26, No. 70(5), pp. 513-28.

EFNS task force on the use of intravenous immunoglobulin in treatment of neurological Diseases: Elovaara, I., Apostolski, S., van Doorn, P., Gilhus, N. E., Hietaharju, A., Honkaniemi, J. I., van Schaik, N., Scolding, N., Soelberg Sψrensen, P. & Udd, B. (2008). EFNS guidelines for the use of intravenous immunoglobulin in treatment of neurological diseases *European Journal of Neurology,* Vol.15, pp. 893–908.

Eftimov, F., Winer J.B., Vermeulen M., de Haan R., van Schaik I.N. (2009). Intravenous immunoglobulin for chronic inflammatory demyelinating polyneuropathy. *Cochrane Database Syst Rev*, Vol. 21:CD001797.

Elovaara, I. & Hietaharju, A. (2010). Can we face the challenge of expanding use of intravenous immunoglobulin in neurology? *Acta Neurologica Scandinavia,* Vol.122, pp. 309–315.

Farbu, E., Rekand, T., Vik-Mo, E., Lygren, H., Gilhus, N.E., Aarli, J.A. (2007). Post-polio syndrome patients treated with intravenous immunoglobulin: a double-blinded randomized controlled pilot study. *European Journal of Neurology,* Vol. 14, pp. 60–65.

Fazekas, F., Lublin, F.D., Li, D. Freedman, M.S., Hartung, H.P., Rieckmann, P., Sorensen P.S., Maas-Enriquez M., Sommerauer B., Hanna, K. PRIVIG Study group. UBC MR/MRI Research group. Intravenous immunoglobulin in relapsing-remitting multiple sclerosis. (2008). A dose finding trial. *Neurology,* Vol. 71, pp. 265–71.

Gajdos, P., Chevret, S., Toyka, K. (2006). Intravenous immunoglobulin for myasthenia gravis. *Cochrane Database Syst Rev,* Vol.19, No.2, CD002277.

Haas, J., Hommes, O.R. (2007). A dose comparison study of IVIG in postpartum relapsing-remitting multiple sclerosis. *Mult Scler,* Vol.13, pp. 900–908.

Hart, I.K., Maddison, P., Newsom-Davis, J., Vincent, A., Mills, K.R. (2002). Phenotypic variants of autoimmune peripheral nerve hyperexcitability. *Brain*, Vol.125, pp.1887-95.

Hughes, R.A., Swan A.V. & van Doorn P.A. (2004). Cytotoxic drugs and interferons for chronic inflammatory demyelinating polyradiculoneuropathy. *Cochrane Database Syst Rev*, Vol. 18, No.4:CD003280.

Hughes, R.A., Raphael J.C., Swan A.V. & van Doorn P.A. (2006). Intravenous immunoglobulin for Guillain-Barre' syndrome, *Cochrane Database Syst Rev,* Vol. 25, No.1,CD002063.

Hughes, R.A., Donofrio, P., Bril V., Dalakas, M.C., Deng C., Hanna K., Hartung H.P., Latov N., Merkies I.S., van Doorn P.A. ICE Study Group. (2008). Intravenous immune globulin (10% caprylate-chromatography purified) for the treatment of chronic inflammatory demyelinating polyradiculoneuropathy (ICE study): a randomised placebo-controlled trial. *Lancet Neurol*, Vol. 7, pp.136–44.

Hughes, R. A. C., Dalakas, M. C., Cornblath D. R., N. Latov, Weksler M. E. & Relkin N. (2009). Clinical applications of intravenous immunoglobulins in neurology, *Clinical and Experimental Immunology*, Vol.158, No. 1, pp. 34–42.

Knudsen, S., Mikkelsen, J.D., Bang, B., Gammeltoft, S. & Jennum P.J. (2010). Intravenous immunoglobulin treatment and screening for hypocretin neuron-specific autoantibodies in recent onset childhood narcolepsy with cataplexy. *Neuropediatrics.* Vol. 41, No. 5, pp. 217-22.

Leger, J.M., Viala, K., Cancalon, F., Maisonobe, T., Gruwez, B., Waegemans, T. & Bouche, P. (2008). Intravenous immunoglobulin as short- and long-term therapy of multifocal motor neuropathy: a retrospective study of response to IVIg and of its predictive criteria in 40 patients. *J Neurol Neurosurg Psychiatry*, Vol.79, pp.93–96.

Lunn, M.P.T. & Nobile-Orazio, E. (2006). Immunotherapy for IgM anti-myelin-associated glycoprotein paraprotein-associated peripheral neuropathies. *Cochrane Database of Systematic Reviews,* CD002827.

Maddison, P. & Newsom-Davis, J. (2005). Treatment for Lambert-Eaton myasthenic syndrome. *Cochrane Database of Systematic Reviews*, Vol. 2: CD003279.

Mori, K., Iijima, M., Koike, H., Hattori, N., Tanaka, F., Watanabe, H., Katsuno, M., Fujita, A., Aiba, I., Ogata, A., Saito, T., Asakura, K., Yoshida, M., Hirayama, M. & Sobue, G. (2005). The wide spectrum of clinical manifestations in Sjφgren's syndrome-associated neuropathy. *Brain,* Vol. 128, No. 11, pp. 2518-2534.

Piepers, S., Van den Berg-Vos, R., Van der Pol, W.L., Franssen, H., Wokke, J. & Van den Berg, L. (2007). Mycophenolate mofetil as adjunctive therapy for MMN patients: a randomized, controlled trial. Brain, Vol.130, pp.2004–10.

Pittock, S.J., Lucchinetti, C.F., Lennon, V.A. (2003). Anti-neuronal nuclear autoantibody type 2: paraneoplastic accompaniments. *Ann Neurol,* Vol. 53, pp.580–587.

Terenghi, F., Cappellari, A., Bersano, A., Carpo, M., Barbieri, S.& Nobile-Orazio, E. (2004). How long is IVIG effective in multifocal motor neuropathy? *Neurology,* Vol. 62, pp. 666–668.

van Doorn P.A., Ruts L. & Jacobs B.C. (2008). Clinical features, pathogenesis, and treatment of Guillain–Barrι syndrome, *Lancet Neurol,* Vol. 7, pp.939-950.

van Schaik, I.N., van den Berg, L.H., de Haan, R., Vermeulen, M. (2005). Intravenous immunoglobulin for multifocal motor neuropathy. *Cochrane Database Syst Rev,* Vol.18, No.2: CD004429.

Vedeler, C.A., Storstein, A.(2009). Autoimmune limbic encephalitis. *Acta neurologica Scandinavica. Supplementum.* Vol.189, pp.63-7

Vucic, S., Black, K.R., Chong, P.S.T., Cros, D. (2004). Multifocal motor neuropathy. Decrease in conduction blocks and reinnervation with long-term IVIG. *Neurology,* Vol.63, pp.1264–1269.

3

Recent Advances in the Treatment of Neurological Autoimmune Disorders

Jagat R. Kanwar*, Bhasker Sriramoju and Rupinder K. Kanwar
*Laboratory of Immunology and Molecular Biomedical Research (LIMBR),
Centre for Biotechnology and Interdisciplinary Biosciences (BioDeakin),
Institute for Technology in Nanomedicine & Research Innovation,
Deakin University Waurn Ponds, Geelong,
Australia*

1. Introduction

Autoimmune diseases are a complex group of diseases arising because of the breakdown of narrow margin that exists between the immunity and tolerance. In simpler terms either T or B-cells or both are activated in the absence of a progressive infection or any other noticeable cause (Davidson & Diamond, 2001). Unable to distinguish self from non self, the renegade immune cells pose a serious threat to self molecules leading to severe destruction. The precise mechanisms that drive this event are still unclear but, most of the studies identified that genetics, environment and infections will have a role in triggering the autoimmune attack (Smith et al., 1999). An approximate of 5% of the population in western countries are currently the victims of these diseases and in this component, a major proportion of them are females displaying a higher risk of incidence (Jacobson, 1997; Kanwar, 2005). Added to this, the general ailments of the humans like atherosclerosis and gastrointestinal disturbances are found to be associated with an autoimmune component, predisposing the risk of developing an autoimmune disease (Ross, 1990, Galperin & Gershwin 1997).The influence of hormones cannot be neglected as preclinical studies have witnessed the role of oestrogen in the emergence of autoimmune diseases while testosterone was found to lower the risk in lupus prone mice (Sakic, 1998; Roubinian et al., 1978). Few epidemiological studies also revealed the preponderance of autoimmune diseases mediated by the nocturnal hormone, melatonin (Cutolo, 2003). In addition, cortisol levels and the secondary events like stress were also found to influence the autoimmune disease generation (Webster et al, 1998). Since ages, the basic principle of immunology has been the concept of clonal deletion of autoreactive immune cells and generation of a mature T & B-cell repertoire that could distinguish self from non self. The formation and survival of mature immune repertoire, always demands prolonged auto antigen exposure acknowledging the physiological importance of autoreactivity (Goldrath & Bevan, 1999; Gu et al., 1991). Though structural resemblances exist between self and non self antigens the attack is directed against self antigens under stimulatory conditions like the presence of infections, cytokines etc (Silverstein & Rose, 2000; Kanwar, 2005; Kanwar et al, 2009). Thus it is always fascinating to find answers for how the physiology of autoimmunity is turned to pathology and how the immune cells enforce their attack. This review focuses on introduction to immunity, pathology of autoimmune diseases and their treatments along with recent advancements.

2. Basics of immune system

The immune system comprises of a complex array of immune cells tailored to defend the body against a variety of substances that are considered as foreign including pathogenic microbes and tumors while remaining nonreactive towards the self. Immune cells are originated from the haematopoietic stem cells and are classified as lymphoid and myeloid cells comprising B & T-lymphocytes, Natural killer cells (NKs), dendritic cells and polymorphonuclear leukocytes, monocytes, mast cells, macrophages respectively (Delves, 2006). The immune cells constantly patrol the body and involve specific and non specific mechanisms in executing immune attack upon finding a foreign substance. The specificity rests particularly with T and B-cells as they display the receptors capable of recognising non self molecules from the self.

The specific attack is also complimented before by the strategic non specific immune responses generated by polymmorphonucelar cells, NKs, macrophages, co-stimulatory molecules like cytokines and serves as the initial site of attack upon finding the foreign entities. The abnormal levels of cytokines have a strong impact in the initiation and progression of autoimmune diseases. Also, therapeutic interventions with exogenous cytokines were found to be associated with the disease process, suggesting their key role in mediating the disease (Hooks et al., 1982; Trembleau et al., 1995; McKall-Faienza et al., 1998; Schattner, 1994; Kanwar et al, 1999; Kanwar et al, 2005; Kanwar et al, 2009). The complex network of immune cells is classified into subpopulations based on the expression of surface markers, functional characteristics, regions where they mature and activate. Likewise, T-cells include helper cells (Th) displaying $CD4^{+}$ marker and involve in modulating the immune responses. Further they comprise subsets of Th1 cells that aid other T-cells and Th2 subtype mediates the antibody generation. Cytotoxic cells (Tc) with $CD8^{+}$ marker are killer cells with lethal effect on intracellular pathogens, infected and tumor cells. Lastly, suppressor cells (Ts) down regulate and monitor the immune reactions. The naive T-cells undergo maturation in the thymus (hence the name T-cells) and are able to respond only to the processed antigens. Most of the nucleated cells of the mammalian system function as the antigen presenting cells (APCs) and dendrites are unique in this category expressing major histocompatibility complex proteins (MHC) and generating co stimulatory gestures for T-cell activation. APCs process the antigen and represent them in association with cell surface MHCs for T-cell recognition. These MHCs categorised as class I and Class II are crucial in the selection process of cytotoxic and helper cells respectively.

The T-cells bear an antigen recognition site on their surface called as T-cell receptor (TCR) and the initiation of T-cell mediated immunity requires the complex association of the antigen, MHC and the TCR. B-cells are specialised immune cells that act as APCs along with a prime function of antibody generation. The immature B-cells initially express a pre-B cell receptor (pre-BCR) on their surface and upon maturation they produce antibodies that act as antigen receptors towards the native antigen (Yang & Santamaria, 2006; Austyn, 2000; Roitt et al., 1998; Janeway & Travers, 1998). Both the T and B-cells express specific receptors for each antigen and this diversity is exhibited by the rearrangement of receptor gene sequences in the somatic cells rather than acquired through the inheritance (Gellert, 2002). In order to mount immune responses, the T and B-cells are activated through corresponding receptors in the presence of co-stimulatory molecules (Crow, 2004; Kanwar et al, 2000; Kanwar et al, 2003; Kanwar et al, 2005). Another essential feature of both these cells is that, upon initial exposure to an antigen both these cells generate memory cells that expand clonally. These memory cells unleash an accelerated immune attack upon antigen re-exposure (Swain, 2003; Bishop et al., 2003).

3. Tolerance

Because of the expression of vast diversity of antigen recognition sites on T and B-cells, molecules that are considered as self also may find chances of binding with the immune cells. Hence, a diverse range of tolerance mechanisms have been developed that train the T & B-cells to differentiate self from nonself. This process is tightly controlled in the primary lymphoid organs and is continuous to inhibit the various modes of auto reactive lymphocyte generation and activation. The basic mechanisms dealt are clonal deletion, clonal anergy and inhibition of self reactive lymphocytes (Yoshida & Gershwin, 1993; Rajewsky, 1996).

3.1 T and B cell tolerance

The tolerance mechanisms that develop in the primary lymphoid organs like thymus and bone marrow respectively for T and B cells constitute central tolerance. The naive T-cells originated from haematopoietic stem cells are devoid of CD4 and CD8 cell surface markers. Once migrated to the thymus, the TCR gene rearranges to develop double positive T-cells that display $CD4^+$ and $CD8^+$. Then these cells are positively selected as $CD4^+$ and $CD8^+$ cells based on their interactions with the MHC class II and Class I respectively. The cells with TCR, that fail to bind or interact MHC with little affinity undergo death and are positively selected based on weaker interactions between TCR and MHC carrying self antigens. T-cells are killed if found to interact strongly with a self antigen displayed by MHC and thus selected negatively (Palmer, 2003; Starr, 2006; Bretscher & Cohn, 1970; Kanwar et al, 2004; Kanwar, 2005). As a matter of enhanced protection from immune attack, the T-cells receiving stronger signals through TCR are deleted and this inactivation is much more sensitive compared to activation of T-cells that demand a stronger interaction between TCR and self antigen-MHC complex (Kappler, 1987; Pircher et al., 1991; Yagi & Janeway, 1990). Similar tolerance mechanisms exist for B-cell repertoire, as they are negatively selected if the BCR is found to interact strongly with the self antigens. However, active investigation is recommended to determine the existence of positive selection for B-cells. Interestingly, successful T-lymphocyte tolerance cuts down the signals for few autoreactive B-cells and thus induces B-cell tolerance (Bretscher & Cohn, 1970). During the course of their maturation, the pre B-cell receptor (BCR) cross links several avid auto-antigens. This event stimulates the rearrangement of light chain genes of the Ig's thus, driving the process of receptor editing where self antigens are replaced with non self ones (Ana et al., 2010). B-cells are deleted by apoptotic mechanism if found to interact strongly with self antigens (this happens mostly in bone marrow) and anergised if bound with little affinity (this happens mostly in periphery) (Monroe et al., 2003; Hodgkin & Basten, 1995). T-cells have a potential role in the generation and progression of chemical and spontaneously induced autoimmune diseases and the same was also demonstrated successfully in the animal studies (Singer & Theofilopoulos, 1990; Druet, 1989; Pettinelli & McFarlin, 1989; Waldor et al., 1985). Few autoreactive T-cells may escape tolerance mechanisms and spread in the periphery but, they are naive and do not hold any threat unless APCs turn active. Potential problem persists incase of molecular mimicry (where pathogenic antigens resemble self antigens) as APCs turn active and trigger T-cell attack that is indiscriminate towards self and nonself. The same also holds true for B-cells (Damian, 1964; Oldstone, 1998). On the whole, generation of autoimmune diseases is based on the narrow margin that exists between tolerance and immunity executed by deletion and survival of self reactive lymphocytes. Too much deletion compromises the immunity and too little deletion follows subsequent autoimmunity. The following figure is an ideal representation of healthy and pathologic immunity and the differentiation between tolerance and autoimmunity.

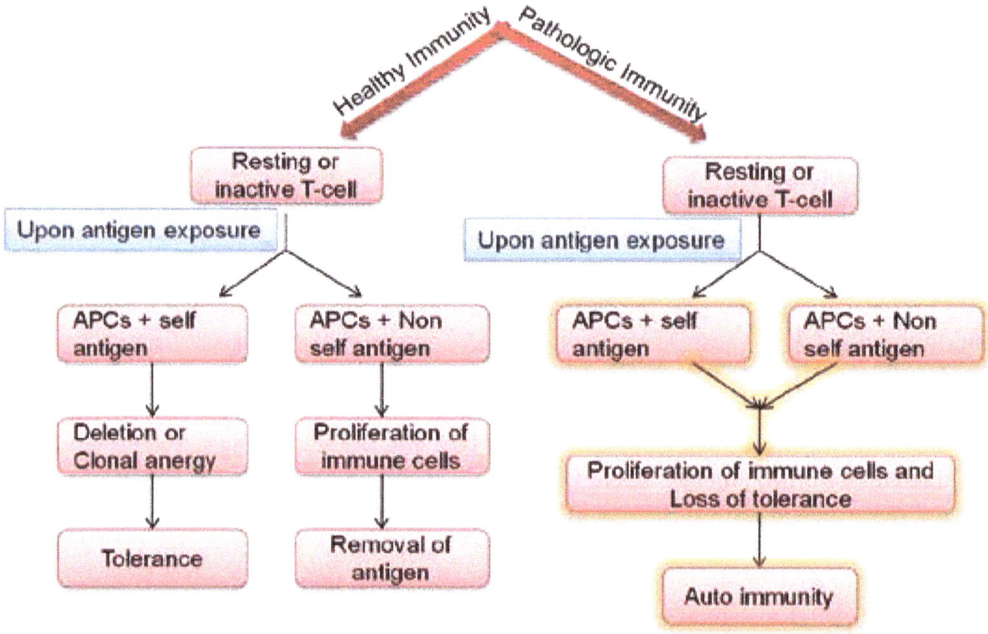

Fig. 1. Showing the comparison of healthy and pathologic immune system. A healthy T-cell upon exposure to self antigens undergo specific mechanisms of inactivation like deletion or clonal anergy constituting peripheral tolerance while an autoreactive T-cell is dysregulated with indiscriminate attack on self and non self antigens because of the lack of tolerance in autoimmunity.

4. Autoimmune triggers

4.1 Genetics

The enhanced knowledge of the mammalian immune system and the genetics lead to understanding the role of genes in autoimmune diseases. In the case of disease pathology, genetic variations are found to affect the MHC and several immunological pathways that in turn lead to the stimulation of autoimmunity. A number of studies have evidenced the potential role of genetics in the disease generation. Twin studies of multiple sclerosis (MS), rheumatoid arthritis (RA), Type- 1 diabetes and systemic lupus erythematosus (SLE) have reported a marked genetic predisposition of which the risk factor was found to be higher for monozygotic twins than the dizygotic twins. The risk of inheriting the systemic autoimmune diseases was also reported and this etiology could be due to the family history associated with the genetic vairaitons. In addition, a variety of MHC and non-MHC susceptible genes are identified in the genome wide studies of MS, SLE and RA while, few studies reported that many autoimmune diseases have a common genetic etiology operating (Glinda, 1999). Likewise, the association of intracellular tyrosine phosphatise, PTPN22 was shared in the pathologies of Type-1diabetes, RA and myasthenia gravis (Bottini, 2004; Begovich, 2004; Vandiedonck et al., 2006). In brief, genetics underscore a significant risk factor for the autoimmune etiology and presents a new area to explore.

4.2 Auto antigens

In the early stages of development some of the self antigens might escape recognition from the T-cell populations. This could happen because, they might not have been formed at the time of T-cell development or they might be separated from T-cell access due to remote anatomical existence (e.g. myelin basic protein) or due to the presence of membrane barriers or they might be inappropriately presented by the MHC proteins (Manoury, 1998). These cryptic antigens hinder the tolerance mechanisms and drive the autoimmune attack if they are encountered by the T-cells upon membrane barrier disruption for e.g. orchiditis upon vasectomy (Flickinger, 1994; Jarow et al., 1994) infections (Type 1 diabetes upon coxsackie B virus infection) or any other mechanism that exposes them (Yoon et al., 1979). A striking feature of auto antigens is that they are not specific to any tissue and form the integral components of all various cell types (Tan et al., 1987).

4.3 Role of infections

Infections have an interesting role to play in the induction of autoimmune diseases and there are several interesting mechanisms where infections mediate them. In the instances of microbial infections, immune cells cannot differentiate antigenic sequences from self proteins if structural similarities are found. This molecular mimicry unleashes the immune attack that is directed towards self and nonself leading to tissue destruction. For e.g. hepatitis B virus polymerase resembles myelin basic protein and generates auto antibodies that destroy myelin leading to multiple sclerosis (Fujinami & Oldstone, 1989; Oldstone, 1998; Fujinami & Oldstone, 1985). Infections are associated with interesting mechanisms that may enhance the severity of autoimmune diseases. Among these, epitope spreading is an instance where in an inflammatory burst, the avid APCs over process and presents the antigens to activate the large T-cell populations lowering the threshold to the disease onset. The other mechanism is termed as polyclonal activation where abundant B-cell populations are activated generating loads of antibodies along with immune complexes that pose serious threat to the tissues. The next mechanism involves the over activation and indiscriminate expansion of self reactive T-cells that are initially considered to be inefficient but can cause the disease in the presence of elevated levels of cytokines. Finally, microbes express super antigens on their surfaces that are unique in coupling T-cells with MHC complexes irrespective of their relativities (Barzilai et al., 2007a, 2007b). On the contrary when correlations were made between autoimmune diseases and infections, the incidences were found to be increased in the subjects who are at reduced risk of infections. The same holds true as autoimmune diseases have a rampant growth in western countries where the infectious incidences are lower compared to less developed nations (Bach, 2002; Patterson et al., 1996) substantiating the concept of hygiene hypothesis which states that the microbial exposure enhances the body's defence mechanisms (Bjorksten B, 1994).

4.4 Role of cell adhesion molecules

The propagation of autoimmune attack desperately needs the in and out migration of the immune cells, in particular T-cells, into the susceptible environment with potent inflammatory mediation. Cell adhesion molecules provide a suitable platform for this setting and are categorised as integrins, immunoglobulins and the selectins (Ziff, 1991). An autoimmune inflammatory setting leads to the enhanced expression of vascular endothelial proteins that constitute mucosal addressin cell adhesion molecule-1 (MAdCAM-1), intercellular adhesion molecule-1 (ICAM-1) and vascular cell adhesion molecule-1 (VCAM-1). Correspondingly, the lymphocytes express the cell surface molecules P-selectin glycoprotein ligand-1 (PSGL-1), leukocyte function-associated antigen-1 (LFA-1) and very late antigen-4 (VLA-4) on their surface facilitating the adherence and entry of the immune traffic into the lesions and further enhancing the autoimmune spread (Dedrick et al., 2003; Kanwar et al., 1999).VLA-4 and LFA-1are specifically expressed by the human B cells (Alter et al, 2003) and therapeutic interventions with anti-adhesion molecule antibodies have witnessed successful termination of autoimmune disease severity in preclinical and clinical models (McMurray, 1996; Kanwar et al, 2000; Kanwar et al 2003; Kanwar, 2005; Kanwar et al 2009).

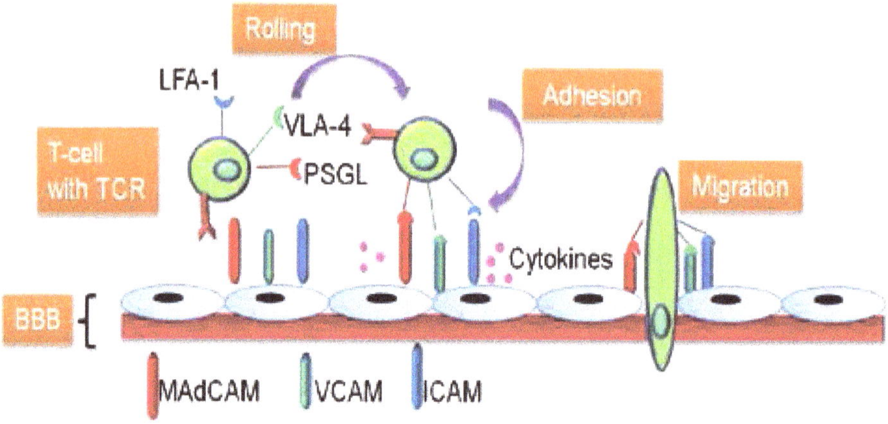

Fig. 2. Showing a typical T-cell exhibiting the phenomenon of rolling, adhesion and migration through the blood brain barrier (BBB) into the CNS. T-cell expresses PSGL-1, VLA-4 and LFA-1 on its cell surface and rolls over to adhere to the corresponding cell adhesion molecules, mucosal addressin cell adhesion molecule (MAdCAM), Vascular cell adhesion molecule (VCAM) and Intracellular cell adhesion molecule, (ICAM) respectively on the blood brain barrier capillary endothelial cells. These cell surface ligands are over expressed in an inflammatory condition facilitating the entry of T-cells into the BBB and thus initiating an autoimmune cascade.

4.5 Long lived plasma cells

The concept of long lived antibody secreting plasma cells were first demonstrated in a mouse model immunized with ovalbumin where in the plasma cells secreted antibodies against ovalbumin and the production was continuous independent of antigen exposure and memory cell assistance (Manz et al., 1997, 1998). The same was also observed in another mouse model infected with lymphocytic choriomeningitis virus (Slifka et al., 1998). The

potential role of long lived plasma cells in the generation of autoimmune diseases was studied in NZB/W mice that served as a model for systemic lupus erythematosis (Hoyer et al, 2004). The differentiation of B-cells leading to the generation of memory cells and antibody secreting plasma cells is guided both by the antigenic and non antigenic stimuli (Tarlinton et al., 2008; Radbruch et al., 2006). However not all antibody secreting plasma cells turn long lived as it entirely depends on the antibody titre maintenance for the generation of secondary immune responses (Manz et al., 2005).
Long lived plasma cells mainly originate from the germinal centre regions and require a close reciprocation of the T and B-cells. But, once generated these cells act independently. In one of the autoimmune pathologies, it was found that self reactive B-cells are not excluded from the germinal centre region allowing the production of long lived plasma cells that were autoreactive (Cappione et al., 2005). This concept of long lived plasma cells is novel and serves as attractive targets for treating autoimmune diseases.

4.6 Auto antibodies

The role of auto antibodies in the pathogenesis of autoimmune diseases is often elusive but considering few autoimmune diseases like myasthenia gravis, the antibodies are specific to cell surface receptors. The basic principle for the autoantibody directed cytotoxicity is the identification of cell surface antigen followed by cell death mechanisms either through complement activated system, antibody dependent cell mediated cytotoxicity (ADCC) or by the macrophage uptake mechanism (Ohishi et al., 1995; Frisoni et al., 2005). Complement activated system is constituted by a collection of specific group of plasma proteins and are considered to be more prevailing in autoimmune diseases. The class of autoimmune haemolytic anaemia, lupus syndrome typically fall under the complement system generated autoimmune diseases (Fang et al., 2009). In the case of classical ADCC, NKs play a prime role in mediating the cell death, after the binding of antibody with the target antigen. NK's binds the Fc portions of these antibodies and induce cell death by free radical generation. Autoimmune thyroid disease is a fine example of ADCC mediated autoimmune disease (Rodien et al., 1996). Finally, macrophages execute the uptake and cell lysis processes once they find the appropriate antibody-antigen interaction (Gehrs & Friedberg, 2002). In general, the auto antibodies are directed to intracellular antigens and this understanding unveils fascinating questions of how they interact with intracellular antigens. The possible explanation could be because of the cross reaction of surface antigens with the intracellular antigens (Frisoni et al., 2005) and the exposure of intracellular components after lysis due to an impaired macrophage phagocytosis (Hansen et al., 2002). The potential significance of auto antibodies in autoimmune diseases were also demonstrated in the foetus as few of the immunoglobulin's (IgG) can cross the placenta and target the cell surface creating a havoc of tissue destruction (Clancy et al., 2004a, 2004b). Also, the apoptotic cells were found to be potent enough to generate autoantibodies if accompanied by other moieties like dendritic cells or Freunds incomplete adjuvant. These dying cells tend to activate Toll like receptors and NF-kB pathway that are associated with inflammation which in turn is linked to generation of autoantibodies (Bondanza et al., 2004), in conclusion it has to keep in mind that, auto antibodies are not always associated with the disease and few of them are valuable diagnostic aids implicated in a clinical setting.

4.7 Stress and autoimmune diseases

Stress of both versions physical and physiological is found to be associated with the disease generation. This was also supported from the several past studies that emotional stress was highly proportionate for predicting the disease onset. These two are related because, stress presumably shoots the neuroendochrine triggers that are predicted to alter the immune function or the cytokine levels ending up with the disease generation (Herrmann et al., 2000; Stojanovich & Marisavljevich, 2008). Also, stress induces the expression of heat shock proteins that are highly immunogenic with a potential of triggering autoimmune diseases (Kanwar et al., 2001). Therefore, therapeutic interventions for these diseases should consider management of emotions and stress.

4.8 Pregnancy and autoimmune diseases

In order to escape the immune attack neither the sperms nor the developing trophoblast bear the MHC proteins of either class. This peculiar feature allows the escape and survival of the sperm from the immune attack to fertilize the ovum (Johnson, 1993). Soon after fertilisation, many protective measures are adopted to protect the developing foetus and likewise it bears the human leucocyte antigen (HLA-G) marker which if otherwise would have been killed by the natural killer cells (VanVoorhis & Stovall, 1997). Also regulatory proteins from the foetus avoid the activation of complement system and its subsequent attack (Holmes & Simpson, 1992). Interesting immunological features are noticed in a pregnant woman, as changes are seen in the immune reactions that shift from Th1 to Th2 type due to the release of cytokines like TGF-beta (Raghupathy, 1997; Lim et al., 1998). This modification has a striking implication in that many of the pregnant woman experience remission of autoimmune diseases like rheumatoid arthritis (RA) and multiple sclerosis that are Th1 mediated (Allebeck et al., 1984; Cutolo & Accardo, 1991). However the risk of systemic lupus erythematosis (SLE) in pregnant woman is much higher compared to non pregnant woman and this also has drastic effects on the survival of the foetus (Khamashta et al., 1997; Cooper et al., 2002; Fraga et al., 1974).

4.9 T and B-cell traffic in the CNS

The migration of T-cells into the CNS adopt the same principles as they enter the peripheral tissues namely, activated T-cells migrate the tissues from the blood where as inactive ones remains in the lymph vessels (Mackay et al., 1990). To demonstrate the migration of T-cells into the CNS, Hickey et al administered labelled T-cells intravenously and observed the appearance of T-cells in the brain parenchyma soon after 3 hrs (Hickey et al., 1991). Also, T-cells in very minute levels were detected in the rat and human brains suggesting the fact that they continuously monitor the CNS (Pender, 1995). Similarly B-cells cross the BBB, perhaps more rapidly than the T-cells and differentiate into the plasma cells in response to an antigen as they do in the periphery (Knopf et al., 1998; Anthony et al., 2003; Kanwar, 2005). The following figure 3 represents the autoreactive T-cell entry and further consequences that lead to the generation of autoimmunity.

4.10 Co-stimulatory molecules

The phenomenon of T-cell activation and the generation of autoimmunity also depend on the involvement of several co-stimulatory molecules like B7-1, B7-2, CD28, inducible co stimulator (ICOS), OX 40 and CD40 ligand that are associated with T-cell activation. Other molecules like cytotoxic T lymphocyte antigen 4 (CTLA-4) and programmed death 1 (PD-1) regulate negative co-stimulation. Hence, effective therapeutics targeting these molecules will have a significant impact in the autoimmune disease control (Racke & Stuart, 2002; Kanwar et al 2004).

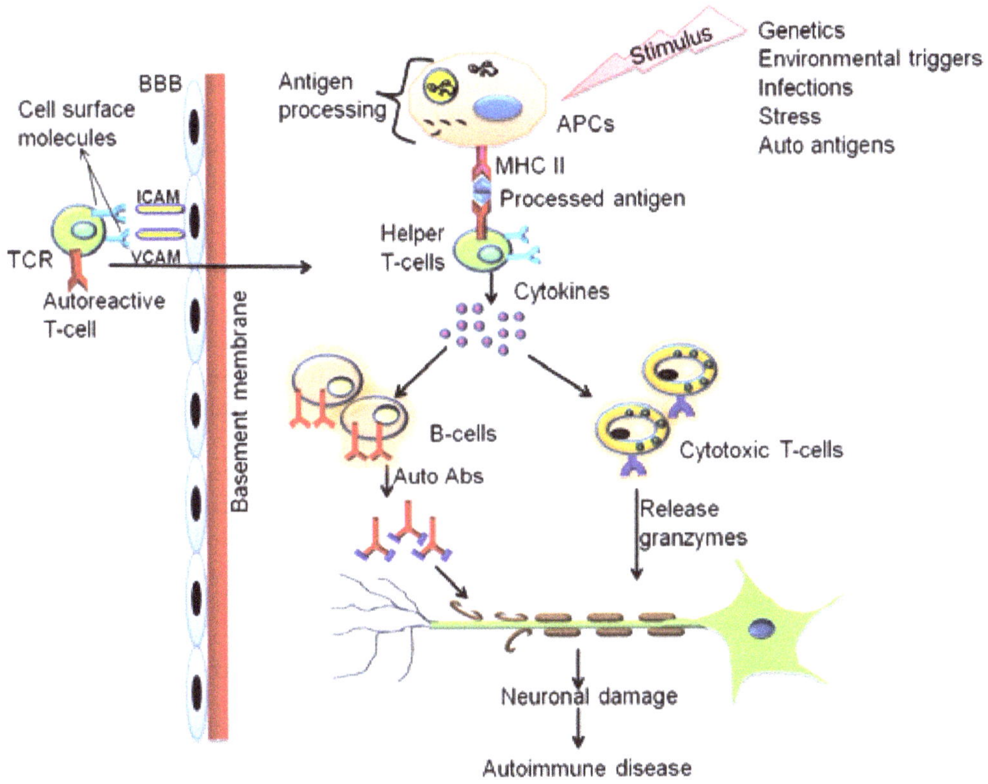

Fig. 3. Schematic representation of autoimmune attack in the CNS APCs-Antigen presenting cells; BBB-Blood brain barrier; ICAM- intercellular cell adhesion molecule; MHC-Major histocompatibility complex; TCR-T-cell receptor; VCAM- Vascular intercellular cell adhesion molecule.

The auto reactive T-cells gain entry into the CNS by the pairing of cell surface molecules leukocyte function-associated antigen-1 (LFA-1) and very late antigen-4(VLA-4) with the cell adhesion molecules, intercellular cell adhesion molecule (ICAM) and vascular cell adhesion molecule (VCAM) expressed on the brain capillary endothelium. Once after entry the helper T-cells (Th) bind with the processed peptide fragments presented along with MHC II by the antigen presenting cells (APCs).The threshold for triggering immune attack is lowered in autoimmune diseases and is stimulated by a variety of factors. The Th cells secrete a variety of cytokines that further activate the cytotoxic T-cells (Tc) and the antibody secreting B-cells. Tc cells, when activated mediate the cytotoxicity by releasing the granzymes while the B-cells differentiate into plasma cells that produce auto antibodies against a variety of targets like the myelin, nicotinic acetylcholine receptors (NAchRs), voltage gated calcium channels (VGCC), voltage gated potassium channels (VGKC), glycolipids etc mediating the corresponding neurological autoimmune disorder.

4.11 Autoimmunity and survivin

In an effort to address issues involved with the treatment of neurodegenerative and autoimmune diseases, the two following strategies can be employed: a neuroprotection strategy and a neuroproliferative strategy. Findings suggest that Bcl2 and IAP inducers are able to inhibit apoptosis for the purpose of neuroprotection in preclinical models (Kanwar, 2010a-d, Baratchi, 2010 a&b). Our understanding of neurodegenerative diseases has improved over the past two decades. Whereas these disorders are initiated due to a range of insults such as reactive oxygen species or misfolded proteins, all of these pathologies end with a common consequence, which is the degeneration and deterioration of neuronal cells (Kanwar et al, 2010a). Despite all of the efforts to understand and treat neurodegenerative diseases, their successful treatment has still not been achieved. A proper treatment should not only protect neural cells but should also increase their proliferation and differentiation so as to provide a promising future for an aging population and families with a history of degenerative disorders, including multiple sclerosis, Parkinson's disease and stroke. The brain's environment is the most protected part of our body and neurons are a unique cell type (Baratchi, 2011a&b). Despite playing an important role in the analysis and transfer of information to the entire body, the lack of neural self-proliferation and repair highlights the importance of their protection and proliferation. To be able to protect these cells from death and to facilitate their proliferation involves mechanisms that still need to be identified. Experimental findings achieved over the past few years have suggested that inhibitors of apoptosis (IAP), which serve a natural role in balancing cell death, might be candidate proteins with a unique potential for drug discovery (Kanwar et al, 2010). Recently we reviewed the exceptional capabilities of survivin (a unique member of IAPs) in both cell cycle and cell death pathways and its unique characteristics related to neuronal cell survival and proliferation (Baratchi, 2010a&b).

Given that this is the first report of a protective effect of SurR9-C84A following an oxidative stress injury, further work should be done to study the effects of SurR9-C84A on *in vivo* models of degenerative diseases. In summary, we reported for the first time, a recombinant, cell-permeable form of the survivin mutant protein (SurR9-C84A) efficiently enters neuronal cells, protects differentiated SK-N-SH cells from the activation of apoptosis induced by H_2O_2, decreases the expression of cell cycle markers, and increases antioxidant activity. Emerging nano-delivery systems could be used to bypass the blood brain barrier, facilitating drug delivery to the damaged brain. Survivin is a member of the IAP family, which has been shown to have a role in early brain development and serves a bifunctional role during mitosis and inhibition of apoptosis (Baratchi et al., 2010a; Kanwar et al., 2010). Different forms of survivin mutants (such as C84A, Δ106 and T34A) have been used for the purpose of targeting survivin overexpression in cancer cells (Cheung, 2010a&b; Kanwar et al, 2010b; (Baratchi, 2010a&b). Among the various survivin mutants, the baculovirus IAP repeat motif (C84A) was initially produced and has since been shown to have proapoptotic effects on human cancer cells. Furthermore, we previously found that SurR9-C84A has protective effects against retinoic acid induced cell toxicity (Baratchi et al., 2011b). We used the SK-N-SH cell line as a culture model of retinoic acid-induced neuronal differentiation (Baratchi, 2010a&b). We showed for the first time, the neuroprotective effect of SurR9-C84A against cytotoxic elements existing in activated T-cell supernatants such as GrB. Because GrB is a powerful pro-apoptotic member of granzymes family and is a very important mediator of damage in progressive MS and other neuro-inflammatory disorders we examined the importance of GrB released from the activated T-cells in an *in-vitro* system and compared the protective effect of SurR9-C84A with GrB inhibitor (Baratchi, 2011a&b). SurR9-C84A can be applied in neuroprotective strategies to protect differentiated neural cells from cell cycle re-entry and apoptosis. Additionally, one important advantage of this mutant over the wild type survivin is that it does not form tumour due to its pro-apoptotic effect in cancer cells. Because the over-expression of survivin has been reported in stimulated T-cells derived from patients with active MS, the neuroprotective ability of SurR9-C84A has the potential to be employed for future neurodegenerative therapies, and may also be further evaluated for targeting stimulated T-cells for the treatment of neurodegenerative diseases such as MS and other brain injuries (Baratchi, 2010a&b).

5. Classification of autoimmune diseases

Autoimmune diseases are characterised by the abnormal activation of the immune responses against our own tissues evidenced by the inability of the immune cells to differentiate self from non self antigens. Hence, mistakenly immune attack is directed towards our own body parts. They are categorised as systemic, involving multi target organ damage (e.g. systemic lupus erythematosis) or they can be localised involving damage to a single organ. (e.g. Type 1 diabetes) (Mackay & Rosen, 2001).
A list of autoimmune neurological diseases are included and described as follows (Dalakas, 2006).

5.1 Multiple sclerosis (MS)

MS is a localised neurological autoimmune disease and is marked by the characteristic inflammation and degradation of the protective nerve lining, the myelin (Lucchinetti et al., 2000; Lassmann, 2000). More than 1 million people are affected by MS with a characteristic presentation of weakness, abnormal senses, ataxia, poor balance, fatigue, vision loss and impaired cognition (Fugger et al., 2009; Kanwar et al 2004; Kanwar, 2005). Based on the histopathology multicentred inflammatory lesions were observed in the patient's brain and the spinal cord (Frohman et al, 2006). Multiple aetiological factors are involved in the preponderance of the disease and are often found to be triggered by a viral infection (Lucchinetti et al., 2000). This initiation by an infection is by the process of molecular mimicry as discussed earlier. It is rather fascinating to study the generation of inflammatory lesions and the entry mechanisms of immune cells in MS. A specific population of activated T-cells that are selective towards myelin crosses the blood brain barrier under the strong influence of chemokines while the resting T-cells are inaccessible towards the BBB due to the unfeasible environment (Charo & Ransohoff, 2006).
The cell surface molecules (integrins, selectins and cadherins) of the T-cells bind with the adhesion molecules expressed on the brain endothelial cells and finally escape into the CNS. Following their entry, the T-cells then direct the immune attack towards myelin antigen presented on their surface by the APCs (Greter et al., 2005). Along with macrophages, dendritic cells, glial cells and astrocytes present the MHC class II expression in the CSF and thus attract the T-cell traffic (Heppner et al., 2005; Greter et al., 2005). Under the influence of activated T-cells the immune attack is boosted up towards the myelin sheath and is executed by recruiting the T-cells and antibody secreting B-cells from the periphery driving the myelin assault leading to demyelination (Cepok et al., 2005; Steinman, 2002). The severity and progression of the demyelination process is influenced significantly by the B-cells as evidenced by the infiltration of macrophages and the deposition of immunoglobulins (Lucchinetti et al., 2000). The same was also supported by the observations made on clonal expansion and the presence of IgG complexes of B-cell populations in the brain and cerebrospinal fluid lesions (Qin et al., 1998; Baranzini et al., 1999; Colombo et al., 2000). The

whole process of immune attack and tissue damage is also encouraged by the active macrophages and glial cells (Brosnan & Raine,1996; Heppner et al., 2005). Interesting results were obtained from the animal model of MS, experimental autoimmune encephalomyelitis where it was found that, the pro-inflammatory T cells of Th1-type were found to be responsible for the disease exacerbations (Wekerle et al., 1986; Gold et al., 2006). There are four subtypes of MS and categorised as relapsing remitting (RR) with majority of the patients displaying recovery symptoms after disability. People who experience RR often complain a second variety of MS termed as secondary-progressive MS where the disability doesn't subside between the cycles of relapses and recoveries. The third form is the primary progressive stage where there is only progression and no remission. The last form of MS is rather rare and termed as Progressive-relapsing MS (PRMS) characterised by the severe attacks and symptoms during the remission period (Mayoclinic, 2008). More than 1 million people are affected by MS with a characteristic presentation of weakness, abnormal senses, ataxia, poor balance, fatigue, vision loss and impaired cognition. Significant contributions are being made for the disease diagnostics and management with the introduction of potential biomarkers. There are findings of glial fibrillary acidic protein (GFAP) and neurofilament light protein (NFL) (the cytoskeletal proteins of astrocytes and axons respectively) release into the CSF during the disease progression (Axelsson et al., 2010).

As per clinical data, the plasma levels of osteopontin was increased well before the induction of lesions with gadolinium (Gd) and similar profiles were observed with 7KC and 15 oxy sterol derivatives of cholesterol in MS patients. Added to this, enhanced antibody binding was reported towards these entities suggesting their potentials as biomarkers (Vogt et al., 2003; Whitaker, 1987). Also in a longitudinal cross sectional study of MS patients, it was found that levels of pentosidine, a well characterised biomarker for advanced glycation end products (AGE) were significantly elevated compared to the healthy controls. It was also observed that patients on treatment showed pentosidine down regulation compared to untreated patients. Thus, this study considers the AGE inhibitors as novel therapeutic interventions against MS. (Sternberg et al., 2011) The recent reports on the associated tissue damage in MS patients found that it is not only limited to axons but also included significant retinal damage (Green et al., 2010).

The current therapeutic strategies for MS include the treatment for disease progression and the symptoms. Interferon's of type I (IFN-1) specifically marked as IFNb1a, IFNb1b and glatiramer acetate are considered as the first line drugs against RR form of MS but have a limited effectiveness. The mechanism of these drugs is that they down regulate the proliferation of T-cells, reduced antigen presentation, T-cell migration (interferon's in particular) and shift the immune response to Th2 type (Clerico et al., 2007; Arnon & Aharoni, 2004). Natalizumab, a humanized monoclonal antibody (mab) is found effective against MS as it inhibits the entry of T-cells into the CNS by acting against the cell surface molecule α-integrins and showed significant reduction in the relapse rate compared to the above treatment strategies (Polman et al., 2006). However, limitation exists on its indiscriminate use as it poses a serious risk of brain infection, progressive multifocal leukoencephalopathy (PML) that even causes death (Clifford et al., 2010). Corticosteroids like prednisone, prednisolone, methyl prednisolone and dexamethasone are also used against the RR and rarely against secondary progressive multiple sclerosis as they act by suppressing the immune system. They are strictly contraindicated for long term use as they are associated with a number of side effects (Merck,). Chemotherapeutics with a potential of suppressing the immune system like mitoxantrone inducing the apoptosis of lymphocytes and cyclophosphamide acting against both the T & B-cell activities, were also tried against RR and secondary progressive MS (Chan et al., 2005; Fauci et al., 1971; Multiple Sclerosis Treatments). The drugs in development for MS are Fingolimod and BG00012 that are in phase II clinical trials. Fingolimod acts by complexing the lymphocytes in the lymph nodes preventing their entry into the CNS and BG00012 is an oral formulation of Fumarate and presumed to act by neuroprotective and anti-inflammatory mechanisms inhibiting the oxidative stress (Lutterotti & Berger, 2010). Drugs in phase III clinical trials for RR form of MS are Laquinimod that acts by shifting the T-cell response to Th2 type and Teriflunomide acts by interrupting pyrimidine synthesis inhibiting the dihydro-orotate dehydrogenase and stops the expansion of T and B cells. Cladribine is efficient against both the resting and dividing T-cells and acts against the adenosine deaminase enzyme (Yang et al., 2004; Warnke et al., 2009). Monoclonal antibodies are also under evaluation and CAMPATH is tried against the CD52 expression on leukocytes. This activity depleted a majority of the lymphocytes, monocytes and dendritic cells in MS patients (Osborne, 2009; Hauser et al., 2008). A similar effect was observed with Rituximab that acts against the CD20 expression.

5.2 Myasthenia Gravis (MG)

In the case of myasthenia gravis the prototypic B cells produce the auto antibodies that are directed against the nicotinic acetylcholine receptor (AchR) in the neuromuscular junction (NMJ) (Drachman, 1994; Ragheb & Lisak, 1998). These antibodies from the peripherally activated B cells infiltrate the end-plate region of NMJ, and down regulate the functionally active Ach receptors either by cross linking the receptor followed by internalization or by initiating the complement-mediated immune destruction or they may make the binding site unavailable for activity (Bufler et al., 1996). Following this, the signal transmission and communication is significantly affected between the neurons and the muscles in NMJ region due to the immune attack.

Based on the symptom severity there are three subtypes of MG, Pure ocular MG characterised by weakness and fatigue of extra ocular muscles, resulting in ptosis and diplopia. Generalized MG, with extensive skeletal muscle weakness and finally myasthenia crisis, with disturbances in swallowing and respiratory failure (Hohlfeld et al., 2003). The exact role of antibodies in the pathogenesis of myasthenia gravis was confirmed from the results that, administration of myasthenic IgG antibodies generated the symptoms while the symptoms were ameliorated upon their removal (Drachman, 1994; Vincent et al., 2000). In a patient subgroup with myasthenia gravis, another variety of autoimmunity was reported with the detection of auto antibodies directed towards the muscle specific kinase. These patients were considered as seronegative to MG. (Vincent et al., 2003). The treatment modalities for MG include the acetylcholinesterase (AchE) inhibitors as the mainstay of treatment as they improve the bioavailability of Ach in the NMJ and the immune modulating agents. The AchE inhibitors of clinical significance are the pyridostigmine and neostigmine. They act by binding with AchE enzyme because of structural resemblance to Ach and slowly get hydrolysed compared to it. This improves the availability and subsequent binding of Ach to the available AchR in the NMJ. The common adverse effects associated are disturbances of GIT, respiratory system, cardiovascular system and glandular secretions (Kumar & Kaminski, 2011).

5.2.1 Agents acting on immune system

Glucocorticosteroids with a potential of strong anti-inflammatory and immunosuppressive activity are tried with a successful outcome. The orally administered glucocorticoids (prednisone in common) show a delayed onset of action and take even months to exhibit maximum therapeutic benefit (Hohlfeld et al., 2003). However, intravenous administration is recommended for the management of exacerbations (Arsura et al., 1985). Long-term treatment is not recommended due to the severe side effects featuring crushing's syndrome, obesity, precipitation of diabetes, gastrointestinal ulcers, opportunistic infections and hypertension etc. In the class of immune suppressive drugs, Azathioprine is the prominent and well tolerated drug tried against MG patients. This is a purine analogue and displays significant decrement in the levels of both T & B-cells thus monitoring the immune attack. Added to its mechanism it also exhibits anti-inflammatory actions by inhibiting promonocyte cell proliferation. It is generally given in combination to lower the dose of glucocorticoids but can also be prescribed alone for long term therapy (Mertens et al., 1981; Gold et al., 2003). Cyclosporine-A acts by binding to an intracellular protein, cyclophilin and forms a cyclosporine-cyclophilin complex. This complex exhibits immunosuppressive activity by inhibiting the phosphatase, calcineurin and prevents the cytokine formation. The clinical significance of this drug was that, it was the first drug tried in a double-blind and placebo-controlled trial MG patient population (Tindall et al., 1987). Patients with refractory MG show better responses towards cyclophosphamide, methotrexate and mycophenolate mofetil (Schneider-Gold et al., 2006). The recent advancements included are the administration of intravenous IgG that has a potential blocking activity against auto antibodies. This treatment is recommended when all the treatment modalities have failed. (Zinman et al., 2007) Advancements are made in the therapeutics of MG with the introduction of SHG2210, a novel entity with a potential to fuse with the α-subunit of the auto antibodies that are directed against AchR. This SHG2210 -autoantibody fusion complex is later cleared by the transferrin receptor mediated cellular uptake (Keefe et al., 2010).

On the whole due to the advancements made in the diagnosis and treatment, MG stands as a rear but treatable autoimmune disease.

5.3 Guillainbarre syndrome (GBS)

GBS is classified as an acute auto immune disease of demyelinating type mostly affecting the peripheral nervous system. Depending upon the target affected by the immune attack it is categorised to 4 subtypes. The first of its kind is the acute inflammatory demyelinating polyneuropathy (AIDP) where the immune attack is directed towards the myelin or schwann cell surface membrane. The next subtype is the acute motor axonal neuropathy (AMAN) targeting the axonal membrane in motor fibres where as both the motor and sensory nerve fibres are targeted in acute motor sensory axonal neuropathy (AMSAN). In the last subtype, distal nerve terminals and nodal regions of the ocular motor nerve are affected and termed as Miller Fisher syndrome (MFS) (Willison et al., 2002; Kuwabara, 2004). GBS is often triggered by an infection of bacterial or viral origin with auto antibodies directed against gangliosides particularly in AMAN where infections with *campylobacter jejuni* produced auto antibodies against GM1, GM1b, GD1 or Ga1NAc-GD1a gangliosides (Ogawara et al., 2000). There were also detectable levels of IgG and complement deposition in the nerves (Hafer-Macko et al., 1996). The distinct involvement of T and B-cells are identified in few subtypes, with the activated complement system playing a prime role in mediating demyelination and impaired conduction but still understanding the pathology of GBS remains rather elusive (Kieseier et al., 2004). The treatment for GBS is often confined to the immunomodulatory therapy where plasmapheresis and intravenous administration of immunoglobulin's IVIg are given the priority (Dalakas, 1999; Hadden et al., 1998).

Plasmapheresis is the plasma exchange where the immunoglobulins and antibodies are removed from the serum with a subsequent separation of the blood cells. Then these blood cells are isolated and added to the fresh plasma or saline to administer back into the patient. IVIg operates through multiple mechanisms that include the inhibition of antibody production, complement binding, macrophage receptor blockade and the abnormal antibody neutralisation. Both these strategies were found to have equal efficiencies in reducing the disease progression (Heather Rachel Davids).. Future therapies for GBS are directed towards the complement inhibitors. (Walgaard et al., 2011)

5.4 Neuromyelitis optica (NMO)

The pathology of this neurological autoimmune disorder is clear with the detection of antibodies against the aquaporin -4 water channels of the endothelial cells in the CNS (Lennon et al., 2005). In the autopsy studies, deposition of Immunoglobulins particularly of the IgM subtype were detected in the lesions with activated complimentary system leading to vascular damage. The predominant immune attack directed in this disorder is of the humoral type with majority of the attack directed towards the optic nerve and the spinal cord (Lucchinetti et al., 2002; Wingerchuk et al., 2004; Bergamaschi, 2007). Immunosuppressive therapeutics like mycophenolate mofetil, mitoxantrone and rituximab are far beneficial rather than immunomodulating agents like interferons in NMO(Bergamaschi, 2007).Eculizumab, is a new molecule under Phase I/II clinical trials and the proposed mechanism for this entity is that it inhibits the complement activation and subsequent destruction (. clinicaltrials.gov.).

5.5 Stiff-Man syndrome (SMS)

Stiff man or Stiff-person syndrome is also a predominant antibody directed autoimmune disease with majority of the auto antibodies directed towards the enzyme, glutamic acid decarboxylase (GAD) that is essential for the synthesis of gamma-amino butyric acid, a principal inhibitory neurotransmitter in the brain. Also, detectable levels of Immunoglobulin belonging to the subtype IgG were found in the CSF confirming the infiltration of B-cells (Dalakas et al., 2001; Ishii, 2010). The recent epidemiological studies report the existence of anti-gephyrin, anti-amphiphysin and anti-gamma-aminobutyric acid A receptor-associated protein (GABARAP) antibodies in the disease pathology. The patients experiencing this disease complain symptoms of muscular rigidity in the legs and trunk region often associated with muscle spasms (Dalakas et al., 2000). The medication for stiff man syndrome initially should begin with the skeletal muscle relaxants benzodiazepine or baclofen. Intrathecal administration of baclofen was even considered in a selected patient group. However great care has to be taken in performing this procedure as it is involved with puncturing the meninges (Duddy & Baker, 2009). Other treatment options considered are plasmapheresis and administration of Intravenous immunoglobulins like Gamimune, Gammagard, Sandoglobulin (Dalakas, 2009; Hayashi et al., 1999).

5.6 Paraneoplastic neurological syndromes (PNS)

The pathology associated with this autoimmune disease is quite peculiar. Antigens that are confined to the nervous system are capable of mediating an immune attack if the same antigens are expressed in the case of pathological conditions such as the breast or ovarian cancers. The immune cells that are activated against these antigens also direct their attack indiscriminately towards the antigens of the CNS that were once considered as self. A diverse range of self-antigens are identified in this setting and within this diversity, multiple epitopes are recognized within each antigen encountered. Thus, stimulated by the cancers, immune drive is targeted against the CNS evidenced by the detection of serum antibodies. The most common serum antibody detected is the anti-Hu antibody in patients coexisting with sensory neuropathy, encephalomyelitis or cerebellar ataxia (Dalmau et al., 1992; Graus et al., 2001; Darnell & Posner, 2003; Maverakis et al., 2011). Other such auto antibodies detected are anti-Yo antibodies in cerebellar degeneration (Peterson et al., 1992) anti-Ma1 and anti-Ma2 antibodies in limbic encephalitis in patients with testicular cancer (Rosenfeld et al, 2001) and antibodies in Lambert-Eaton myasthenic syndrome in small cell lung cancer patients (Carpentier & Delattre, 2001). In the paraneoplastic autoimmune CNS disorders, immune cells penetrate the blood-brain barrier and the antibody mediated destruction serves as the dominant mode of immune attack as evidenced by the localised synthesis of antibodies by the B cells (Darnell & Posner, 2003 & Pranzatelli et al., 2004). However, defining the precise mechanisms of cellular and humoral pathways in the pathophysiology is still unclear and the immune system adapts the elusive mode to identify the intracellular antigens.

The treatment for this disorder should be aimed at treating the underlying tumor with standard anticancer therapeutic regimen while the immune mediated disorder is treated by plasmapheresis or administration of immune suppressive drugs like Cyclosporine and glucocorticoids. Cyclosporine acts against both the cell and humoral mediated immune reactions and glucocorticoids are the potent anti-inflammatory and immune suppressive agents as discussed. Immune reaction suppression is even achieved by the administration of IVIg and Antithymocyte globulin is recommended in this case. It is a polyclonal IgG antibody particularly effective against T-lymphocytes and reduces the count to 85-90% (Buchwald et al., 2005; Koski & Patterson, 2006).

5.7 Lambert-Eaton Myasthenic Syndrome (LEMS)

Lambert-Eaton syndrome is a muscular disorder characterised by the autoantibody generation against the voltage gated calcium channels in the presynaptic nerve terminals. The communication is drastically affected between the nerves and muscles due to the inability of the nerve cells to release Ach required for muscular contraction. Hence, the symptoms of muscular rigidity and weakness are experienced in the patient population. The difference noticed between MG and LEMS is that in the latter form of the disease, with repeated contractions the muscle gets stronger for a shorter span of time instead of turning weaker (Lambert-Eaton syndrome, 2000). The primary treatment for LEMS aims to enhance the levels of Ach either by increasing its release or by inhibiting its metabolism thus making it available at the NMJ. The agents that are considered effective in this regard are Pyridostigmine bromide, 3,4-Diaminopyridine (DAP) and guanidine HCl. Pyridostigmine is an AchE inhibitor and shows symptomatic relief, while DAP and guanidine HCL acts by enhancing the release of Ach with noticeable improvement in the muscular strength. Patients who are refractory to the above treatment are prescribed with the immunosuppressive drugs as mentioned earlier (McEvoy et al., 1989; Sanders, 1995).

5.8 Neuromyotonia (NM)

Neuromyotonia, is a rare autoimmune disorder with antibodies directed against the voltage gated K^+ channels of the Shaker-type (Kv1). Based on the symptoms observed the disease is categorised as acquired neuromyotonia (NMT) with peripheral nerve hyperexcitability, fasciculations and muscle stiffness. Morvan's syndrome is associated with the symptoms of NMT along with encephalopathy and sleep disorders. The last subtype is the limbic encephalitis characterised by the CNS involvement with encephalopathic seizures, hyponatremia and abnormal electroencephalographic abnormalities. The antibodies noticed in this immune disorder were pathogenic and were confirmed by the observations of electrophysiological changes in mice, upon administration of IgG derived from patients (Kleopas et al., 2006; Buckley & Vincent, 2005; Merchut, 2010). Recently, a novel pathology was attributed to limbic encephalitis in which auto antibodies were identified against leucine-rich glioma-inactivated 1 (LGI1) protein. Previously, these auto antibodies were assumed to be acting against K^+ channels and hence, this disorder is now termed as limbic encephalitis associated with LGI1 antibodies (Lai et al., 2010).

Most of the patients with these disorders fairly respond when treated with immunosuppressive drugs like glucocorticosteroids. Also other recommendations include plasmapheresis and IVIg (Merchut, 2010).

5.9 Polyneuropathies (PN)

Polyneuropathies are divided into 3 subtypes as chronic inflammatory demyelinating polyneuropathy (CIDP), multifocal motor neuropathy (MMN) and IgM anti-myelin-associated glycoprotein (MAG) demyelinating neuropathy (Kornberg & Pestronk, 2003; Czaplinski & Steck, 2004; Kieseier et al., 2004). Both the T and B-cell mediated immune havoc is noticed in CIDP with the majority of antibodies directed towards the glycolipids GM1 (Yan et al., 2000). Similar type of antibody production is identified against GM1 in half of the patient population in MMN but the pathogenecity of these antibodies are left unidentified (Nobile-Orazio, 2001). On the contrary, the IgM antibodies generated against the myelin associated glycoprotein in anti-MAG neuropathies are identified as pathogenic with a successful transfer of the disease to the animals. The normal cellular interactions were also found to be disturbed by these anti-MAG antibodies by the complement activation towards the myelin lamellae (Latov, 1994; Dalakas & Quarles, 1996; Quarles & Weiss, 1999). The treatment options considered are mainly immunosuppressive in nature and administration of glucocorticosteroids, plasmapheresis and IVIg are in use (Shy, 2007). Figure 4 summarises the pathologies of all the neurological autoimmune diseases.

6. What's in the pipeline?

The role of B-cells in the autoimmune disorders is inevitable and considering this concrete paradigm researchers have now focussed targeting them with the mainstay of B-cell depletion. The targets identified were the B-lymphocyte stimulator (BLyS) protein and the CD20 expression on B-cells. Belimumab, is the humanised anti-BLyS monoclonal antibody and showed effective inhibition of invitro B-cell proliferation. (Baker et al, 2003) Also, phase I clinical trials of belimumab in SLE was well tolerated and further results are yet to be reported (Stohl, 2004). Rituximab, a chimeric anti-CD20 monoclonal antibody has the ability to deplete B-cells by multiple mechanisms and results are encouraging when it was tried against a variety of autoimmune disorders (Wylam et al., 2003; Ruegg et al., 2004; Stuve et al., 2005).. In extension ocrelizumab, a humanized version of rituximab is currently in the developing stage for targeting several autoimmune disorders (Genovese et al., 2008). The same also holds true for Epratuzumab, a humanised mab that acts by blocking CD22 and

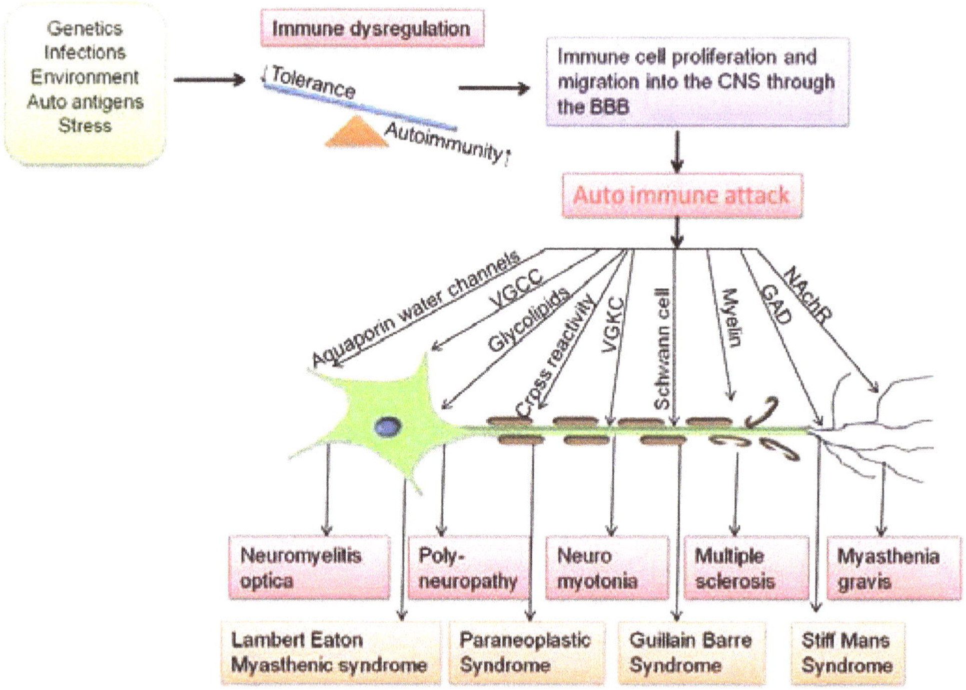

GAD-Glutamicacid decarboxylase; NAchR-Nicotinic acetylcholine receptors; VGCC- Voltage gated calcium channels; VGKC- Voltage gated potassium channels

Fig. 4. Representing the various triggers of autoimmune diseases and the different targets involved in the generation of neurological autoimmune diseases.

thereby depletes B-cell population (Dalakas, 2008). Targeting the T-cell antigens was always an area of intense interest. Researchers have made significant contributions with the development of anti-CD3 MAbs that displayed not only potent immunosuppressive activities but also the ability to restore self tolerance (Chatenoud, 2003). Progress was also presumed with the introduction of T-lymphocyte subsets, the invariant natural killer T (iNKT) cells. These unique cells stimulate a diverse range of cytokines that regulate the activities of various immune cells and thus prove to be handy for autoimmune disease therapeutics (Gabriel et al., 2010). The preclinical studies of methyl thioadenosine, a natural metabolite was found effective with its immunomodulatory activity in MS model. The results of this study showed an enhanced efficiency when it was combined with interferon's or glatiramer acetate (Moreno et al., 2010). Midkine (MK) a cytokine that binds heparin is generally involved in inflammation by promoting T-cell traffic and cytokine up regulation. The MK inhibitors are assumed to be very valuable for treating MS as an aptamer to MK was found to repress experimental autoimmune encephalitis (Muramatsu, 2011). Histone deacetylase inhibitors were also found to have a potential against MS as they are found to interfere the immune system activation empowered with neuroprotective activities (Faraco et al., 2011). Recent advancements include the application of autologous and allogenic stem cell transplantations following intense immunoablation and the former application has lower toxicities compared to the latter. Encouraging results were obtained in a group of MS patients when treated with autologous stem cells compared to the existing therapies. However, further trials are warranted for the effective use (Marmont, 2000).

S. No	Disorder	Immune attack directed to	Current therapy	Future drugs
1	MS	Myelin	IFNb1a, IFNb1b, (Clerico et al., 2007) glatiramer acetate, (Arnon & Aharoni, 2004) natalizumab, (Polman et al., 2006) glucocorticosteroids (Merck) and chemotherapeutics (Chan et al., 2005)	Fingolimod, BG00012, (Lutterotti & Berger, 2010) Laquinimod Teriflunomide Cladribine (Yang et al., 2004; Warnke et al., 2009) Rituximab (Hauser et al., 2008) CAMPATH (Osborne, 2009) Midkine (Muramatsu, 2011) Methylthio-adenosine (Moreno et al., 2010) MAdCAM-1) antibody (Kanwar et al., 2004) Histone deacetylase inhibitors (Faraco et al., 2011)
2	MG	Nicotinic acetylcholine receptor and muscle specific kinase	AchE inhibitors, (Kumar & Kaminski, 2011) Glucocorticosteroids, (Hohlfeld et al., 2003) Azathioprine, (Mertens et al., 1981). cyclosporine, (Tindall et al., 1987) Cyclophosphamide and mycophenolate mofetil (Schneider-Gold et al., 2006)	SHG2210 (Keefe et al., 2010)
3	GBS	Myelin and axonal membrane in motor and sensory fibres	immunomodulatory therapy with plasmapheresis and IVIg (Dalakas, 1999; Hadden et al., 1998)	Complement inhibitors (Walgaard et al., 2011)
4	NMO	Aquaporin -4 water channels	interferons , mycophenolate mofetil, mitoxantrone and rituximab (Bergamaschi, 2007)	Eculizumab (clinicaltrials.gov)

5	SMS	Glutamic acid decarboxylase enzyme	skeletal muscle relaxants, (Duddy & Baker, 2009) Plasmapheresis and IVIg (Dalakas, 2009; Hayashi et al., 1999)	-------
6	PNS	Hu, Yo,Ma1 & Ma2 antibodies	Cyclosporine, glucocorticoids and Antithymocyte globulin (Buchwald et al., 2005; Koski & Patterson, 2006)	-------
7	LEMS	Voltage gated calcium channels	Pyridostigmine bromide, 3,4-Diaminopyridine, guanidine HCl and immunosuppressive agents (McEvoy et al., 1989; Sanders, 1995)	-------
8	NM	Voltage gated K+ channels and leucine-rich glioma-inactivated 1 protein	Glucocorticosteroids, Plasmaoheresis and IVIg (Merchut, 2010)	-------
9	PN	Glycolipid GM1 and myelin associated glycoprotein	Glucocorticosteroids, Plasmapheresis and IVIg (Shy, 2007)	-------

Multiple sclerosis=MS; Myasthenia gravis=MG; Guillain-Barre syndrome=GBS; Neuromyelitis optica=NMO; Stiff-Man syndrome =SMS; Paraneoplastic neurological syndromes=PNS; Lambert-Eaton myasthenic syndrome=LEMS; Neuromyotonia=NM and Polyneuropathies=PN

Table 1. showing the disease mechanisms, current and future therapeutics for neurological autoimmune diseases.

Targeting the immune cell entry is considered to be an ideal approach and based on this concept we noticed a significant blockade of lymphocyte traffic and eventual recovery in EAE mouse model when administered with mucosal addressin cell adhesion molecule (MAdCAM-1) antibody that binds with the integrins on the lymphocyte cell surface. We also developed a combinatorial approach for this model to protect the neurons against glutamate mediated damage with the α-amino-3-hydroxy-5-methyl-4-isoxazolepropionate (AMPA)/ Kainate receptor antagonist 2,3-dihydroxy -6- nitro-7- sulfamoylbenzo (f)quinoxaline (NBQX), and the N-methyl D-aspartate (NMDA) receptor antagonist GPE(neuro protector glycine-proline-glutamic acid;N-terminal tripeptide of insulin like growth factor). This combinatorial therapy also helps in reducing the infiltrating immune cells at the site of inflammation in the brain (Kanwar et al, 2004).. We have also patented the treatment of demyelinating diseases by administering GPE (WIPO).In addition, there are reports on the highly conserved BARF1 epitopes of Epstein Barr Virus with potent neuroprotective and mitogenic activities (Wynne et al., 2010). We, therefore anticipate conjugating antibodies with such neuroprotectors that would be definitely fruitful for treating a group of neurological autoimmune diseases. Application of nanotechnology also has a tremendous potential for their treatment, as the conjugation of nanoparticles with neuroprotectors and other therapeutics will significantly enhance the targeted delivery, bioavailability and efficacy. Finally introduction of locked nucleic acids (LNAs) has opened a new boom in the area of gene silencing. These LNAs are valuable nucleic acid analogues with striking abilities to regulate gene expression both *in vitro* and *in vivo* (Kauppinen et al., 2005). Thus, in the near future they can be suitably modified to control the genetically mediated autoimmune diseases. Table 1 shows the comparison of current and future drugs.

7. Conclusion

Further to conclude, the immunosuppressive and anti-inflammatory treatments considered for treating autoimmune diseases pose serious side effects upon long term administration. Hence, it is rather expected, than to hope that emerging therapies based on the advancements made in T and B-cell targeting would definitely complement or if not replace the existing therapies. It is worth mentioning to find many new novel entities that are in clinical trials for MS and other neurological autoimmune diseases. Inspite of these attractive therapeutic strategies strenuous efforts are to be made to identify the best possible candidates for effective disease control benefiting the patient population.

8. References

Allebeck, P., Ahlboom, A., Ljungstrom, K. & Allander, E. (1984). Do oral contraceptives reduce the incidence of rheumatoid arthritis? *Scand.J. Rheumatol*, Vol.13, pp. 140-146.

Alter, A., Duddy, M., Hebert, S., Biernacki, K., Prat, A. & Antel, J. P. (2003). Determinants of human B cell migration across brain endothelial cells. *J Immunol*, Vol.170, pp. 4497-4505.

Anthony, I.C., Crawford, D.H. & Bell, J.E. (2003). B lymphocytes in the normal brain: contrasts with HIV-associated lymphoid infiltrates and lymphomas. *Brain*, Vol.126, pp. 1058-1067.

Arnon, R. & Aharoni, R. (2004). Mechanism of action of glatiramer acetate in multiple sclerosis and its potential for the development of new applications. *Proc Natl Acad Sci USA*, Vol.101, Suppl.2, pp. 14593-14598.

Arsura, E., Brunner, N.G., Namba, T. & Grob, D. (1985). High-dose intravenous methylprednisolone in myasthenia gravis. Arch Neurol, *Vol.42, pp. 1149-1153.*

Austyn, J.M. (2000). Antigen-presenting Cells Experimental and Clinical Studies of Dendritic Cells. *American Journal of Respiratory and Critical Care Medicine*, Vol.162, pp.(146-150). Axelsson, M., Malmeström, C., Nilsson, S., Haghighi, S., Rosengren, L. & Lycke, J. (2010). Glial fibrillary acidic protein: a potential biomarker for progression in multiple sclerosis. *Journal of Neurology*, pp. 1-7.

Bach, J.F. (2002).The effect of infections on susceptibility to autoimmune and allergic diseases. *N Engl J Med*, Vol.347, pp. 911-920.

Baker, K.P., Edwards, B.M., Main, S.H., Choi, G.H., Wager, R.E. & Halpern, W.G. (2003). Generation and characterization of LymphoStat-B, a human monoclonal antibody that antagonizes the bioactivities of B lymphocyte stimulator. *Arthritis Rheum*, Vol.48, pp. 3253-3265.

Baranzini, S. E., Jeong, M. C., Butunoi, C., Murray, R. S., Bernard, C. C. & Oksenberg, J. R. (1999). B cell repertoire diversity and clonal expansion in multiple sclerosis brain lesions. *J Immunol*, Vol.163, pp. 5133-5144.

Baratchi, S., Kanwar, R.K., Cheung, C.H. & Kanwar, J.R. (2010a). Proliferative and protective effects of SurR9-C84A on differentiated neural cells. *J Neuroimmunol*, Vol.8, No.227, pp. 120-32.

Baratchi, S., Kanwar, R.K. & Kanwar, J.R. (2010b). Survivin: a target from brain cancer to neurodegenerative disease. *Crit Rev Biochem Mol Biol*, Vol.45, No.6, pp. 535-554.

Baratchi, S., Kanwar, R.K. & Kanwar, J.R. (2011a). Novel survivin mutant protects differentiated SK-N-SH human neuroblastoma cells from activated T-cell neurotoxicity. *J Neuroimmunol*, Vol.233, No.1-2, pp. 18-28.

Baratchi, S., Kanwar, R.K. & Kanwar, J.R. (2011b). Survivin mutant protects differentiated dopaminergic SK-N-SH cells against oxidative stress. *PLoS One,* Vol.10, No.6, pp. e15865.

Barzilai, O., Ram, M. & Shoenfeld, Y. (2007a). Viral infection can induce the production of autoantibodies. *Curr Opin Rheumatol,* Vol.19, pp. 636-643.

Barzilai, O., Sherer, Y., Ram, M., Izhaky, D.,Anaya, J.M. & Shoenfeld, Y. (2007b). Epstein-Barr virus and cytomegalovirus in autoimmune diseases: are they truly notorious? A preliminary report. *Ann N Y Acad Sci*, Vol.1108, pp. 567-577.

Begovich, A.B., Carlton, V.E., Honigberg, L.A., Schrodi, S.J. & Chokkalingam, A.P. (2004). Amissense singlenucleotide polymorphism in a gene encoding a protein tyrosine phos,phatase (PTPN22) is associated with rheumatoid arthritis. *Am. J. Hum. Genet*, Vol.75, pp. 330-337.

Bergamaschi, R. (2007).Immune agents for the treatment of Devic's neuromyelitis optica. *Neurol Sci* , Vol.28, pp. 238-240.

Bottini, N., Musumeci, L., Alonso, A., Rahmouni, S. & Nika, K. (2004). A functional variant of lymphoid tyrosine phosphatase is associated with type I diabetes. *Nat. Genet,* Vol.36, pp. 337-338.

Bishop, G.A., Haxhinasto, S.A., Stunz, L.L. & Hostager, B.S. (2003). Antigen-specific B-lymphocyte activation. *Crit. Rev. Immunol,* Vol.23, pp. 149-197.

Bretscher, P. & Cohn, M. A. (1970). Theory of self-nonself discrimination. *Science,* Vol.169, pp. 1042-1049.

Bjorksten, B. (1994). Risk factors in early childhood for the development of allergic disease. *Allergy,* Vol.49, pp. 400-407.

Bondanza, A., Zimmermann, V.S., Antonio, G.D., Cin, E.D., Balestrieri, G., Tincani, A., Amoura, Z., Piette, J.C., Sabbadini, M.G., Querini, P.R. & Manfred, A.A. (2004). Requirement of Dying Cells and Environmental Adjuvants for the Induction of Autoimmunity. *ARTHRITIS & RHEUMATISM,* Vol.50, No. 5, pp. 1549-1560.

Brosnan, C.F. & Raine, C.S, (1996). Mechanisms of immune injury in multiple sclerosis. *Brain Pathol,* Vol.6, pp. 243-257.

Buchwald, B., Ahangari, R., Weishaupt, A. & Toyka, K.V. (2005). Presynaptic effects of immunoglobulin G from patients with Lambert-Eaton myasthenic syndrome: their neutralization by intravenous immunoglobulins. *Muscle Nerve,* Vol.31, No.4, pp. 487-494.

Buckley, C. & Vincent, A. (2005). Autoimmune Channelopathies. *Nature Clin Pract Neurol,* Vol.1, pp. 22-32.

Bufler, J., Kahlert, S., Tzartos, S., Toyka, K.V., Maelicke, A. & Franke, C. (1996). Activation and blockade of mouse muscle nicotinic channels by antibodies directed against the binding site of the acetylcholine receptor. *J Physiol,* Vol.492, pp. 107-114.

Cappione, A., Anolik, J.H., Pugh-Bernard, A., Barnard, J., Dutcher, P., Silverman, G. & Sanz, I. (2005). Germinal center exclusion of autoreactive B cells is defective in human systemic lupus erythematosus. *J. Clin. Invest,* Vol.115, pp. 3205-3216.

Carpentier, A.F. & Delattre, J.Y. (2001). The Lambert-Eaton myasthenic syndrome, *Clin Rev Allergy Immunol,* Vol.20, pp. 155-158.

Cepok, S., Rosche., Grummel, V., Vogel, F., Zhou, D., Sayn, J., Sommer,N., Hartung, H.P. & Hemmer, B. (2005). Short-lived plasma blasts are the main B cell effector subset during the course of multiple sclerosis. *Brain,* Vol.128, pp. 1667-1676.

Chan, A., Weilbach, F.X., Toyka, K.V. & Gold, R. (2005). Mitoxantrone induces cell death in peripheral blood leucocytes of multiple sclerosis patients. *Clin Exp Immunol,* Vol.139, pp. 152-158.

Charo, I.F. & Ransohoff, R.M. (2006). The many roles of chemokines and chemokine receptors in inflammation. *N. Engl. J. Med,* Vol.354, pp. 610-621.

Chatenoud, L. (2003). CD3-specific antibody-induced active tolerance:from bench to bedside. *Nat. Rev. Immunol,* Vol.3, pp. 123-132.

Cheung, C.H., Chen, H.H., Cheng, L.T., Lyu, K.W., Kanwar, J.R. & Chang, J.Y. (2010). Targeting Hsp90 with small molecule inhibitors induces the over-expression of the anti-apoptotic molecule, survivin, in human A549, HONE-1 and HT-29 cancer cells. *Mol Cancer,* Vol.15, No.9, pp. 77.

Cheung, C.H., Sun, X., Kanwar, J.R., Bai, J.Z., Cheng, L. & Krissansen, G.W. (2010b). A cell-permeable dominant-negative survivin protein induces apoptosis and sensitizes prostate cancer cells to TNF-α therapy. *Cancer Cell Int,* Vol.1, No.10, pp. 36.

Clancy, R.M., Backer, C.B., Yin, X., Chang, M.W., Cohen, S.R. & Lee, L.A. (2004a). Genetic association of cutaneous neonatal lupus with HLA class II and tumor necrosis factor alpha: implications for pathogenesis. *Arthritis Rheum,* Vol.50, pp. 2598-2603.

Clancy, R.M., Kapur, R.P., Molad, Y., Askanase, A.D. & Buyon, J.P. (2004b). Immunohistologic evidence supports apoptosis, IgG deposition, and novel macrophage/fibroblast crosstalk in the pathologic cascade leading to congenital heart block. *Arthritis Rheum,* Vol.50, pp. 173-182.

Clerico, M., Contessa, G. & Durelli, L. (2007). Interferon-beta1a for the treatment of multiple sclerosis. *Expert Opin Biol Ther,* Vol.7, No.4, pp. 535-542.

Clifford, D.B., De Luca, A., Simpson, D.M., Arendt, G., Giovannoni, G. & Nath, A. (2010). Natalizumabassociated progressive multifocal leukoencephalopathy in patients with multiple sclerosis: lessons from 28 cases. *Lancet Neurol, Vol.9,* pp. 438-446.

Colombo, M., Dono, M., Gazzola, P., Roncella, S., Valetto, A. & Chiorazzi, N. (2000). Accumulation of clonally related B lymphocytes in the cerebrospinal fluid of multiple sclerosis patients. *J Immunol,* Vol.164, pp. 2782-2789.

Cooper, G.S., Dooley, M.A., Treadwell, E.L., St Clair, E.W. & Gilkeson, G.S. (2002). Hormonal and reproductive risk factors for development of systemic lupus erythematosus: results of a population-based, casecontrol study. *Arthritis Rheum*, Vol.46, pp. 1830–1839.

Crow, M.K. (2004). Costimulatory molecules and T-cell–B-cell interactions. *Rheum. Dis. Clin. North Am*, Vol.30, pp. 175–191.

Cutolo, M. & Accardo, S. (1991). Sex hormones and rheumatoid arthritis. *Clin. Exp. Rheumatol*, Vol.9, pp. 641–646.

Cutolo, M. (2003). Solar light effects on onset/relapses and circannual/circadian symptomatology in rheumatoid arthritis. *Clin Exp Rheumatol*, Vol.21, pp. 148–150.

Czaplinski, & Steck, A.J. (2004). Immune mediated neuropathies: an update on therapeutic strategies. *J Neurol*, Vol.251, pp. 127–137.

Dalakas, M.C. & Quarles, R.H. (1996). Autoimmune ataxic Neuropathies (sensory ganglionopathies): are glycolipids the responsible autoantigens?. *Ann Neurol*, Vol39, pp. 419–422.

Dalakas, M.C. (1999). Intravenous immunoglobulin in the treatment of autoimmune neuromuscular diseases: present status and practical therapeutic guidelines. *Muscle Nerve*, Vol.22, No.11, pp. 1479-1497.

Dalakas, M.C., Fujii, M., Li, M. & McElroy, B. (2000). The clinical spectrum of anti-GAD antibody-positive patients with stiff-person syndrome. *Neurology*, Vol.55, pp. 1531–1535.

Dalakas, M.C., Li, M., Fujii, M. & Jacobowitz, D.M. (2001). Stiff-person syndrome: quantification, specificity and intrathecal synthesis of GAD65 antibodies. *Neurology*, Vol.57, pp. 780–785.

Dalakas, M.C. (2006). B cells in the pathophysiology of autoimmune neurological disorders: A credible therapeutic target. *Pharmacology & Therapeutics*, Vol.112, No.1, pp. 57-70.

Dalakas, M.C. (2008). B cells as therapeutic targets in autoimmune neurological disorders. *Nat Clin Pract Neurol*, Vol.4, No.10, pp. 557-567.

Dalakas, M.C. (2009). Stiff person syndrome: advances in pathogenesis and therapeutic interventions. Curr Treat Options Neurol, Vol.11, No.2, pp. *102-110.*

Dalmau, F., Graus, M.K., Rosenblum, & Posner, J.B. (1992). Anti-Hu-associated paraneoplastic encephalomyelitis/sensory neuropathy: a clinical study of 71 patients. *Medicine (Baltimore)*, Vol.71, pp. 59–72.

Damian, R.T. (1964). Molecular mimicry: antigen sharing by parasite and host and its consequences. *Am. Naturalist*, Vol.XCVIII, pp. 129–149.

Darnell, R.B. & Posner, J.B. (2003). Paraneoplastic syndromes involving the nervous system, *N Engl J Med*, Vol.349, pp. 1543–1554.

Davidson, A. & Diamond, B. (2001). Advances in Immunology. *N Engl J Med*, Vol. 345, No. 5, pp. 340-350.

Dedrick, R.L., Bodary, S. & Garovoy, M.R. (2003). Adhesion molecules as therapeutic targets for autoimmune diseases and transplant rejection. Expert Opin Biol Ther, Vol.3, No.1, pp. 85-95.

Delves, P.J. (2006). Structural and functional aspects of the innate and adaptive systems of immunity. In: Rose, NR and Mackay, IR, (eds.) *The autoimmune diseases*. pp. 9-21. Elsevier: San Diego.

Drachman, D.B. (1994). Myasthenia gravis, *N Engl J Med*, Vol.330, pp. 1797–1810.

Druet, P. (1989). Contributions of immunological reactions to nephrotoxicity. *Toxicol Lett*, Vol.46 pp. 55-64.

Duddy, M.E. & Baker, M.R. (2009). Stiff person syndrome. *Front Neurol Neurosci*, Vol.26, pp. 147-165.

Fang, C., Zhang, X., Miwa, T. & Song, W.C. (2009). Complement promotes the development of inflammatory T-helper 17 cells through synergistic interaction with Toll-like receptor signaling and interleukin-6 production. *Blood*, Vol.114, pp. 1005–1015.

Faraco, G., Cavone, L. & Chiarugi, A. (2011). The Therapeutic Potential of HDAC Inhibitors in the Treatment of Multiple Sclerosis. *Mol Med.* Feb 25. [Epub ahead of print].

Fauci, A.S., Wolff, S.M. & Johnson, J.S. (1971). Effect of cyclophosphamide upon the immune response in Wegener's granulomatosis, *N Engl J Med*, Vol.285, pp. 1493-1496.

Flickinger, C.J., Baran, M.L., Howards, S.S. & Herr, J.C. (1994). Epididymal obstruction during development results in antisperm autoantibodies at puberty in rats. *J Androl*, Vol.19, pp. 136-144.

Fraga, A., Mintz, G. & Orozco, J. (1974). Sterility and fertility rates, fetal wastage and maternal morbidity in SLE. *J. Rheumatol*, Vol.1, pp. 293–298.

Frisoni, L., McPhie, L., Colonna, L., Sriram, U., Monestier, M. & Gallucci, S. (2005). Nuclear autoantigen translocation and autoantibody opsonization lead to increased dendritic cell phagocytosis and presentation of nuclear antigens: a novel pathogenic pathway for autoimmunity? *J Immunol*, Vol.175, pp. 2692–2701.

Frohman, E.M., Racke, M.K. & Raine, C.S. (2006). Multiple sclerosis-the plaque and its pathogenesis. *N. Engl. J. Med*, Vol.354, pp. 942–955.

Fugger, L., Friese, M.A. & Bell, J.I. (2009). From genes to function: The next challenge to understanding multiple sclerosis. *Nat Rev Immunol*, Vol.9, No.6, pp. 408–417.

Fujinami, R.S. & Oldstone, M.B. (1989). Molecular mimicry as a mechanism for virus-induced autoimmunity. *Immunol Res*, Vol.8, pp. 3-15.

Fujinami, R.S.& Oldstone, M.B. (1985). Amino acid homology between the encephalitogenic site of myelin basic protein and virus: mechanism for autoimmunity. *Science*, Vol.230,No.4729, pp. 1043-1045.

Gabriel, C.L., Wu, L., Parekh, V.V. & Van Kaer, L. (2010). Invariant natural killer t cell-based therapy of autoimmune diseases. *Current Immunology Reviews*, Vol.6, No.2, pp. 88-101.

Gehrs, B.C. & Friedberg, R.C. (2002). Autoimmune hemolytic anemia. *Am J Hematol*, Vol.69, pp. 258–271.

Gellert, M. (2002). V(D)J recombination: RAG proteins, repair factors, and regulation. *Annu. Rev. Biochem*, Vol.*71*, pp. 101–132.

Genovese, M.C., Kaine, J.L., Lowenstein, M.B., Del Giudice, J., Baldassare, A., Schechtman, J., Fudman, E., Kohen, M., Gujrathi, S., Trapp, R.G., Sweiss, N.J., Spaniolo, G. & Dummer, W. (2008). Ocrelizumab, a humanized anti-CD20 monoclonal antibody, in the treatment of patients with rheumatoid arthritis: a phase I/II randomized, blinded, placebo-controlled, dose-ranging study. *Arthritis Rheum*, Vol.58, No.9, pp. 2652-2661.

Gold, R., Dalakas, M.C. & Toyka, K.V. (2003). Immunotherapy in autoimmune neuromuscular disorders. *Lancet Neurol*, Vol.2, pp. 22-32.

Gold, R., Linington, C. & Lassmann, H. (2006). Understanding pathogenesis and therapy of multiple sclerosis via animal models: 70 years of merits and culprits in experimental autoimmune encephalomyelitis research. *Brain*, Vol.129, pp. 1953-1971.

Goldrath, A.W. & Bevan, M.J. (1999). Selecting and maintaining a diverse T-cell repertoire. *Nature*, Vol.402, pp. 255-262.

Graus, F., Keime-Guibert, F., Rene, R., Benyahia, B., Ribalta, T. & Ascaso, C. (2001). Anti-Hu-associated paraneoplastic encephalomyelitis: analysis of 200 patients. *Brain*, Vol.24, pp. 1138-1148.

Green, A.J., McQuaid, S., Hauser, S.L., Allen I.V. & Lyness, R. (2010). Ocular pathology in multiple sclerosis: retinal atrophy and inflammation irrespective of disease duration, *Brain*, Vol.133, pp. 1591-1601.

Greter, M., Heppner, F.L., Lemos, M.P., Odermatt, B.M., Goebels, N., Laufer, T., Noelle, R.J. & Becher, B. (2005). Dendritic cells permit immune invasion of the CNS in an animal model of multiple sclerosis. *Nat. Med*, Vol.11, pp. 328-334.

Gu, H., Tarlinton, D., Muller, W., Rajewsky, K. & Forster, I. (1991). Most peripheral B cells in mice are ligand selected. *J Exp Med*, Vol.173, pp. 1357-1371.

Hadden, R.D., Cornblath, D.R., Hughes RA., Zielasek, J., Hartung, H.P., Toyka, K.V. & Swan, A.V. (1998). Electrophysiological classification of Guillain-Barre syndrome: clinical associations and outcome. Plasma Exchange/Sandoglobulin Guillain-Barre Syndrome Trial Group. *Ann Neurol*, Vol.44, No.5, pp. 780-788.

Hafer-Macko, C. E., Sheikh, K. A., Li, C. Y., Ho, T. W., Cornblath, D. R. & McKhann, G. M.. (1996). Immune attack on the Schwann cell surface in acute inflammatory demyelinating polyneuropathy. *Ann Neurol*, Vol.39, pp. 625-635.

Hauser, S.L. (2008). Multiple lessons for multiple sclerosis. *N Engl J Med*, Vol.359, No.17, pp. 1838-1841.

Hauser, S.L., Waubant, E., Arnold, D.L., Vollmer, T., Antel, J., Fox, R.J., Bar-Or, A., Panzara, M., Sarkar, N., Agarwal, S., Langer-Gould, A. & Smith, C.H. (2008) B-cell depletion with rituximab in relapsing-remitting multiple sclerosis. *N Engl J Med*, Vol.358, No.7, pp. 676-688.

Hayashi, A., Nakamagoe, K., Ohkoshi, N., Hoshino, S. & Shoji, S. (1999). Double filtration plasma exchange and immunoadsorption therapy in a case of stiff-man syndrome with negative anti-GAD antibody. *J Med*, Vol.30, No.(5-6), pp. 321-327.

Heather Rachel Davids, (Mar, 2010), Guillain-Barre Syndrome: Treatment & Medication In: *emedicine*,16.03.2011,Available from URL: emedicine.medscape.com/article/315632-treatment.

Hennies, C., Sternberg, D., Bistulfi, G.L., Kazim, L., Benedict, R.H.B., Chadha, K., Leung, C., Weinstock-Guttman, B., Munschauer, F. & Sternberg, Z. (2011). Plasma pentosidine: A potential biomarker in the management of multiple sclerosis. *Multiple Sclerosis*, Vol.17, No.2, pp. 157-163

Heppner, F.L., Greter, M., Marino, D., Falsig, J., Raivich, G., Hovelmeyer, N., Waisman, A., Rulicke, T., Prinz, M., Priller, J., Becher, B. & Aguzzi, A. (2005). Experimental autoimmune encephalomyelitis repressed by microglial paralysis. *Nat Med*, Vol.11, No.2, pp. 146-152.

Herrmann, M., Sholmerich, J. & Straub, R.H. (2000). Stress and rheumatic disease. *Rheum Dis Clin North Am*, Vol.26, No.4, pp. 737-763.

Hickey, W. F., Hsu, B. L. & Kimura, H. (1991). T-lymphocyte entry into the central nervous system. *J. Neurosci. Res*, Vol.28, pp. 254-260.

Hodgkin, P.D. & Basten, A.B. (1995). Cell activation, tolerance and antigenpresenting function. *Curr Opin Immunol*, Vol.7, pp. 121-129.

Hohlfeld, R., Melms, A., Schneider, C., Toyka, K.V. & Drachman, D.B. (2003). Therapy of myasthenia gravis and myasthenic syndromes. Brandt, T., Caplan, L.R., Dichgans, J., Diener, H.C. & Kennard, C. In: *Neurological disorders: course and treatment*, Elsevier, Stuttgart, pp. 1341-1362.

Holmes, C.H. & Simpson, K.L. (1992). Complement and pregnancy. New insights into the immunobiology of the feto maternal relationship. *Ballières Clin. Obstet. Gynecol,*Vol.6, pp.(439–460).

Hooks, J.J., Jordan, G.W., Cupps, T., Moutsopoulos, H.M., Fauci, A.S. & Notkins, A.L.. (1982). Multiple interferons in the circulation of patients with systemic lupus erythematosus and vasculitis. *Arthritis Rheum,* Vol.25, pp. 396-400.

Hoyer, B.F., Moser, K., Hauser, A.E., Peddinghaus, A., Voigt, C., Eilat, D., Radbruch, A., Manz, R.A. & Hiepe, F. (2004). Short-lived plasmablasts and long-lived plasma cells contribute to chronic humoral autoimmunity in NZB/w mice. *J. Exp.Med,* Vol.199, pp. 1577–1584.

Ishii, A. (2010). Stiff-person syndrome and other myelopathies constitute paraneoplastic neurological syndromes. *Brain Nerve,* Vol.62, No.4, pp. 377-385.

Jacobson, D.L. (1997). Epidemiology and estimated population burden of selected autoimmune disease in the United States. *Clin Immunol Immunopathol,* Vol.84, pp. 223-243.

Janeway, C. Jr. & Travers, P. (1998) Immunobiology. In: *The Immune System in Health and Disease,* pp 625-640. Garland Publishing Inc, New York Jarow, J.P., Goluboff, E.T., Chang, T.S. & Marshall, F.F. (1994). Relationship between antisperm antibodies and testicular histologic changes in humans after vasectomy. *Urology,* Vol.43, pp. 521-524.

Johnson, P.M. (1993). Reproductive and maternofetal relations, In: Gell, P.G.H. & Coombs, R.R.A, *Clinical Aspects of Immunology,* Blackwell Johnson, Oxford, pp. 755–767.

Kanwar, J.R., Harrison, J.E.B., Wang, D., Leung, E., Mueller, W., Wagner, N. & Krissansen, G.W. (1999). β7 integrins contribute to demyelinating disease of the central nervous system. *Journal of Neuroimmunology,* Vol.103, No.2000, pp. 146–152.

Kanwar, J.R., Kanwar, R.K., Wang, D. & Krissansen, G.W. (2000). Prevention of a chronic progressive form of experimental autoimmune encephalomyelitis by an antibody against mucosal addressin cell adhesion molecule-1, given early in the course of disease progression. *Immunology and Cell Biology,* Vol.78, pp. 641–645.

Kanwar, R.K., Kanwar, J.R., Wang, D., Ormrod, D.J. & Krissansen, G.W. (2001). Temporal Expression of Heat Shock Proteins 60 and 70 at Lesion-Prone Sites. *Arterioscler Thromb Vasc Biol,* Vol.21, pp. 1991-1997.

Kanwar, J.R., Berg, R.W., Yang, Y., Kanwar, R.K., Ching, L.M., Sun, X. & Krissansen, G.W. (2003). Requirements for ICAM-1 immunogene therapy of lymphoma. *Cancer Gene Ther,* Vol.10, No.6, pp. 468-476.

Kanwar, J.R., Kanwar, R.K. & Krissansen, G.W. (2004). Simultaneous neuroprotection and blockade of inflammation reverses autoimmune encephalomyelitis. *Brain,* Vol.127, No.6, pp. 131313-131331.

Kanwar. J.R. (2005). Anti-inflammatory immunotherapy for multiple sclerosis/experimental autoimmune encephalomyelitis (EAE) disease. *Curr Med Chem,* Vol.12, No.25, pp. 2947-2962.

Kanwar, J.R, Kanwar, R.K., Burrow, H. & Baratchi, S. (2009). Recent advances on the roles of NO in cancer and chronic inflammatory disorders. *Curr Med Chem*, Vol.16, No.19, pp. 2373-2394.

Kanwar, J.R., Kamalapuram, S.K. & Kanwar, R.K. (2010a). Targeting survivin in cancer: patent review. *Expert Opin Ther Pat*, Vol.20, No.12, pp. 1723-37.

Kanwar, J.R, Mahidhara, G. & Kanwar, R.K. (2010b). MicroRNA in human cancer and chronic inflammatory diseases. *Front Biosci (Schol Ed*, Vol.1, No.2, pp. 1113-1126.

Kanwar, J.R., Mohan, R.R., Kanwar, R.K., Roy, K. & Bawa, R. (2010c). Applications of aptamers in nanodelivery systems in cancer, eye and inflammatory diseases. *Nanomedicine*,Vol.5, No.9, pp. 1435-45.

Kanwar, R.K., Cheung, C.H., Chang, J.Y. & Kanwar, J.R. (2010d). Recent advances in anti-survivin treatments for cancer. *Curr Med Chem*, Vol.17, No.15, pp. 1509-1015.

Kappler, J.W., Roehm, N. & Marrack, P. (1987). T cell tolerance by clonal elimination in the thymus. *Cell,* Vol.49, pp. 273–280.

Kauppinen, S., Vester, B. & Wengel, J. (2005). Locked nucleic acid (LNA): High affinity targeting of Complementary RNA for diagnostics and therapeutics. *Drug Discovery Today: Technol*, Vol.2, pp. 287.

Keefe, D., Parng, C., Lundberg, D., Ray, S., Martineau-Bosco, J., Leng, C., Tzartos, S., Powell, J., Concino, M., Heartlein, M., Lamsa, J. & Josiah, S. (2010). In vitro characterization of an acetylcholine receptor–transferrin fusion protein for the treatment of myasthenia gravis. *Autoimmunity,* Vol.43, No.8, pp. 628–639.

Khamashta, M.A., Ruiz-Irastorza, G. & Hughes, G.R. (1997). Systemic lupus erythematosus flares during pregnancy. *Rheum. Dis. Clin. N. Am*, Vol.23, pp. 15–30.

Kieseier, B.C., Kiefer, R., Gold, R., Hemmer, B., Willison, H.J. & Hartung, H. P. (2004). Advances in understanding and treatment of immune-mediated disorders of the peripheral nervous system. *Muscle Nerve,* Vol.30, pp. 131–156.

Kleopas, A.K., Elman, L.B., Lang, B., Vincent, A. & Scherer, S.S. (2006). Neuromyotonia and limbic encephalitis sera target mature Shaker-type K+ channels: subunit specificity correlates with clinical manifestations. *Brain,* Vol.129, pp. 1570–1584.

Knopf, P. M., Harling-Berg, C. J., Cserr, H. F., Basu, D., Sirulnick, E. J. & Nolan, S. C. (1998). Antigen-dependent intrathecal antibody synthesis in the normal rat brain: tissue entry and local retention of antigen-specific B cells. *J Immunol,* Vol.161, pp. 692–701.

Kornberg, A.J. & Pestronk, A. (2003). Antibody-associated polyneuropathy syndromes: principles and treatment. *Semin Neurol,* Vol.23, pp. 181–190.

Koski, C.L. & Patterson, J.V. (2006). Intravenous immunoglobulin use for neurologic diseases. *J Infus Nurs,* Vol.29, Suppl.3, pp. S21-8.

Kumar, V. & Kaminski, H.J. (2011). Treatment of Myasthenia Gravis. *Curr Neurol Neurosci Rep,* Vol.11, pp. 89–96.

Kuwabara, S. (2004). Guillain-Barré syndrome: epidemiology, pathophysiology and management. *Drugs,* Vol.64, pp. 597–610.

Lai, M., Huijbers, M.G.M., Lancaster, E., Graus, F., Bataller, L., Balice-Gordon, R., Cowell, J.K. & Dalmau, J. (2010). Investigation of LGI1 as the antigen in limbic encephalitis previously attributed to potassium channels: A case series *The Lancet Neurology,* Vol.9, No.8, pp. 776-785.

Lambert-Eaton syndrome, In: *PubMed Health*,09.03.2011,Available from URL: www.ncbi.nlm.nih.gov/pubmedhealth/PMH0001729/.

Lennon, V.A., Kryzer, T.J., Pittock, S.J., Verkman A.S. & Hinson, S.R. (2005). IgG marker of optic-spinal multiple sclerosis binds to the aquaporin-4 water channel, *J Exp Med,* Vol.202, pp. 473-477.

Leung, E., Kanwar, R.K., Kanwar, J.R. & Krissansen, G.W. (2003). Mucosal vascular addressin cell adhesion molecule-1 is expressed outside the endothelial lineage on fibroblasts and melanoma cells. *Immunol Cell Biol,* Vol.81, No.4, pp. 320-327.

Lim, K.J.H., Odukoya, O.A. & Ajjan, R.A. (1998). Profile of cytokine mRNA expression in peri-implantation human endometrium. *Mol.Hum. Reprod,* Vol.4, pp. 77-81.

Lleo, A., Invernizzi, P., Gao, B., Podda, M. & Gershwin, M.E. (2010). Definition of human autoimmunity – autoantibodies versus autoimmune disease. *Autoimmunity Reviews,* Vol.9, pp. 259-266.

Lucchinetti, C., Bruck, W., Parisi, J., Scheithauer, B., Rodriguez, M. & Lassmann, H. (2000). Heterogeneity of multiple sclerosis lesions: implications for the pathogenesis of demyelination. *Ann Neurol,* Vol.47, pp. 707-717.

Lucchinetti, C.F., Mandler, R.N., McGavern, D., Bruck, W., Gleich, G. & Ransohoff R.M. (2002). A role for humoral mechanisms in the pathogenesis of Devic's neuromyelitis optica, *Brain,* Vol.125, pp. 1450-1461.

Lutterotti, A. & Berger, T. (2010). Advances in Multiple Sclerosis Therapy: New Oral Disease-Modifying Agents, *CML - Multiple Sclerosis,* Vol.2, No.1, pp. 1-10.

Mackay, C. R., Marston, W. L. & Dudler, L. (1990). Naive and memory T cells show distinct pathways of lymphocyte recirculation. *J. Exp. Med,* Vol. 171, No.3, pp. 801-817. Mackay, R. & Rosen, F.S. (2001). Autoimmune Diseases. *N Engl J Med,* Vol.345, pp. 340-350.

Manoury, B, Hewitt, E.W, Morrice, N, Dando, P.M, Barrett, A.J. & Watts, C. (1998). An asparaginyl endopeptidase processes a microbial antigen for class II MHC presentation. *Nature,* Vol.396, pp. 695-699.

Manz, R.A., Thiel, A. & Radbruch, A. (1997). Lifetime of plasma cells in the bone marrow.*Nature,* Vol.388, pp. 133-134.

Manz, R.A., Löhning, M., Cassese, G., Thiel, A. & Radbruch, A. (1998). Survival of long-lived plasma cells is independent of antigen. *Int. Immunol,* Vol.10, pp. 1703-1711.

Manz, R.A., Hauser, A.E., Hiepe, F. & Radbruch, A. (2005). Maintenance of serum antibody levels. *Annu. Rev. Immunol,* Vol.23, pp. 367-386.

Marmont, A.M. (2000). New horizons in the treatment of autoimmune diseases: immunoablation and stem cell transplantation. *Annu Rev Med,* Vol.51, pp. 115-134.

Maverakis, E., Goodarzi, H., Wehrli, L.N., Ono, Y. & Garcia, M.S. (2011). The Etiology of Paraneoplastic Autoimmunity. *Clin Rev Allergy Immunol,* Jan 19 [Epub ahead of print].

MayoClinic, *Multiple Sclerosis,* 25.02.2011, Available from URL: www.mayoclinic.org/multiple-sclerosis/

McEvoy, K.M., Windebank, A.J., Daube, J.R. & Low, PA. (1989). 3,4-Diaminopyridine in the treatment of Lambert-Eaton myasthenic syndrome. N Engl J Med, Vol.321, No.23, pp. 1567-1571.

McKall-Faienza, K.J., Kawai, K., Kundig, T.M., Odermatt, B., Bachmann, M.F., Zakarian, A., Mak, T.W. & Ohashi, P.S. (1998). Absence of TNFRp55 influences virus-induced autoimmunity despite efficient lymphocytic infiltration. *Int Immunol,* Vol.10, pp. 405-412.

McMurray, R.W. (1996). Adhesion molecules in autoimmune disease. *Semin Arthritis Rheum,* Vol.25, No.4, pp. 215-33.

Merchut, M.P. (2010). Management of voltage-gated potassium channel antibody disorders. *Neurologic Clinics*, Vol.28, No.4, pp. 941-959.

Merck, *Multiple Sclerosis (MS),* 27.02.2011, Available from URL: www.merckmanuals.com/home/sec06/ch092/ch092b.html

Mertens, H.G., Hertel, G., Reuther, P. & Ricker, K. (1981). Effect of immunosuppressive drugs (azathioprine). *Ann NY Acad Sci,* Vol.377, pp. 691-699.

Monroe, J.G., Bannish, G., Fuentes-Panana, E.M., King, L.B., Sandel, P.C., Chung, J. & Sater, R. (2003). Positive and negative selection during B lymphocyte development. *Immunol. Res,* Vol.27, pp. 427-442.

Moreno, B., Fernandez-Diez, B., Di Penta, A. & Villoslada, P. (2010). Preclinical studies of methylthioadenosine for the treatment of multiple sclerosis. *Mult Scler,* Vol.16, No.9, pp. 1102-1108.

Muramatsu, T. (2011). Midkine: a Promising Molecule for Drug Development to Treat Diseases of the Central Nervous System. *Curr Pharm Des,* Mar 4. [Epub ahead of print]. *Multiple Sclerosis Treatments,* 27.02.2011, Available from URL: www.mult-sclerosis.org/mstreatments.html Nobile-Orazio, E. (2001). Multifocal motor neuropathy. *J Neuroimmunol,* Vol.115, pp. 4-18.

Latov, N. (1994). Antibodies to glycoconjugates in neuropathy and motor neuron disease. *Prog Brain Res,* Vol.101, pp. 295-303.

Ogawara, K., Kuwabara, S., Mori, M., Hattori, T., Koga, M. & Yuki, N. (2000). Axonal Guillain-Barré syndrome: relation to anti-ganglioside antibodies and Campylobacter jejuni infection in Japan. *Ann Neurol,* Vol.48, pp. 624-631.

Ohishi, K., Kanoh, M., Shinomiya, H., Hitsumoto, Y. & Utsumi, S. (1995). Complement activation by cross-linked B cell-membrane IgM. *J Immunol,* Vol.154, pp. 3173-3179.

Oldstone, M.B.A. (1998). Molecular mimicry and immune-mediated diseases. *FASEB J,* Vol.12, pp. 1255-1265.

Osborne, R. (2009). Buzz around Campath proof-of-concept trial in MS. *Nat Biotechnol,* Vol.27, No.1, pp. 6-8.

Palmer, E. (2003). Negative selection - clearing out the bad apples from the T-cell repertoire. *Nat. Rev. Immunol,* Vol.3, pp. 383-391.

Patterson, C.C., Carson, D.J. & Hadden, D.R. (1996). Epidemiology of childhood IDDM in Northern Ireland 1989e1994: low incidence in areas with highest population density and most household crowding. *Diabetologia,* Vol.39, pp. 1063-1069.

Pender, M.P. (1995). An introduction to neuroimmunology, In: *Autoimmune neurological diseases,*Pender, M.P & McCombe, P.A, pp.16. cambridge university press.

Peterson, K., Rosenblum, M.K., Kotanides, H. & Posner, J.B. (1992). Paraneoplastic cerebellar degeneration: I. A clinical analysis of 55 anti-Yo antibody positive patients, *Neurology,* Vol.42, pp. 1931-1937.

Pettinelli, C.B. & McFarlin, D.E. (1981). Adoptive transfer of experimental allergic encephalomyelitis in SJL/J mice after in vivo activation of lymph node cells by myelin basic protein: requirement for Lyt-1+2- T lymphocytes. *J Immunol,* Vol.127, pp. 1420-1423.

Pircher, H., Rohrer, H.U., Moskophidis, D., Zinkernagel, R.M. & Hengartner, H. (1991). Lower receptor avidity required for thymic clonal deletion than for effector T cell function. *Nature,* Vol.351, pp. 482-485.
Polman, C.H., O'Connor, P.W., Havrdova, E., Hutchinson, M., Kappos, L. & Miller, D.H. (2006). A randomized, placebo-controlled trial of natalizumab for relapsing multiple sclerosis. *N Engl J Med, Vol.*354, pp. 899-910.
Pranzatelli, M.R., Travelstead, A.L., Tate, E.D., Allison, T.J., Moticka, E.J., Franz, D.N., Nigro, M.A., Parke, J.T., Stumpf, D.A. & Verhulst, S.J. (2004). B- and T-cell markers in opsoclonus-myoclonus syndrome: immunophenotyping of CSF lymphocytes, *Neurology,* Vol.62, pp. 1526-1532.
Qin, Y., Duquette, P., Zhang, Y., Talbot, P., Poole, R. & Antel, J. (1998). Clonal expansion and somatic hypermutation of VH genes of B cells from cerebrospinal fluid in multiple sclerosis. *J Clin Invest,* Vol.102, pp. 1045-1050.
Quarles, R.H. & Weiss, M.D. (1999). Autoantibodies associated with peripheral neuropathy. *Muscle Nerve,* Vol.22, pp. 800-822.
Racke, M.K & Stuart, R.W. (2002). Targeting T cell costimulation in autoimmune disease. *Expert Opin Ther Targets,* Vol.6, No.3, pp. 275-89.
Radbruch, A., Muehlinghaus, G., Luger, E.O., Inamine, A., Smith, K.G., Dörner, T. & Hiepe, F. (2006). Competence and competition: the challenge of becoming a long-lived plasma cell. *Nat. Rev. Immunol,* Vol.6, pp. 741-750.
Ragheb. & Lisak, R.P. (1998). Immune regulation and myasthenia gravis. *Ann N Y Acad Sci,* Vol.841, pp. 210-224.
Raghupathy, R. (1997). Th-1 type immunity is incompatible with successful pregnancy. *Immunol. Today,* Vol.18, pp. 478-482.
Rajewsky, K. (1996). Clonal selection and learning in the antibody system. *Nature,* Vol.381, pp.(751-758).
Rodien, P., Madec, A.M., Ruf, J., Rajas, F., Bornet, H. & Carayon, P. (1996). Antibody-dependent cell-mediated cytotoxicity in autoimmune thyroid disease: relationship to antithyroperoxidase antibodies. *J Clin Endocrinol Metab,* Vol.81, pp. 2595-2600.
Roitt, I, Brostoff, J & Male, D. (1998). Immunology, Mosby, London UK, pp. 410- 425.
Rosenfeld, M.R., Eichen, J.G., Wade, D.F., Posner, J.B. & Dalmau, J. (2001). Molecular and clinical diversity in Paraneoplastic immunity to Ma proteins. *Ann Neurol,* Vol.50, pp. 339-348.
Ross, R. (1990). Mechanisms of atherosclerosis-a review. *Adv Nephrol Necker Hosp,*Vol.19, pp.79-86.
Galperin, C & Gershwin, ME. (1997). Immunopathogenesis of gastrointestinal and hepatobiliary diseases. *JAMA,*Vol.278, pp. 1946-1955.
Roubinian, J.R., Talal, N., Greenspan, J.S., Goodman, J.R. & Siiteri, P.K. (1978).Effect of castration and sex hormone treatment on survival,anti-nucleic acid antibodies, and glomerulonephritis in NZB/NZW F1 mice. *J Exp Med,* Vol.147, pp. 1568-1583.
Ruegg, S.J., Fuhr, P. & Steck, A.J. (2004). Rituximab stabilizes multifocal motor neuropathy increasingly less responsive to IVIg. *Neurology,* Vol.63, pp. 2178-2179.
Sakic, B., Szechtman, H., Denburg, J.A., Gomy, G., Kolb, B. & Whishaw IQ. (1998).Progressive atrophy of pyramidal neuron dendrites in autoimmune MRL/lpr mice. *J Neuroimmunol,* Vol.87, pp. 162-170.

Sanders, D.B. (1995). Lambert-Eaton myasthenic syndrome: clinical diagnosis, immune-mediated mechanisms, and update on therapies. *Ann Neurol*, Vol.37, Suppl 1, pp. 63-73.

Schattner, A. (1994). Lymphokines in autoimmunity-a critical review. *Clin Immunol Immunopathol*, Vol.70, pp. 177-189.

Schneider-Gold, C., Hartung, H.P. & Gold, R. (2006). Mycophenolate mofetil and tacrolimus: New therapeutic options in neuroimmunological diseases. *Muscle & Nerve*, Vol.34, pp.284-291.

Shy, M.E. (2007). Peripheral neuropathies, Goldman L, Ausiello D. In: *Cecil Medicine*, Elsevier, Philadelphia, Pa: Saunders, pp.446.

Silverstein, A.M. & Rose, N.R. (2000).There is only one immune system! The view from immunopathology. *Semin Immunol*, Vol.12, No.173, No.8, pp. 257-344.

Singer, P.A. & Theofilopoulos, A.N. (1990).T cell receptor V) repertoire expression in murine models of SLE. *Immunol Rev*, Vol.118, pp. 103-127.

Slifka, M.K., Antia, R., whitmire, J.K. & Ahmed, R. (1998). Humoral immunity due to long-lived plasma cells. *Immunity*, Vol.8, pp. 363-372.

Smith, D.A. & Dori, R. (1999). Introduction to Immunology and Autoimmunity. *Environmental Health Perspectives*, Vol.107, Supplement. 5, pp. 661-665.

Starr, T.K., Jameson, S.C. & Hogquist, K.A. (2003). Positive and negative selection of T cells. *Annu. Rev. Immunol*, Vol.21, pp. 139-176.

Steinman, L. (2002). A few autoreactive cells in an autoimmune infiltrate control a vast population of nonspecific cells: a tale of smart bombs and the infantry. *Proc. Natl. Acad. Sci. U. S. A*, Vol.93, pp. 2253-2256.

Stohl, S.W. (2004). Targeting B lymphocyte stimulator in systemic lupus erythematosus and other autoimmune rheumatic disorders. *Expert Opin Ther Targets*, Vol.8, pp. 177-189.

Stojanovich, L. & Marisavljevich, D. (2008). Stress as a trigger of autoimmune disease *Autoimmun Rev*, Vol.7, No.3, pp. 209-213.

Stuve, O., Cepok, S., Elias, S., Saleh, A., Hartung, H.P., Hemmer, B. & Kieseier, B.C. (2005). Clinical stabilization and effective bB-lymphocyte depletion in the cerebrospinal fluid and peripheral blood of a patient with fulminant relapsing-remitting multiple sclerosis, *Arch Neurol*, Vol.62, pp. 1620-1623.

Swain, S.L. (2003). Regulation of the generation and maintenance of T-cell memory: a direct, default pathway from effectors to memory cells. *Microbes. Infect*, Vol.5, pp. 213-219

Tan, M.E., Reimer, G. & sullivan, K.(1987).Itracellularv antigens:diagnostic fingerprints but aetiological dilemmas, Evered, D & Whelan, J. In: *autoimmunity and autoimmune disease*. John Wiley & Sons Ltd, Chichester,UK, pp. 25-30.

Tarlinton, D., Radbruch, A., Hiepe, F. & Dörner, T. (2008). Plasma cell differentiation and survival. *Curr.Opin. Immunol*, Vol.20, pp. 162-169.

Tindall, R.S., Rollins, J.A., Phillips, J.T., Greenlee, R.G., Wells, L. & Belendiuk, G. (1987). Preliminary results of a double-blind, randomized, placebo-controlled trial of cyclosporine in myasthenia gravis. *N Engl J Med*, Vol.316, pp. 719-724.

Trembleau, S., Germann, T., Gately, M.K. Z. & Adorini, L. (1995).The role of IL-12 in the induction of organ-specific autoimmune diseases. *Immunol Today*, Vol.16, pp. 383-386.

Vandiedonck, C., Capdevielle, C., Giraud, M., Krumeich, S. & Jais, J.P. (2006). Association of the PTPN22*R620W polymorphism with autoimmune myasthenia gravis. *Ann. Neuro,* .Vol.59, pp. 404-407.

VanVoorhis, B.J. & Stovall, D.W. (1997). Autoantibodies and fertility: a review of the literature. *J. Reprod. Immunol.*Vol.33, pp. 239-256.

Vincent, A., Beeson, D. & Lang, B. (2000). Molecular targets for autoimmune and genetic disorders of neuromuscular transmission. *Eur J Biochem,* Vol.267, pp. 6717-6728.

Vincent, A., Bowen, J., Newsom-Davis, J. & McConville, J. (2003). Seronegative generalised myasthenia gravis: clinical features, antibodies and their targets. *Lancet Neurol,* Vol.2, pp. 99-106.

Vogt, M.H., Lopatinskaya, L., Smits, M., Polman, C.H. & Nagelkerken, L. (2003). Elevated osteopontin levels in active relapsing-remitting multiple sclerosis. *Ann Neurol,* Vol.53, No.6, pp. 819-822.

Waldor, M.K., Sriram, S., Hardy, R., Herzenberg, L.A., Herzenberg, L.A., Lanier, L., Lim, M. & Steinman, L. (1985). Reversal of experimental allergic encephalomyelitis with a monoclonal antibody to a T cell subset marker (L3T4). *Science,* Vol.15, pp. 417

Walgaard, C., Jacobs, B.C. & Van Doorn, P.A. (2011). Emerging drugs for Guillain-Barr? Syndrome. *Expert Opin Emerg Drugs,* Vol.16, No.1, pp. 105-120.

Warnke, C., Meyer, H.G., Hartung, H.P., Stuve, O. & Kieseier, B.C. (2009). Review of teriflunomide and its potential in the treatment of multiple sclerosis. *Neuropsychiatr Dis Treat,* Vol.5, pp. 333-340.

Webster, E.L., Torpy, D.J., Elenkov, I.J. & Chrousos, G.P. (1998). Corticotropinreleasing hormone and inflammation. *Ann NY Acad Sci,* Vol.840, pp. 21-32.

Wekerle, H., Linington, C., Lassmann, H. & Meyermann, R, (1986). Cellular immune reactivity within the CNS. *Trends Neurosci,* Vol.9, pp. 271-277.

Whitaker, J.N. (1987). The presence of immunoreactive myelin basic protein peptide in urine of persons with multiple sclerosis. *Ann Neurol,* Vol.22, No.5, pp. 648-655.

Willison, H. J. & Yuki, N. (2002). Peripheral neuropathies and anti-glycolipid antibodies. *Brain,* Vol.125, pp. 2591-2625.

Wingerchuk, D.M. (2004). Neuromyelitis optica: current concepts, *Front Biosci,* Vol.9, pp. 834-840.

WIPO, 28.03.2011, Available from URL: www.wipo.int/pctdb/en/fetch.jsp?LANG=ENG&DBSELECT=PCT&SERVER_TYPE=19-10&SORT=11316447-KEY&TYPE_FIELD=256&IDB=0&IDOC=1324445&C=10&ELEMENT_SET=B&RESULT=5&TOTAL=7&START=1&DISP=25&FORM=SEP-0/HITNUM,B-ENG,DP,MC,AN,PA,ABSUM-ENG&SEARCH_IA=US2001032198&QUERY=%28PA%2fJagat+AND+PA%2fKanwar%29+]

Wylam, M.E., Anderson, P.M., Kuntz, N.L. & Rodriguez, V. (2003). Successful treatment of refractory myasthenia gravis using rituximab: a pediatric case report. *J Pediatr,* Vol.143, pp. 674-677.

Wynne, A., Kanwar, R.K., Khanna, R. & Kanwar, J.R. (2010). Recent Advances on the Possible Neuroprotective Activities of Epstein- Barr Virus Oncogene BARF1 Protein in Chronic Inflammatory Disorders of Central Nervous System. *Current Neuropharmacology,* Vol.8, pp. 268-275.

Yagi, J. & Janeway, C.A. (1990). Ligand thresholds at different stages of T cell development. *Int. Immunol,* Vol.2, pp. 83–89.

Yan, W.X., Taylor, J., Andrias-Kauba, S. & Pollard, J.D. (2000). Passive transfer of demyelination by serum or IgG from chronic inflammatory demyelinating polyneuropathy patients. *Ann Neurol,* Vol.47, pp. 765–775.

Yang, J.S., Xu, L.Y., Xiao, B.G., Hedlund, G. & Link, H. (2004). Laquinimod (ABR-215062) suppresses the development of experimental autoimmune encephalomyelitis, modulates the Th1/Th2 balance and induces the Th3 cytokine TGF-beta in Lewis rats. *J Neuroimmunol,* Vol.56, pp. 3–9.

Yang, Y. & Santamaria, P. (2006). T cells and autoimmunity. In: Rose, N.R. & Mackay, I.R. *The Autoimmune Diseases,* Elsevier Academic Press, San Diego, pp. 59-82.

Yoon, J.W., Austin, M., Onodera, T. & Notkins, A.L. (1979).Virus-induced diabetes mellitus. Isolation of a virus from the pancreas of a child with diabetic ketoacidosis. *N Engl J Med,* Vol.300, pp. 1173-1179

Yoshida, S. & Gershwin M.E. (1993). Autoimmunity and selected environmental factors of disease induction. *Semin Arthritis Rheum,* Vol.22, pp. 399-419.

Ziff, M. (1991). Role of the endothelium in chronic inflammatory synovitis. *Arthritis Rheum,* Vol.34, pp. 1345-1352.

Zinman, L., Ng, E. & Bril, V. (2007). IV immunoglobulin in patients with myasthenia gravis - A randomized controlled trial. *Neurology,* Vol.68, pp. 837-841.

An Open Label Study of the Effects of Eculizumab in Neuromyelitis Optica, In: *clinical trials.gov,* 7.03.2011, Available from URL: clinicaltrials.gov/ct2/show/NCT00904826

4

Cellular Based Therapies for the Treatment of Multiple Sclerosis

James Crooks[1], Guang-Xian Zhang[2] and Bruno Gran[1]
[1]*University of Nottingham,*
[2]*Thomas Jefferson University, Philadelphia,*
[1]*United Kingdom*
[2]*USA*

1. Introduction

Multiple sclerosis (MS) is a chronic inflammatory autoimmune disease of the central nervous system (CNS) and the primary cause of non-traumatic neurologic disability in the western world. Infiltration of myelin-specific effector T cells into the CNS is thought to cause demyelination and loss of axons resulting in deficient signal conduction and clinical onset of the disease. Although previously thought to be initiated by T helper 1 (Th1) cells, it has become evident that Th17 cells are also involved (Cua 2003). In addition, CD8+ T cells, macrophages, and B cells are also found in inflammatory infiltrates in the CNS of affected individuals. During the initial phases of the disease, once the myelin-specific peripherally activated T cells penetrate the CNS, they are re-activated by antigen presenting cells presenting their target antigen within the CNS and act to cause damage to axonal myelin through the activation of macrophages and the release of myelin toxic substances (Aktas, Waiczies et al. 2007).

One of the main obstacles to recovery and to the treatment of MS is the relatively low efficiency of spontaneous remyelination of axons by oligodendrocytes. In the majority of cases during the early phases of the disease a large amount of oligodendrocytes and their precursors are preserved within the characteristic demyelination plaques and retain the ability to remyelinate. Despite this resident population of remyelinating cells it has been shown that over time remyelination becomes incomplete and fails, resulting in the irreversible neurological damage associated with the disease (Franklin 2002).

The direct cause of MS remains unknown but it seems most likely to be a mixture of both genetic susceptibility and environmental factors. Genetic factors had been long suspected to affect the chances of an individual developing MS. It has been known for some time that there is a familial link to the disease with a sharp increase in disease probability if a family member has the disease (Dyment, Ebers et al. 2004), with a direct correlation between how closely related the affected individual is and the probability of developing the disease. The importance of genetic factors was underscored by the fact that adopted children have no statistically significant increase in there disease susceptibility compared to the general population, even if any of their adoptive family members have the disease. Other genetic factors such as gender and race have also been shown to have an effect (Sospedra and Martin 2005).

More recently environmental factors have been highlighted by an increase in MS cases in westernised society as opposed to that of other less developed areas of the world. It is thought this may be due to the lack of exposure to infection during adolescence and childhood and has been highlighted in places such as Japan (Li, Chu et al. 2007) where a strong link may exist between the number of MS cases and the increase in sanitation. Among infectious environmental factors, Epstein Barr and other human Herpes viruses have received most attention in recent years (Levin, Munger et al. 2010). Other non-infectious environmental factors, such as latitude and sun exposure have also been linked to the disease (Sospedra and Martin 2005).

Current treatments for MS include IFN-β, glatiramer acetate and mitoxantrone which show some degree of efficacy and have potential side effects (Markowitz 2010). New more effective treatments for MS are highly desirable, in particular those able to slow disease progression in addition to reducing the frequency of clinical exacerbations. Although several pharmacological therapies are in clinical trials or have recently been approved (such as the immunosuppressive drug Fingolimoid, (Cohen and Chun 2011)), cellular treatments are attractive alternatives. They may theoretically possess the ability to modulate the immune response but also enhance spontaneous remyelination of damaged axons and thus limit or even reverse the irreversible neurological damage associated with MS. The challenge is making this theoretical potential become a reality.

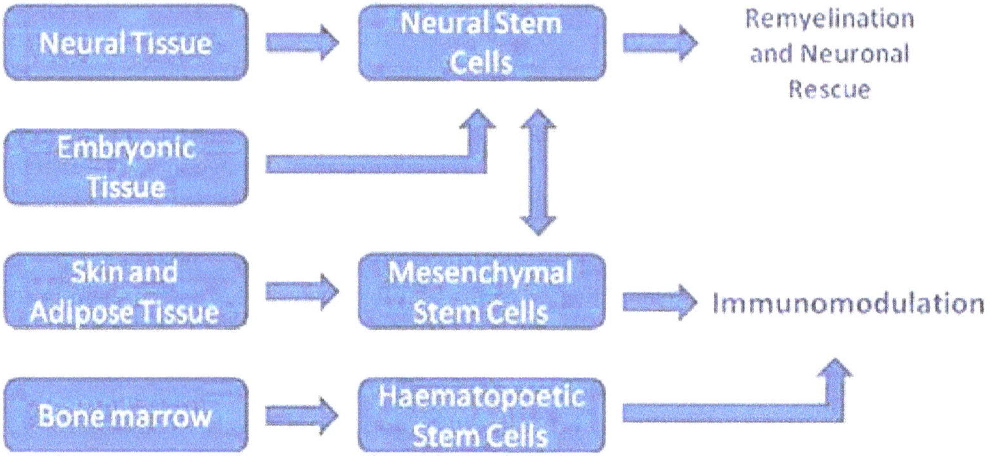

Fig. 1. Potential roles for different types of stem cells in the treatment of MS [Adapted from (Martino, Franklin et al. 2010)].

2. Stem cell therapies

Stem cells are the most promising treatment option in cellular therapy as they have the potential to differentiate into a multitude of cells. There are several types of stem cells which are isolated from different types of tissue which include embryonic, mesenchymal, hematopoietic and neuronal stem cells along with the relatively new discovery of fibroblast derived induced pluripotent stem cells (IPS). These different phenotypes of stem cells hold great potential in the treatment of a variety of different conditions and potentially have a range of positive effects on MS and a range of other inflammatory, traumatic and neurodegenerative CNS conditions. The fact that stem cells possess the theoretical ability, under the right conditions, to differentiate into any type of cell in the body makes them a very desirable treatment option. However significant issues arise with their use including ethics, access to the cells, and their potential side effects.

2.1 Embryonic stem cells

Of all the different types of stem cells, embryonic stem cells (ESC) have the largest differentiating potential and are also the best categorised but despite this their use has come up against a variety of practical and ethical hurdles due to their embryonic source. Theoretically embryonic stem cells can provide an unlimited supply of cells with vast differentiation potential. In animal models and in the right environment, they can be directed into differentiating into oligodendrocytes and successfully undertaking remyelination (Nistor, Totoiu et al. 2005). This remyelination has been shown in a number of animal models following the infusion of ESC derived glial precursors leading to a significant degree of remyelination in both the spinal column and the brain (Brustle, Jones et al. 1999). It has also been noted that the time of infusion with these cells is crucial, with some studies showing that, in the case of spinal injury, remyelination is much more effective if the embryonic stem cell derived cells are introduced soon after the damage (7 days) as opposed to later after the event (10 months) (Keirstead, Nistor et al. 2005). This suggests that in the case of neurodegenerative disease these cells may be more effective if transplanted in the earlier stages of the condition.

Not only do embryonic stem cells show the potential to remyelinate but also have an effect on EAE through the modulation of the immune system, with a number of animal models showing a down regulation of the auto-immune T-lymphocyte response against self antigen (Fandrich, Lin et al. 2002). This immunomodulatory potential has been proposed to be through both contact-dependent mechanisms and the release of soluble factors. For example PGE_2 was identified as one of these factors in murine models in which embryonic stem cells had been used to dampen the immune response in organ transplantation (Imberti, Casiraghi et al. 2011).

Despite the promising potential of embryonic stem cells as a therapy for multiple diseases and conditions there are several hurdles which realistically may never be fully overcome. The first of these are the ethical ramifications of work involving embryonic stem cells. The fact that embryonic stem cells would most likely have to be sourced from human embryos has raised serious concerns about the use of sources of 'potential life' as a research tool. To date, much of the work in stem cell research has been conducted using unwanted embryos originally produced for IVF treatment. However, if this became a main stream treatment embryos would have to be produced for the specific purpose of producing appropriate stem cells, which many see as unethical (de Wert and Mummery 2003). Another ethical hurdle would be the production of autologus stem cells where the nucleus from the cell of the patient would be infused into a de-nucleated oocyte in order to create a strain of stem cells specific to the patient which would help to bypass the issue of rejection (de Wert and Mummery 2003). Many believe the specific use of embryonic stem cells is not the issue; it is the precedent it would set. The ethical debate surrounding ESC is unlikely to be easily resolved.

Another issue surrounding embryonic stem cells is safety. The use of heterologus embryonic stem cells carries the risk of the formation of teratoma (tumour) within the specific organ of transplantation (Bjorklund, Sanchez-Pernaute et al. 2002; Blum and Benvenisty 2008). Altering the cells to reduce this risk may prove very difficult and may also have a detrimental effect on the cells' ability to exert the therapeutic purpose for which they are intended. This issue can be avoided with the use of autologus stem cells (mentioned above) but this leads to not only ethical but also practical issues, with every patient being treated having to be cloned to produce the stock of autologous cells for treatment.

2.2 Adult neuronal stem cells

Adult neural stem cells (aNSC) do not carry the same ethical burden as embryonic stem cells and have shown the ability to both remyelinate demyelinated axons and modulate the autoimmune response. These cells are generally isolated from the adult mammalian sub ventricular zone (SVZ), which makes them difficult to extract and use for clinical purposes. They can be maintained for extended periods in vitro and still retain the ability to differentiate and proliferate (Nunes, Roy et al. 2003). In EAE it has been documented that aNSC can act to aid the disease both through remyelination and through an immunomodulatory effect. In terms of remyelination, aNSC have been proposed as treatments for a multitude of different conditions such as neurodegenerative disorders including MS (Magalon, Cantarella et al. 2007), CNS traumas (Iwanami, Kaneko et al. 2005) and malignant tumours. Transplanted cells have been shown to migrate from the area of infusion to the area of inflammation (Ben-Hur, Einstein et al. 2003) especially within the white matter of the CNS, with the labelling of infused cells showing that 80% of lesions contain labelled cells within 24 hours of infusion (Politi, Bacigaluppi et al. 2007). aNSC are also seen to be durable within the body with labelled cells still detected within lesions 20 days after infusion (Politi, Bacigaluppi et al. 2007). Along with the detection of aNSC presence and migration visualised by cell labelling, remyelination and cell replacement have also been visualised in EAE with the use of electron microscopy (Pluchino, Quattrini et al. 2003). aNSC's have been shown to migrate to areas of demyelination (and not to areas of normal looking brain and CNS matter) and differentiate into oligodendrocytes capable of remyelination and thus attenuate the clinical symptoms of EAE within the tested animals.

In terms of the immunomodulatory effects of aNSC on neurodegenerative diseases such as MS there has been some debate. It has been shown that animals given an IV injection of aNSCs in the early stages of EAE show a significant immunosuppressive effect. Animals treated with aNSCs were shown to have a gathering of the infused cells at the spleen and lymph nodes and here had a profound effect on the immune response to self CNS antigen through their interaction with the T-cell populations in these areas (Einstein, Fainstein et al. 2007). T-cells isolated from the lymph nodes of mice that had been infused with aNSC's showed no activation in the presence of either CNS specific antigens or other non-specific stimulus (Einstein, Fainstein et al. 2007). It is evident that these cells, when injected intravenously at the early stages of the disease, do not penetrate the CNS or get attracted to areas of inflammation like aNSC's injected at the height of the disease but travel to areas of immune regulation such as the spleen and lymph nodes where they have an dampening effect on the peripheral immune response (Ben-Hur 2008).

The key to the use of aNSC's in therapy will be optimising the technique to allow both the immunomodulatory and the remyelinating features of the treatment to work in tandem and thus have a greater effect on the symptoms of the disease. aNSCs have several advantages over other forms of stem cells, including fewer ethical burdens, maintaining differential and proliferative ability over long periods of time, and having both immunomodulatory and remyelinating potential. Therefore, they are one of the more promising avenues of investigation into MS treatments. They also seem to pose little risk of tumour formation, which is in stark contrast to a number of other stem cell types. In all the aNSC transplant studies in both healthy and diseased animals there have been no instances of tumour formation which suggests that the potential use of this treatment in vivo would carry little if any risk in the way of tumour development.

2.3 Mesenchymal stem cells

Mesenchymal stem cells are stromal stem cells which can be isolated from a variety of adult tissues but predominantly from the bone marrow. The therapeutic effect of these cells on neurodegenerative diseases has previously been based mainly on immunomodulation, but recently it has been proposed that these cells may be able to induce axon remyelination. However, this is yet to be unequivocally proven. In terms of immunomodulation, bone marrow isolated mesenchymal stem cells are known to have a dampening effect of the autoimmune response to CNS self antigens in EAE. The mesenchymal cells are shown to have an inhibitory effect on the activation of encephalitogenic T cells primed against self CNS antigen, thus reducing disease severity (Kassis, Grigoriadis et al. 2008). T-cells isolated from MSC-treated animals show a reduced ability to produce inflammatory cytokines (such as IFN-γ and TNF-α) and do not proliferate in the presence of the EAE-inducing CNS self antigen (Gerdoni, Gallo et al. 2007). In addition to reducing T-cell function, MSCs can also modulate the proliferation and maturation of antigen presenting cells (APC) (Beyth, Borovsky et al. 2005), which in turn affect T-cell priming to self antigens.

The potential for the infusion of mesenchymal bone marrow derived stem cells to induce a degree of remyelination in animal models of MS has been reported in a few studies. Such cells removed from the bone marrow of donor mice and cultured in vitro were infused into damaged EAE spinal cords and induce both central and peripheral myelination (Akiyama, Radtke et al. 2002).

Bone marrow stem cells can also be used as a source of neural cells, bone marrow-derived neural stem cells. These cells are phenotypically identical to aNSC isolated from the SVC and express the neural stem cell marker nestin. Like aNSC's and unlike other stem cells isolated from the bone marrow, these cells show the ability to migrate into the CNS and differentiate into both oligodendrocytes and neurons at sites of CNS damage, such as inflammatory CNS lesions in MS (Kabos, Ehtesham et al. 2002). However, their differentiation into cells capable of remyelination is not the only way these cells are said to act in the repair of damaged axons. They may also promote remyelination by pre-existing cells through the release of growth factors. Bone marrow derived neuronal cells also seem to have significant immunomodulatory properties, such as in vitro suppression of T cells, B cells and natural killer (NK) cells.

2.4 Haematopoietic stem cells

Hematopoietic stem cells (HSC) have been extensively studied for immune replacement therapy in aggressive forms of MS. There are a number of advantages to this form of stem cell which is why research into it has been so thorough. The isolation process compared to that of other stem cells is less invasive and more ethically acceptable as the CD34+ cells can be easily isolated from peripheral blood. HSC transplantation (HCST) may be one of the most potent available forms of immunotherapy; however issues of safety have limited the advance of this approach into clinical use. Useful predictors of good therapeutic outcomes after HSCT include rigorous selection of the most suitable patients for this type of treatment and the specific treatment protocol. Patients with low to intermediate level of disability experiencing active relapses despite treatments with IFN-beta or with more potent immunosuppressive drugs, such as mitoxantrone, may show a better risk/benefit ratio than those with advanced, secondary progressive disease with higher disability (Muraro, Cassiani Ingoni et al. 2003; Burt, Cohen et al. 2005). The regime of treatment is also vital to the success of the treatment with early studies, which used myeloblative transplantation regimes, suffering high levels of toxicity and mortality (Burt, Cohen et al. 2005). The use of revised, non myeloblative HSCT conditioning protocols, seems to have had a positive effect on the mortality rates associated with the previous treatment regimes.

There are many issues when using hematopoietic stem cells as a treatment option in MS involving both ethics and safety. The risk involved in HSCT is relatively high although safety has increased over recent years. An example is the drop in mortality rate in patients suffering from autoimmune conditions treated with autologus hematopoietic stem cell transplantation, which was 7.3% between 1995 and 2000 and dropped to 1.3% in the period from 2001-2007 (Schippling, Heesen et al. 2008). The direct effect of the hematopoietic stem cells in giving rise to malignant tumours is an obvious risk but another major issue is the level of immunosupression needed during a stem cell transplantation, which leaves the patient particularly vulnerable to infections. The risk factors in this type of immunosuppressive therapy make it a last resort, with patients and treating physicians having to assess and discuss the risk/benefit ratios of such a treatment before undertaking it. Considering that many patients with MS live for many years and can, to some degree, manage and slow the progression of their illness with pharmaceutical treatments, it may be hard to justify a therapy such as AHSCT. However, as the methods and techniques involved in AHSCT improve and the favourable outcomes seen in animal models are translated into human studies (this has already been seen in the limited number of humans successfully treated with the method), this treatment could in time become a key immunomodulation technique in treating MS. As these issues are overcome large scale, long term, controlled studies will be necessary to test the true efficacy of the treatment (Mancardi and Saccardi 2008) after which HSCT treatment may be deemed safe for larger scale use.

2.5 Induced pluripotent stem cells

Induced pluripotent stem cells (IPS) are possibly the most exciting development in the field of stem cell therapy for the last few years. A group in Japan has shown that it is possible to generate pluripotent stem cells from fibroblast cultures with the addition of just 4 transcription factors (Oct 3/4, Sox2, Klf4 and c-Myc) under ESC culturing conditions (Takahashi, Tanabe et al. 2007). These cells represent a significant step forward as they share the morphology and many functional properties with ESCs but can be generated from fibroblasts in the laboratory. The accessibility of fibroblasts, the comparatively straight forward techniques involved in generating IPS and the removal of important ethical burdens suggests an enormous treatment potential for such a type of stem cells. These cells could become a valid treatment option in regenerative medicine not only in MS but a variety of other inflammatory, neurodegenerative, and traumatic diseases including spinal cord injury, juvenile diabetes (Thomson, Itskovitz-Eldor et al. 1998) and potentially many others.

Despite their enormous potential, IPS do raise a number of safety concerns which must be overcome before they are considered as a valid treatment in humans. Due to a large number of retroviral integration sites (retroviruses are used to insert the relevant transcription factors into target cells to induce IPS) on IPS for each of the stimulating factors they may be prone to tumourigenesis. Mouse studies showed around 20% rate of tumour formation which is thought to be due to the reactivation of the c-Myc oncogene by retrovirus (Okita, Ichisaka et al. 2007). Tumour formation caused by retroviral integration is a serious issue which must be solved before this treatment is considered in the clinic.

Other problems must be resolved as well. The yield of IPS cells from human fibroblast cultures is very low, which could represent a practical obstacle to the development of IPS as a treatment. The precise nature of IPS and their origin is still a matter of debate. Different theories suggest that the cells induced into IPS are actually undifferentiated stem cell-like cells within the fibroblast cultures. It is also possible that undetectable genetic alterations in the cells of origin may be required for IPS induction (Takahashi, Tanabe et al. 2007). For now these cells are a very useful tool within the process of understanding disease mechanisms and toxicology ex-vivo however the ultimate goal must be to develop this therapy to a point where it can be used to treat human conditions. Considering that these cells were only discovered in 2007, research into this form of pluripotent cells is still at an early stage. As time progresses it is likely some of the issues surrounding these cells will be overcome, and along with a better understanding of the mechanisms behind these cells they may become a valid treatment option in human medicine.

In summary, stem cells treatments are, and have been for some time, one of the most promising and exciting potential treatment options within human medicine. Thus far, they have failed to fulfil this immense promise having been held back by many ethical, practical and safety related hurdles. Nevertheless, stem cell research is constantly moving forward. With the discovery of new treatment protocols and new types of promising cells, such as IPS, the time when stem cells become a front line treatment for immunomodulation and neural regeneration in MS may be closer than ever.

3. Non-stem cell cellular therapies

It is not only stem cells which have been identified as a potential treatment option for patients suffering from MS. There are a range of possible cellular treatments which involve the infusion of cells isolated from the body with aims varying from halting the progression of the disease through immunomodulation to the active re-myelination of affected axons. Non-stem cell treatments would include the infusion of peripheral nervous system myelinating Schwann cells into the CNS as well as the use of ex vivo cultured oligodendrocytes, olfactory ensheathing cells and even cells isolated from the body's immune system such as T-cells.

3.1 Oligodendrocyte and oligodendrocyte precursor cells

Myelination of axons within the CNS is typically the task of oligodendrocytes and their precursors during development and in response to damage, however it has been shown that a significant proportion of these cells are lost or are deemed functionally inactive in MS, particularly in chronic phases of disease. It has been suggested that the reason for this decrease in numbers of oligodendrocytes is due to either the lack of differentiation of precursor cells into mature oligodendrocytes or the death of the oligodendrocytes once they reach a certain point within the developmental process (Wolswijk 2000).

There is a degree of debate over the stage at which oligodendrocyte precursor cells (OPC) are most effective at myelinating axons along there maturation process. It is thought that oligodendrocyte progenitor cells are responsible for generating the largest amount of myelin over the widest area and are more proficient than mature oligodendrocytes (Franklin 2002; Wolswijk 2002). There is evidence that mature oligodendrocytes when infused into a demyelinated CNS environment are less capable of migration and division at the site of demyelination than the more motile and proliferative oligodendrocyte progenitor cell. Another advantage of OPCs is their ability to react to their microenvironment. The path of maturation of these cells is affected by cytokines, chemokines and growth factors causing their maturation to a cell with remyelinating potential "in the right place at the right time", which is also aided by enhancement of the signalling matrix and removal of phagocytic debris by inflammatory cells (Zawadzka and Franklin 2007).

3.2 Schwann cells

Schwann cells, typically responsible for myelination within the peripheral nervous system, are seen as an alternative to oligodendrocytes and OPCs in the cellular treatment of MS and have been shown to be capable of a significant degree of axonal remyelination within the CNS of MS patients (Lavdas, Papastefanaki et al. 2008). Despite the issues surrounding the use of these cells, such as their inability to interact with astrocytes and limited survivability within the CNS, their ability to remyelinate axons and improve axonal conduction in damaged axons is not in doubt. The question is whether they can do so to such a degree that it is an effective and worthwhile treatment option for patients with MS. Schwann cells have been proposed as a treatment for CNS damage not only for MS but for other pathological conditions including the repair of spinal cord injury (Oudega 2007) where their proposed function to aid the remyelination of damaged axons remains the same. There are many positive and negative aspects to Schwann cells as a potential cellular treatment option in MS, with the main advantage being the ease of accessibility from peripheral nerve biopsies and thus the relatively simple task of culturing autologus populations of these cells. Another positive aspect is that they are less likely than oligodendrocytes to be prone to MS related autoimmune attack as this tends to be against the CNS myelinating cells due to being targeted towards mature oligodendrocyte antigens (Kohama, Lankford et al. 2001). On this note, the myelin they produce is also less likely to be susceptible to autoimmune attack due the slight differences in its make up as compared with the myelin produced by oligodendrocytes. Due to the autoimmune attack in the CNS being focused against antigens within the oligodendrocyte produced myelin, the subtle differences in the makeup of Schwann cell myelin makes it a less likely target.

As we have explained, the fact that Schwann cells are not usually resident within the CNS has its advantages in terms of not being recognised in an autoimmune attack, however the fact that these cells are out of their usual environment also has some negative ramifications. Schwann cells do not tend to migrate to areas of inflammation within the white matter of the CNS due to the inhibitory effect that astrocytes have on them. Schwann cells and astrocytes cannot coexist which poses huge problems in the treatment of MS as the majority of demyelinated plaques contain large numbers of astrocytes. Astrocytes have a number of detrimental effects on Schwann cells, effecting both their successful migration into the CNS white matter (Iwashita, Fawcett et al. 2000) and their ability to remyelinate and survive (Shields, Blakemore et al. 2000) within damaged astrocyte rich areas. It is proposed that this negative effect on Schwann cells in mediated by the release of soluble factors from the astrocytes (astrocyte conditioned medium reduced Schwann cell proliferation and remyelination (Guenard, Gwynn et al. 1994)) such as Ephrins (Afshari, Kwok et al. 2010) and also through a prolonged contact interaction between Schwann cells and the astrocytes mediated by N-Cadherin (Wilby, Muir et al. 1999). This limited ability to function within the CNS is a major drawback for the use of Schwann cells as a remyelinating treatment as any effect they do have will be short lived due to the short time span they can survive within the appropriate system. If Schwann cells are to become a widely used remyelinating treatment option in the treatment of MS work will have to be done to produce a Schwann cell-based therapy capable of migrating to sites of CNS inflammation and able to survive in the presence of astrocytes. Efforts are being made to improve the chances of Schwann cells surviving interaction with astrocytes through methods such as genetically altering the cells (Papastefanaki, Chen et al. 2007).

3.3 Olfactory ensheathing cell

Another type of cell that has been proposed for the remyelination of axons in multiple sclerosis is the olfactory ensheathing cell (OEC). These are a form of unique glial cell found only in the olfactory system close to the first cranial nerve. These cells are favourable over other cell based therapies for a number of properties, one of which is their ability to survive in the presence of astrocytes. Astrocytes are found around areas of MS induced CNS inflammation and as previously discussed are a major problem for Schwann cell therapy. OEC's can survive in conjunction with astrocytes and can also make the environment around the CNS inflammation more hospitable to the migration and survival of endogenous Schwann cells (Boyd, Lee et al. 2004).

Despite this ability to survive and retain function in the presence of astrocytes there are also some disadvantages to the OEC in the treatment of MS. Despite their ability to remyelinate axons and partially regenerate nerve fibres (Richter and Roskams 2008) they do not seem to have a great deal of the ability to cross the MS associated lesion and or to reconnect with neurons on the opposite side of the lesion. It is thought that due to this process of repair not being overly apparent most of the benefit for the use of OEC comes from the promotion of the growth of intact fibres. However, in the case of spinal injury it has been shown that, to at least some degree, these cells have the ability to stimulate neuroprotection, activate angiogenesis and stimulate axon re-growth as well as remyelination (Richter and Roskams 2008). Another benefit of these cells is that in some cases they have been suggested to restore a degree of functions lost due to the CNS lesions. However, there is very little immunological data to support this conclusion, which was derived mainly from behavioural tests (Barnett and Riddell 2004). It is thought that the most useful way to utilise this type of cells may be to use them in parallel with other synergistic treatments. This would produce a combination treatment with the potential to regenerate axons but also reconnect the damaged connections across the compromised areas of the CNS which OEC alone are unable to do (Barnett and Riddell 2007).

3.4 T-cell therapy

Another cellular treatment for MS which differs from all the previous treatments as it does not involve remyelinating cells is T-cell therapy. When thinking of ways to tackle autoimmunity one of the most obvious candidates for cellular therapy has to be regulatory T-cells due to their role in maintaining immunological self tolerance within the body. This CD4+CD25+ cell surface marker positive family of cells within the body is in part to control the immune response and therefore seem an obvious choice for cellular therapy for MS. It is known that in the peripheral blood of patients with MS there is a significant decrease in the functionality of T-regulatory cells (Viglietta, Baecher-Allan et al. 2004) when compared to healthy controls, which shows this may be a causative mechanism behind the disease and readdressing this balance may go some way to alleviating autoimmunity.

It has been shown in animal models that adoptive transfer of such T-regulatory cells has a positive effect on models of autoimmune disease (Jiang, Lechler et al. 2006), in some cases offering a significant degree of protection from the disease (Kohm, Carpentier et al. 2002) and therefore poses a degree of therapeutic potential in the treatment of MS. The therapeutic potential of these cells is based on their ability to suppress the function of auto reactive T helper cells in-vitro and to show a significant potential for in-vivo treatment as well. There is also the possibility of targeting these cells in-vivo with other drugs in an attempt to expand an antigen specific population of these cells to tackle the autoimmune response in the MS patients.

Another form of T cell therapy which has been proposed is the use of inflammatory CD4+ T cells. These cells have long been thought to have little therapeutic potential in CNS autoimmunity but it has been proposed by a group in Israel that a lack of CD4+ immune cells recruited to the CNS may affect the immunological balance in the CNS further and exacerbate inflammation within the system (Schwartz and Shechter 2010). Their theory is that these CD4+ T cells must be recruited to the CNS to modify areas of local inflammation and also to aid the protective process through the recruitment of blood-borne monocytes (Schwartz, London et al. 2009). Many current therapies for MS involve treatment with immunosuppressive drug regimes which will strongly inhibit the ability of these inflammatory T cells to perform the proposed protective function and it has thus been proposed that a boost of such a T cell response to carefully chosen CNS proteins may act to improve and not hinder the immunological response against the localised inflammation.

In summary, although cellular therapies for MS are often focused around stem cells, it is evident that non stem cell therapies have an important role to play. They do in most cases provide a safer, more ethical and more practical option of treatment compared to stem cells but may not posses as much treatment potential. However, this is not to say they are less effective than the treatments currently available. Like stem cells, the different types of these cells give non stem cell cellular therapies both remyelination and immunomodulatory potential. These cells have the potential to be used on their own or in combination with other therapies. With steps being taken to improve their efficacy (such as genetic alteration in the case of Schwann cells), they could become mainstream treatments in the fight against MS.

4. Conclusion

The devastating effect MS has on the lives of affected individuals and those close to them demands that this field of research be at the forefront of treatment development. The lack of current effective and curative therapies for this disease makes the advancement of cellular treatments all the more important as a new more effective line of treatment. The outstanding potential of cellular therapies to cover all bases in terms of treatment of MS including immunomodulation, neuroprotection and remyelination makes them impossible to ignore as they realistically have the most potential of any field of treatment currently available. Their potential is almost limitless with the variety of different effects the different cellular treatments can have on the disease and how these could fit the needs of individual patients and their specific disease circumstances.

The challenge to take these cellular therapies from being full of potential to being effective treatment options is one thousands of researchers around the world are working on every day. They strive to remove the issues which at the moment are holding back the clinical potential of these 'shining light' treatments in order to be able to offer patients diagnosed with MS hope that it may be possible to restore the myelin architecture within their CNS and to overcome the disease. The treatment options for MS are currently insufficient but the encouraging point is that the field is constantly moving forwards. With cellular based therapies at the forefront of this advancement it will give sufferers of the disease hope that better treatments and better prognosis may be just around the corner.

5. References

Afshari, F. T., J. C. Kwok, et al. (2010). "Astrocyte-produced ephrins inhibit schwann cell migration via VAV2 signaling." *J Neurosci* 30(12): 4246-4255.

Akiyama, Y., C. Radtke, et al. (2002). "Remyelination of the rat spinal cord by transplantation of identified bone marrow stromal cells." *J Neurosci* 22(15): 6623-6630.

Aktas, O., S. Waiczies, et al. (2007). "Neurodegeneration in autoimmune demyelination: recent mechanistic insights reveal novel therapeutic targets." *J Neuroimmunol* 184(1-2): 17-26.

Barnett, S. C. and J. S. Riddell (2004). "Olfactory ensheathing cells (OECs) and the treatment of CNS injury: advantages and possible caveats." *J Anat* 204(1): 57-67.

Barnett, S. C. and J. S. Riddell (2007). "Olfactory ensheathing cell transplantation as a strategy for spinal cord repair--what can it achieve?" *Nat Clin Pract Neurol* 3(3): 152-161.

Ben-Hur, T. (2008). "Immunomodulation by neural stem cells." *J Neurol Sci* 265(1-2): 102-104.

Ben-Hur, T., O. Einstein, et al. (2003). "Transplanted multipotential neural precursor cells migrate into the inflamed white matter in response to experimental autoimmune encephalomyelitis." *Glia* 41(1): 73-80.

Beyth, S., Z. Borovsky, et al. (2005). "Human mesenchymal stem cells alter antigen-presenting cell maturation and induce T-cell unresponsiveness." *Blood* 105(5): 2214-2219.

Bjorklund, L. M., R. Sanchez-Pernaute, et al. (2002). "Embryonic stem cells develop into functional dopaminergic neurons after transplantation in a Parkinson rat model." *Proc Natl Acad Sci U S A* 99(4): 2344-2349.

Blum, B. and N. Benvenisty (2008). "The tumorigenicity of human embryonic stem cells." *Adv Cancer Res* 100: 133-158.

Boyd, J. G., J. Lee, et al. (2004). "LacZ-expressing olfactory ensheathing cells do not associate with myelinated axons after implantation into the compressed spinal cord." *Proc Natl Acad Sci U S A* 101(7): 2162-2166.

Brustle, O., K. N. Jones, et al. (1999). "Embryonic stem cell-derived glial precursors: a source of myelinating transplants." *Science* 285(5428): 754-756.

Burt, R. K., B. Cohen, et al. (2005). "Hematopoietic stem cell transplantation for multiple sclerosis." *Arch Neurol* 62(6): 860-864.

Cohen, J. A. and J. Chun (2011). "Mechanisms of fingolimod's efficacy and adverse effects in multiple sclerosis." *Ann Neurol* 69(5): 759-777.

Cua, D. J. (2003). "Interleukin-23 rather than Interleukin-12 is the critical cytokine for autoimmune inflammation of the brain." *Nature* 421: 744-748.

de Wert, G. and C. Mummery (2003). "Human embryonic stem cells: research, ethics and policy." *Hum Reprod* 18(4): 672-682.

Dyment, D. A., G. C. Ebers, et al. (2004). "Genetics of multiple sclerosis." *Lancet Neurol* 3(2): 104-110.

Einstein, O., N. Fainstein, et al. (2007). "Neural precursors attenuate autoimmune encephalomyelitis by peripheral immunosuppression." *Ann Neurol* 61(3): 209-218.

Fandrich, F., X. Lin, et al. (2002). "Preimplantation-stage stem cells induce long-term allogeneic graft acceptance without supplementary host conditioning." *Nat Med* 8(2): 171-178.

Franklin, R. J. (2002). "Remyelination of the demyelinated CNS: the case for and against transplantation of central, peripheral and olfactory glia." *Brain Res Bull* 57(6): 827-832.

Franklin, R. J. (2002). "Why does remyelination fail in multiple sclerosis?" *Nat Rev Neurosci* 3(9): 705-714.

Gerdoni, E., B. Gallo, et al. (2007). "Mesenchymal stem cells effectively modulate pathogenic immune response in experimental autoimmune encephalomyelitis." *Ann Neurol* 61(3): 219-227.

Guenard, V., L. A. Gwynn, et al. (1994). "Astrocytes inhibit Schwann cell proliferation and myelination of dorsal root ganglion neurons in vitro." *J Neurosci* 14(5 Pt 2): 2980-2992.

Imberti, B., F. Casiraghi, et al. (2011). "Embryonic stem cells, derived either after in vitro fertilization or nuclear transfer, prolong survival of semiallogeneic heart transplants." *J Immunol* 186(7): 4164-4174.

Iwanami, A., S. Kaneko, et al. (2005). "Transplantation of human neural stem cells for spinal cord injury in primates." *J Neurosci Res* 80(2): 182-190.

Iwashita, Y., J. W. Fawcett, et al. (2000). "Schwann cells transplanted into normal and X-irradiated adult white matter do not migrate extensively and show poor long-term survival." *Exp Neurol* 164(2): 292-302.

Jiang, S., R. I. Lechler, et al. (2006). "CD4+CD25+ regulatory T-cell therapy." *Expert Rev Clin Immunol* 2(3): 387-392.

Kabos, P., M. Ehtesham, et al. (2002). "Generation of neural progenitor cells from whole adult bone marrow." *Exp Neurol* 178(2): 288-293.

Kassis, I., N. Grigoriadis, et al. (2008). "Neuroprotection and immunomodulation with mesenchymal stem cells in chronic experimental autoimmune encephalomyelitis." *Arch Neurol* 65(6): 753-761.

Keirstead, H. S., G. Nistor, et al. (2005). "Human embryonic stem cell-derived oligodendrocyte progenitor cell transplants remyelinate and restore locomotion after spinal cord injury." *J Neurosci* 25(19): 4694-4705.

Kohama, I., K. L. Lankford, et al. (2001). "Transplantation of cryopreserved adult human Schwann cells enhances axonal conduction in demyelinated spinal cord." *J Neurosci* 21(3): 944-950.

Kohm, A. P., P. A. Carpentier, et al. (2002). "Cutting edge: CD4+CD25+ regulatory T cells suppress antigen-specific autoreactive immune responses and central nervous system inflammation during active experimental autoimmune encephalomyelitis." *J Immunol* 169(9): 4712-4716.

Lavdas, A. A., F. Papastefanaki, et al. (2008). "Schwann cell transplantation for CNS repair." *Curr Med Chem* 15(2): 151-160.

Levin, L. I., K. L. Munger, et al. (2010). "Primary infection with the Epstein-Barr virus and risk of multiple sclerosis." *Ann Neurol* 67(6): 824-830.

Li, Y., N. Chu, et al. (2007). "Increased IL-23p19 expression in multiple sclerosis lesions and its induction in microglia." *Brain* 130(Pt 2): 490-501.

Magalon, K., C. Cantarella, et al. (2007). "Enriched environment promotes adult neural progenitor cell mobilization in mouse demyelination models." *Eur J Neurosci* 25(3): 761-771.

Mancardi, G. and R. Saccardi (2008). "Autologous haematopoietic stem-cell transplantation in multiple sclerosis." *Lancet Neurol* 7(7): 626-636.

Markowitz, C. E. (2010). "The current landscape and unmet needs in multiple sclerosis." *Am J Manag Care* 16(8 Suppl): S211-218.

Martino, G., R. J. Franklin, et al. (2010). "Stem cell transplantation in multiple sclerosis: current status and future prospects." *Nat Rev Neurol* 6(5): 247-255.

Muraro, P. A., R. Cassiani Ingoni, et al. (2003). "Hematopoietic stem cell transplantation for multiple sclerosis: current status and future challenges." *Curr Opin Neurol* 16(3): 299-305.

Nistor, G. I., M. O. Totoiu, et al. (2005). "Human embryonic stem cells differentiate into oligodendrocytes in high purity and myelinate after spinal cord transplantation." *Glia* 49(3): 385-396.

Nunes, M. C., N. S. Roy, et al. (2003). "Identification and isolation of multipotential neural progenitor cells from the subcortical white matter of the adult human brain." *Nat Med* 9(4): 439-447.

Okita, K., T. Ichisaka, et al. (2007). "Generation of germline-competent induced pluripotent stem cells." *Nature* 448(7151): 313-317.

Oudega, M. (2007). "Schwann cell and olfactory ensheathing cell implantation for repair of the contused spinal cord." *Acta Physiol (Oxf)* 189(2): 181-189.

Papastefanaki, F., J. Chen, et al. (2007). "Grafts of Schwann cells engineered to express PSA-NCAM promote functional recovery after spinal cord injury." *Brain* 130(Pt 8): 2159-2174.

Pluchino, S., A. Quattrini, et al. (2003). "Injection of adult neurospheres induces recovery in a chronic model of multiple sclerosis." *Nature* 422(6933): 688-694.

Politi, L. S., M. Bacigaluppi, et al. (2007). "Magnetic-resonance-based tracking and quantification of intravenously injected neural stem cell accumulation in the brains of mice with experimental multiple sclerosis." *Stem Cells* 25(10): 2583-2592.

Richter, M. W. and A. J. Roskams (2008). "Olfactory ensheathing cell transplantation following spinal cord injury: hype or hope?" *Exp Neurol* 209(2): 353-367.

Schippling, S., C. Heesen, et al. (2008). "Stem cell transplantation in multiple sclerosis." *J Neurol* 255 Suppl 6: 43-47.

Schwartz, M., A. London, et al. (2009). "Boosting T-cell immunity as a therapeutic approach for neurodegenerative conditions: the role of innate immunity." *Neuroscience* 158(3): 1133-1142.

Schwartz, M. and R. Shechter (2010). "Systemic inflammatory cells fight off neurodegenerative disease." *Nat Rev Neurol* 6(7): 405-410.

Shields, S. A., W. F. Blakemore, et al. (2000). "Schwann cell remyelination is restricted to astrocyte-deficient areas after transplantation into demyelinated adult rat brain." *J Neurosci Res* 60(5): 571-578.

Sospedra, M. and R. Martin (2005). "Immunology of multiple sclerosis." *Annu Rev Immunol* 23: 683-747.

Takahashi, K., K. Tanabe, et al. (2007). "Induction of pluripotent stem cells from adult human fibroblasts by defined factors." *Cell* 131(5): 861-872.

Thomson, J. A., J. Itskovitz-Eldor, et al. (1998). "Embryonic stem cell lines derived from human blastocysts." *Science* 282(5391): 1145-1147.

Viglietta, V., C. Baecher-Allan, et al. (2004). "Loss of functional suppression by CD4+CD25+ regulatory T cells in patients with multiple sclerosis." *J Exp Med* 199(7): 971-979.

Wilby, M. J., E. M. Muir, et al. (1999). "N-Cadherin inhibits Schwann cell migration on astrocytes." *Mol Cell Neurosci* 14(1): 66-84.

Wolswijk, G. (2000). "Oligodendrocyte survival, loss and birth in lesions of chronic-stage multiple sclerosis." *Brain* 123 (Pt 1): 105-115.

Wolswijk, G. (2002). "Oligodendrocyte precursor cells in the demyelinated multiple sclerosis spinal cord." *Brain* 125(Pt 2): 338-349.

Zawadzka, M. and R. J. Franklin (2007). "Myelin regeneration in demyelinating disorders: new developments in biology and clinical pathology." *Curr Opin Neurol* 20(3): 294-298.

5

Application of Novel Quantitative Proteomic Technologies to Identify New Serological Biomarkers in Autoimmune Diseases

Soyoung Lee, Satoshi Serada, Minoru Fujimoto and Tetsuji Naka
National Institute of Biomedical Innovation, Laboratory of Immune Signal
Japan

1. Introduction

Autoimmune diseases comprise a wide variety of systemic or organ-specific inflammatory diseases, characterized by aberrant activation of immune cells that target self tissues due to misrecognizing tissue-derived proteins as foreign antigens (Hueber and Robinson, 2006; Prince, 2005). The prevalence of autoimmune diseases is approximately 2,000 ~ 3,000 per 100,000, although the prevalence varies depending on the diseases, ethnic groups and regions (Prieto and Grau, 2010). The etiology and exact pathogenesis of autoimmune diseases remain poorly understood. However, both genetic factors and environmental triggers are profoundly involved in the pathogenesis of autoimmune diseases. Notably, clinical manifestations of autoimmune disease may be different among patients, even though they have the same diagnosis, depending on the affected organs of each patient. Therefore, careful evaluation of the clinical manifestations combined with the examination of laboratory tests is required for proper diagnosis of autoimmune diseases and subsequent monitoring of the disease activity during therapy. In addition, therapeutic choices for these diseases have been limited so far and conventional therapeutics include non-steroidal anti-inflammatory drugs (NSAID), glucocorticoids, cytotoxic drugs and disease modifying anti rheumatoid drugs (DMARDs). For these reasons, autoimmune diseases have been considered to be intractable and the goal of the treatment is to control disease activity rather than to achieve remission or cure.

Recently, however, the advent of biological agents has led to the marked improvement in the treatment of rheumatoid arthritis (RA) and other inflammatory autoimmune diseases. These agents greatly contribute to improve health-related quality or daily life of patients with autoimmune diseases (Han et al., 2007; Keystone et al., 2008; Laas et al., 2009; Strand and Singh, 2007). Nevertheless, biological agents are not effective for all patients with autoimmune diseases and current biomarkers are not helpful to select an effective biological agent for individual patients. In addition, conventional inflammatory biomarkers are often inadequate to evaluate the disease activity in patients treated with biological agents. Thus, there is a growing need for the development of new biomarkers that can predict individual treatment response before starting biological therapy and evaluate the disease activity and therapeutic efficacy during therapy. In this chapter, we first outline the clinical usage and current understanding of biological agents for the treatment with autoimmune diseases and then describe our attempt to identify new biomarkers in autoimmune diseases by taking advantage of a new proteomic approach.

2. Biological agents for the treatment of autoimmune diseases

2.1 Biological agents for autoimmune therapy in clinics

The immune response is a highly coordinated process and involves complex interactions of diverse molecules including cytokines and various cell types such as lymphocytes (Figure 1). Dysregulation in immune response such as overproduction of cytokines and aberrant activation of immune cells is implicated in autoimmune disorders. Therefore, these molecules and/or cells involved in immune response have been targeted to develop therapies in autoimmune disorders (Figure 1).

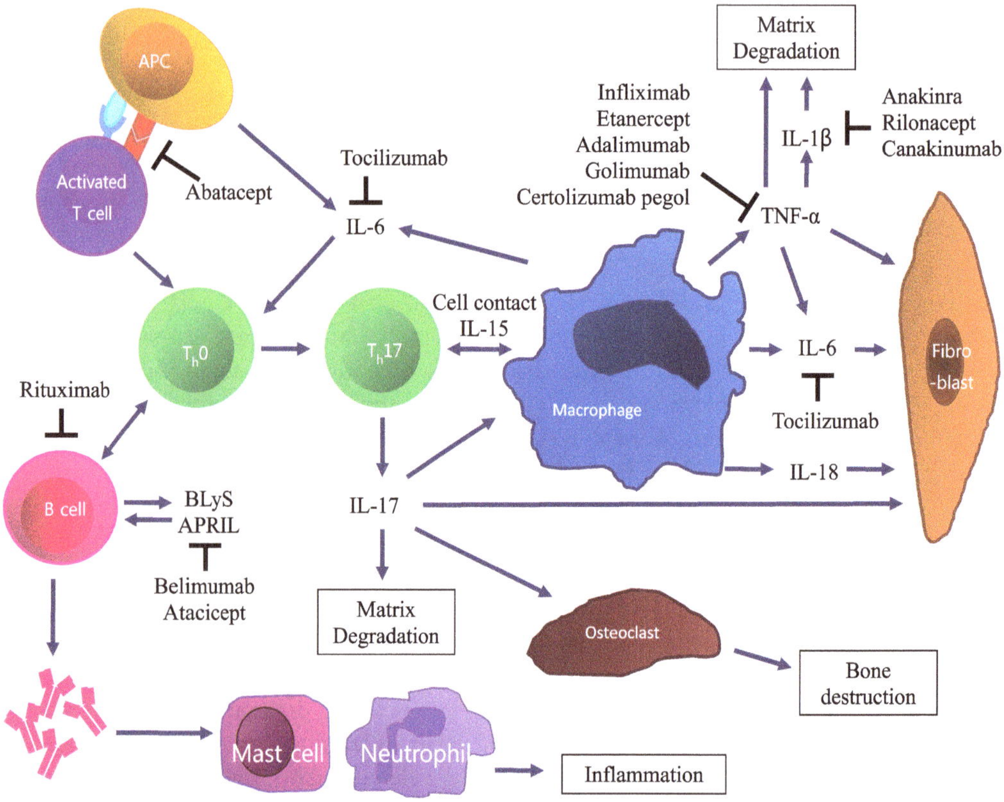

This figure summarizes the cellular interactions in the pathogenesis of RA and the interaction among antigen presenting cells (APCs), T cells, B cells, macrophages, hematopoietic cells (neutrophil, mast cell) and nonhematopoietic cells (fibroblast, connective tissue cell, and bone). These interactions are facilitated by the actions of cytokines released from the activated cells then induce the production of other pro-inflammatory and inflammatory cytokines, which contribute to the pathogenesis of RA. Also, this figure shows therapeutic biological agents proved as a RA treatment (Brennan and McInnes, 2008; McInnes and Schett, 2007).

Fig. 1. An overview of the pathogenesis of rheumatoid arthritis (RA) and the cytokine targets.

Every biological agent used in clinics today has its own specific targets and can be grouped as follows according to its aims: 1) tolerance induction, 2) inhibition of MHC, antigen, and T cell receptor interaction, 3) Inhibition of cellular function and cell-cell interaction, 4) Interference with cytokines, 5) apoptosis (Table 1). Among them, the anticytokine biological

Strategy	Biologic Agent	Molecule	Target	Indication
Tolerance induction	Abetimus	ds-DNA	Anti-ds-DNA	SLE
Inhibition of MHC, antigen, and T cell receptor interaction		Under studying		
Inhibition of cellular unction and cell-cell interaction	Abatacept	CTLA4-Ig	CD80/86	RA, JIA
	Rituximab	mAb to CD20	B cells	RA, JIA
	Belimumab	mAb to BLyS	BLyS	SLE
Interference with cytokines	Etanercept	TNFRII/FcIgG1	TNF-α, TNF-β	RA, PsA, Ps, AS, JIA
	Infliximab	mAb to TNF-α	TNF-α	RA, PsA, Ps, AS, JIA, IBD, uveitis
	Golimumab	mAb to TNF-α	TNF-α	RA, PsA, AS
	Adalimumab	mAb to TNF-α	TNF-α	RA, PsA, Ps, AS, JIA, IBD, uveitis
	Certolizumab pegol	Pegylated mAb to TNF-α	TNF-α	CD, RA
	Anakinra	IL-1 Ra	IL-1	RA, sJIA
	Rilonacept	IL-1R/IL-1AcP/IgG1	IL-1	CAPS, sJIA
	Canakinumab	mAb to IL-1	IL-1	CAPS, sJIA
	Tocilizumab	mAb to IL-6R	IL-6	JIA
Apoptosis		mAb to Fas	Fas	

AS: Ankylosing spondylitis, CAPS: Cryoprin-associated periodic syndrome, CD: Crohn's disease, ds-DNA: double strand-DNA, IBD: Inflammatory bowel disease, JIA: Juvenile idiopathic arthritis, mAb: Monoclonal antibody, Ps: Psoriasis, PsA: Psoriatic arthritis, RA: Rheumatoid arthritis, sJIA: Systemic-typed JIA, SLE: Systemic lupus erythematosus. (Textbook of Pediatric Rheumatology, 6th ed. 2011, Saunders)

Table 1. Summary of biological agents

agents that suppress the action of proinflammatory cytokines such as TNF, IL-1 and IL-6 are well-known and widely used in clinics. These agents were developed as therapies in RA and recommended for the treatment of patients whose disease does not respond to conventional therapies (Gomez-Reino and Carmona, 2006). RA patients treated with the anticytokine biological agents show dramatic improvement of their clinical symptoms and the levels of inflammatory biomarkers such as C-reactive protein (CRP) and erythrocyte sedimentation rate (ESR). Subsequently, these agents have been applied to the treatment of other inflammatory autoimmune diseases and have had a significant impact on patients' prognosis and survival (Andreakos et al., 2002; Efthimiou and Markenson, 2005; Maini et al., 2006; Nishimoto et al., 2009; Yokota et al., 2008).

However, it has been reported that substantial numbers of patients with autoimmune diseases still do not respond to one or more anticytokine biological agents. Among biological agents, TNF inhibitors have been extensively investigated with regard to the frequency of inadequate responders (Launois et al., 2011; Lovell et al., 2008; Maini et al., 2006; Yokota et al., 2008), because anti-TNF antibodies were the first agents approved as the therapy of RA. For example, 20~40 % of patients treated with a TNF inhibitor failed to achieve an improvement of 20 % in American College of Rheumatology criteria (Emery et al., 2008; Rubbert-Roth and Finckh, 2009). More patients lose efficacy during therapy, as shown by a report that 21 % of RA patients initially treated with etanercept no longer receive this therapy after 24 months (Feltelius et al., 2005).

Recently, patients who had an inadequate response or adverse events with one anticytokine agent are often treated with another biologic agent (Gomez-Reino and Carmona, 2006; Hyrich et al., 2007; Karlsson et al., 2008; Rubbert-Roth and Finckh, 2009). In the case of the treatment failure with the first TNF inhibitor, one survey reported that over 94 % of practicing rheumatologists in the United States of America have switched from one TNF inhibitor to another (Yazici et al., 2009). Interestingly, while some surveys reported that the efficiency of second TNF inhibitors is less than that of the first TNF inhibitor (Gomez-Reino and Carmona, 2006; Hyrich et al., 2007; Karlsson et al., 2008; Rubbert-Roth and Finckh, 2009), a large cohort study from the UK revealed that patients who switched their therapy from an initial TNF inhibitor continued to receive the second TNF inhibitor for mean length of 6 months and only 16 % of patients stopped it again due to poor response (Hyrich et al., 2007). This observation indicates that biological agents that share the common target do not always show the same effect on patients. One reason for the inefficacy of the first TNF inhibitor but not of the second one is the development of neutralizing antibody against the first agent, which may not interfere with the action of the second TNF inhibitor. Nevertheless, this observation also raises the possibility that these agents may have their own mode of action. Supporting the latter notion, there are differences in the efficacy between TNF inhibitors depending on diseases (Ackermann and Kavanaugh, 2007; Nash and Florin, 2005; Ramos-Casals et al., 2008; Sfikakis et al., 2007; Triolo et al., 2002; Veres et al., 2007). For example, while anti-TNF antibodies are effective for both RA and Crohn's disease, TNF receptor-Fc fusion protein (TNFR-Fc) is effective for RA but not for Crohn's disease.

The other treatment option after the failure with TNF inhibitors is to switch from TNF inhibitors to other biological agents with different targets. The Abatacept Trial in Treatment of Anti-TNF INadequate responders (ATTAIN) study investigated the effect of abatacept (CTLA4-Ig), an inhibitor of T cell co-stimulatory signal, on patients with active RA and an inadequate response to previous anti-TNF therapy. At 6 months, the ACR20 response rate was

50.4% in the abatacept group versus 19.5% in the placebo group and sustained improvements in ACR responses were achieved after 2 years of threatment with abatacept (Genovese et al., 2005; Rubbert-Roth and Finckh, 2009). In Randomized Evaluation of Long-Term Efficacy of Rituximab in RA (REFLEX) trial, B cell-depleting anti-CD20 antibody, rituximab, was administered to active RA patients with an inadequate response to TNF inhibitor. Among 208 patients treated with rituximab, 51 % of patients achieved an ACR20 response compared to 18 % of patients treated with placebo (Cohen et al., 2006). In addition, the patients treated with rituximab, by themselves, reported clinically meaningful and statistically improvements of pain, functional disability, and health-related quality of life (Keystone et al., 2008).
Recently, the Research on Actemra Determining efficacy after Anti-TNF failures (RADIATE) study examined the efficacy and safety of anti-IL-6 receptor (IL-6R) antibody, tocilizumab, in patients with active RA who had failed TNF inhibitor. Especially, 50.0 % of patients treated with tocilizumab at the 8 mg/kg of dose achieved ACR20 as well as rapid and sustained improvement of RA symptoms compared to 10.1 % of patients treated with placebo achieved ACR20 (Emery et al., 2008) (Figure 2). These findings are in accordance with the supposition that biological agents targeting different molecules have distinctive mechanism of action and show different effects on patients.

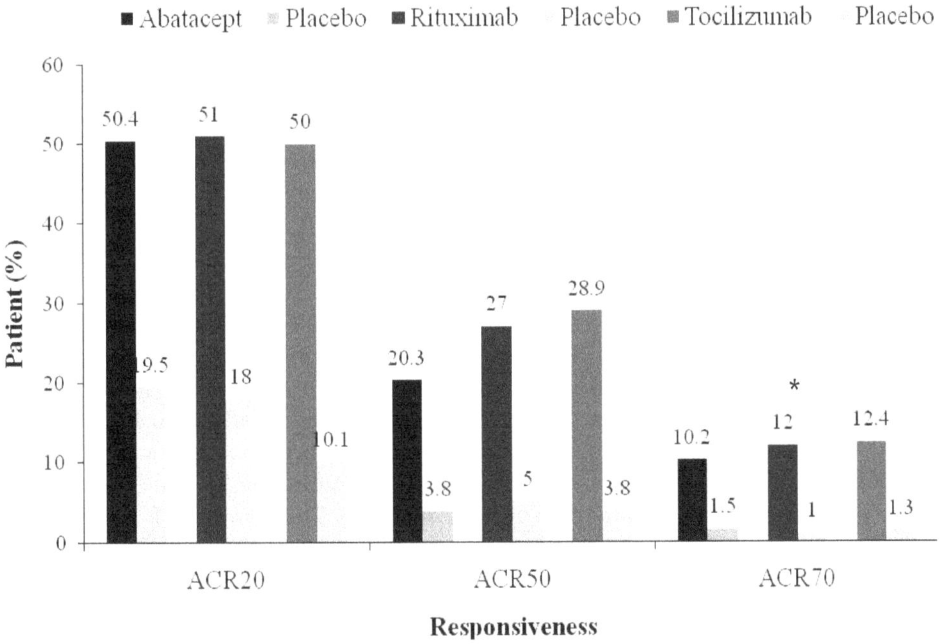

The second biological agents with other mechanisms with TNF inhibitors such as abatacept, rituximab and tocilizumab were used for patients who failed to initial TNF inhibitors. Bars show percentages of patients achieving a response according to the American College of Rheumatology 20% improvement criteria (ACR20), 50% improvement criteria (ACR50), and 70% improvement criteria (ACR70). The ACR20, ACR50, ACR70 responses in patients treated with abatacept, rituximab and tocilizumab were significantly higher than patients treated with placebo ($p<.001$, *$p=.003$).

Fig. 2. Responsiveness of treatment with the second biological agents in the patients with RA refractory to initial TNF inhibitors.

2.2 Biological therapeutic agents tested in animal models of autoimmune disorders

The analyses on murine disease models have contributed greatly to gain insight into pathogenesis and therapeutic strategy of autoimmune disorders. These models are also useful to clarify the detailed mechanisms of action of biological agents. We have recently investigated several disease models and reveled that anticytokine biological agents have different mechanism of action and show different effects on clinical manifestations of disease models (Fujimoto et al., 2008; Terabe et al., 2011).

We analyzed the effect of two anticytokine agents, anti-IL-6R monoclonal antibody (mAb) and TNFR-Fc, on collagen-induced arthritis (CIA), a murine model of human RA (Fujimoto et al., 2008). In accordance with the pivotal proinflammatory role of IL-6 and TNF in this arthritis model, both agents could inhibit the development of arthritis. However, while anti-IL-6R mAb potently inhibited the differentiation of Th17 cells, a highly inflammatory subset of T helper cells, TNFR-Fc exhibited no effect on Th17 cells. This observation suggests that these two agents have different action points: IL-6 blockade acts on initial phase of adoptive immune response and regulates T helper cell differentiation, whereas TNF inhibitors act much later, presumably at inflamed sites. Our study also suggests that IL-6 inhibitors may be applicable to other Th17-related autoimmune diseases. Indeed, anti-IL-6R mAb suppressed disease in a murine model of multiple sclerosis via the inhibition of Th17 cell differentiation (Serada et al., 2008). The different modes of action in anti-IL-6R mAb and TNF inhibitors may explain the difference in their efficiency in a murine model of uveoretinitis. Anti-IL-6R mAb treatment had a significant protective effect in experimental autoimmune uveoretinitis (EAU) mice, but either TNFR-Fc or anti-TNF mAb treatment did not (Hohki et al., 2010). Interestingly, in the EAU model, anti-IL-6R mAb not only suppressed Th17 cell differentiation but also suppressed autoantigen-specific Th1 cells via the generation of induced regulatory T cells, supporting the notion that IL-6 inhibitors act on initial phase of adoptive immune response (Haruta et al., 2011).

Confusingly, biological agents may act differently on different autoimmune diseases. Indeed, anti-IL-6R mAb and anti-TNF mAb, but not TNFR-Fc exerted similar effect on a murine inflammatory bowel disease (IBD) model (Terabe et al., 2011). This model is a T cell dependent colitis and is induced by the transfer of purified naïve CD4 T cells into lymphopenic mice. Both anti-IL-6R mAb and anti-TNF mAb successfully inhibited colitis, whereas TNFR-Fc did not show any protective effect on colitis. In addition, anti-IL-6R mAb and anti-TNF mAb could comparably inhibit the expansion of colitogenic T cells in this model, although like in other models, anti-IL-6R mAb additionally could modulate the profile of T helper cell differentiation (Terabe et al., 2011). Thus, anti-IL-6R mAb and anti-TNF mAb may share a similar mode of action in the inhibition of IBD. It is also notable that TNFR-Fc failed to inhibit inflammation in this colitis model (Terabe et al., 2011). Similar discrepancy in the effect of anti-TNF mAb and TNFR-Fc has been observed in human IBD. Many mechanisms have been proposed so far to explain the difference of action between these two agents. For example, anti-TNF mAb binds not only to soluble TNF-α, but also to membrane-bound TNF-α, leading to the induction of antibody-dependent and complement dependent cytotoxicity (Maini, 2004). The anti-TNF mAb may also have more capacity than TNFR-Fc to induce apoptosis via reverse signaling with cross-linking by binding firmly to transmembrane TNF(Terabe et al., 2011). Nevertheless, these hypotheses are still controversial and it remains to be explained why anti-TNF mAb and TNFR-Fc have differential effectiveness in some autoimmune diseases such as Crohn's disease. We believe that further study on this murine IBD model is useful for elucidation of this issue.

3. Biomarkers

3.1 A need for new biomarkers in the era of biological agents

Given the difference in mechanism and therapeutic effect of each biologic agent, it is desirable to select an effective biological agent on each patient before initiating therapy or after failure of the initial therapy. However, no reliable guidance is available at present for the selection of biological therapies. There is a growing need for the development of biomarkers that predict individual treatment response before therapy.

In addition, in patients treated with biological agents in whom immune response is substantially suppressed, conventional laboratory biomarkers such as CRP and ESR do not always reflect disease activity. In particular, since serum CRP is primarily dependent on liver by circulating IL-6, CRP is unable to reflect disease activity in patients treated with IL-6 inhibitors. Moreover, conventional markers may also be inadequate for the detection of inflammation unrelated to original diseases. In RA patients after joint surgery, anti-IL-6R mAb tocilizumab completely suppressed the increase in CRP and partially suppressed the rise in body temperature (Hirao et al., 2009). More importantly, biological agents may mask typical symptoms of bacterial infection and inhibit the elevation of serum biomarkers. Indeed, RA patients treated with tocilizumab did not present characteristic clinical symptoms and typical elevation of serum CRP after bacterial pneumonia and septic shock (Fujiwara et al., 2009). Even without biologic treatment, current inflammatory biomarkers are not useful to distinguish infection from flares of autoimmune diseases. This is an important issue in clinical settings, because therapeutic strategies for infection and disease flares are completely opposite. Infection must be treated primarily with antibiotics and discontinuation of biological agents should be considered. In contrast, disease flares should be treated intensively with the same or alternative biological agents. Thus, new biomarkers are needed for the detection and discrimination of inflammation by either infection or disease flares.

Even after the successful repression of disease with biologic therapies, it remains unknown yet whether biological agents can be terminated safely without disease recurrence. Therefore, a biomarker that indicates clinical remission or cure of autoimmune diseases is helpful to determine the timing to stop biological agents.

Collectively, the development of a number of novel biomarkers, such as those that can help to select biological agents before therapy, can precisely evaluate disease activity and therapeutic effect during the therapy or can instruct the timing of therapy completion after achievement of remission, are warranted for the appropriate clinical management of patients receiving biological therapies.

3.2 Serum proteome analysis using the new technology iTRAQ

The pathogenesis of autoimmune diseases involves alterations in the expression of genes that control pathways regulating self tolerance. However, gene transcripts may not faithfully reflect their protein levels. In addition, post-translational modifications are not amenable to the study of transcriptional profiling (Hueber and Robinson, 2006). Recently, there has been the remarkable improvement of the proteomic approaches as represented by the development of sophisticated methods of protein sample preparation and the improvement of the sensitivity, accuracy and resolution in mass spectrometer. Therefore, direct proteomic measurement may provide greater utility for the discovery of new biomarkers monitoring autoimmune diseases in the post genomic era. Current efforts to

identify autoimmune disease biomarkers have focused on three groups of proteins reflective of the autoimmune disease process. These groups include 1) degradation products arising from destruction of the affected tissues, 2) enzymes that play a role in tissue degradation, and 3) cytokines and other proteins associated with immune system activation and the inflammatory response (Prince, 2005). Recent proteomics technologies have enabled us to screen these markers from proteins extracted from tissues and sera from patients (Hueber and Robinson, 2006). Accordingly, there are many proteomic studies that analyzed protein profiles and searched new biomarkers in autoimmune diseases (Dwivedi et al., 2009; Ferraccioli et al., 2010; Ling et al., 2010; Serada et al., 2010; Takeuchi et al., 2007).
The quantitative proteome analysis by mass spectrometry (MS) usually involves differential isotope labeling of proteins and peptides metabolically, enzymatically or chemically using

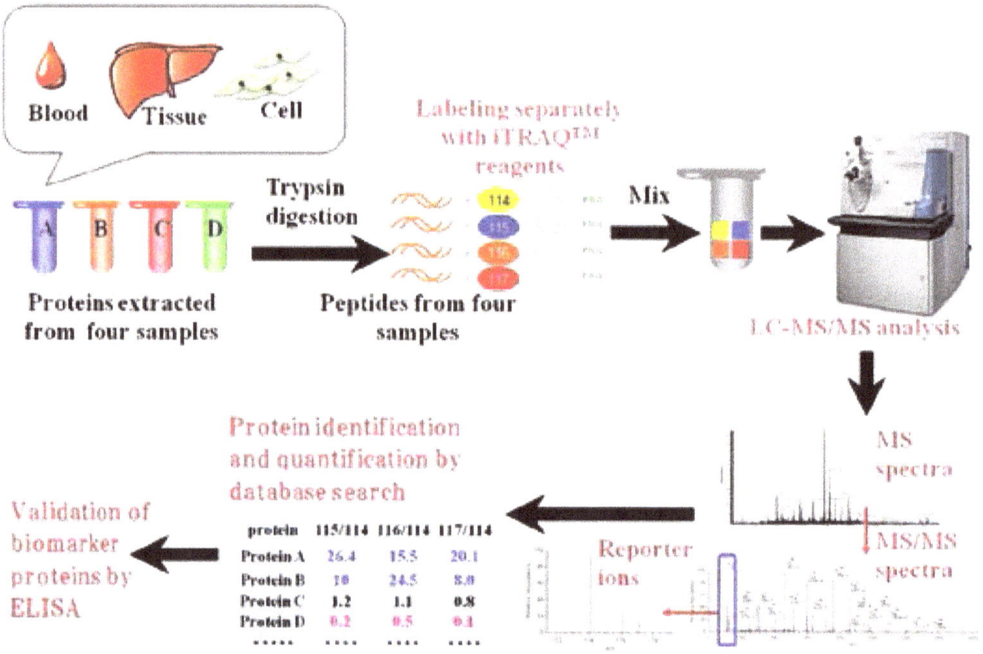

In a single experiment of iTRAQ analysis, 4 to 8 samples differentially labeled with iTRAQ reagents can be quantitatively analyzed by mass spectrometry (this figure shows a four-plex reagent experiment). First, proteins extracted from cells, tissue and/or body fluid such as blood are reduced, alkylated and digested with trypsin. Second, obtained peptides in each sample are labeled with each iTRAQTM reagent at N-terminal amino group or epsilon amino group from lysine. The iTRAQ tags are isobaric and the labeling with iTRAQ reagents results in the uniform increase in molecular weight of peptides in every sample. After labeling, samples are mixed into one tube and analyzed by liquid chromatography-tandem mass spectrometry (LC-MS/MS). Mass spectrometry is performed by full scan MS, followed by MS/MS spectra of peptides. In MS/MS spectra, iTRAQ tag-specific reporter ions (114.1, 115.1, 116.1, 117.1 in the figure) are detected in low m/z region, and these reporter ion intensities represent the abundance of the peptide from each sample. Peptide sequence information is obtained from high m/z region of MS/MS spectra and the protein is identified by database search after comparing obtained MS/MS spectra with theoretical MS/MS spectra in the database. Usually, candidate biomarker proteins obtained by iTRAQ analysis are further verified by other methods such as ELISA analysis.

Fig. 3. Flowchart of iTRAQ analysis

external reagent tags. These methods address some of the limitations faced in traditional gel-based proteomic approaches. However, these approaches still suffer from some limitations such as inability to multiplex and to quantify zero protein expression level. In contrast, a novel quantitative proteomic technology, isobaric tagging of peptides enable simultaneous identification and quantification of peptides by tandem MS and permit parallel proteome analysis of more than two samples (Aggarwal et al., 2006).

The isobaric tags for relative and absolute quantitation (iTRAQ), which is one such method commercialized, uses four amine specific isobaric reagents to label the primary amines of peptides from four to eight different biological samples. The labeled peptides from each sample are mixed, separated using two-dimensional liquid chromatography and analyzed using MS and tandem mass spectrometry (Figure 3). The isobaric tagging strategy provides multiple independent measures of the relative abundance of a protein. The capability of iTRAQ for protein quantitation has been verified by analyzing standard mixtures of proteins of known proportions (Aggarwal et al., 2006). The iTRAQ approach has now been successfully used to identify and quantify the proteins in variety of prokaryotic and eukaryotic samples (Aggarwal et al., 2006; Cong et al., 2006; DeSouza et al., 2005; Dwivedi et al., 2009; Hardt et al., 2005; Zhang et al., 2005).

3.3 Leucin-rich-α-2 glycoprotein as a novel biomarker

We reported for the first time that the iTRAQ technology is applicable to identify novel biomarkers in sera from patients with autoimmune diseases (Serada et al., 2010). Before we publish our results, a study was published and reported the serum proteome of RA patients treated with anti-TNF mAb therapy. They provided evidence that iTRAQ strategy can be used to obtain quantitative data that reflect changes in the serum proteome after targeted therapeutic interventions (Dwivedi et al., 2009).

We used iTRAQ technology to obtain profiles of serum proteome in RA patients before and after TNF inhibitor treatment. We then listed serum proteins that declined remarkably after treatment. Our strategy was verified by the detection of familiar biomarkers including CRP and serum amyloid A (SAA) as reduced serum proteins after treatment. Among the candidate proteins that declined after therapy, we focused on an uncharacterized protein called leucine-rich-α-2 glycoprotein (LRG) and examined further on this protein using other methods such as Western blot and ELISA. Indeed, taking advantage of ELISA analysis of many serum samples from RA patients, we found that serum levels of LRG significantly declined after therapy with TNF inhibitors and correlate well with disease activity of RA patients. In addition, LRG levels were significantly high in patients with other autoimmune diseases such as Crohn's disease and Behcet disease. As expected, the LRG correlated well with a conventional biomarker CRP in patients with these autoimmune inflammatory diseases. Interestingly, however, while CRP correlated with serum IL-6 levels, LRG did not. In accordance with this, in some Crohn's disease patients with active disease, CRP levels remained low but serum LRG concentrations were significantly elevated. Thus, LRG exhibits similarity with CRP but also has a unique property. Moreover, because serum LRG concentrations of Crohn's disease patients before starting therapy were higher in the non-responders to anti-TNF therapy than in the responders, LRG may predict therapeutic responses to TNF inhibitors in Crohn's disease patients (Serada et al., 2010).

Until now, LRG has been reported to be expressed by liver cells and neutrophils, and regulated by multiple factors and produced at local inflammatory sites. According to the previous reports, it seems that LRG is not a unique biomarker in autoimmune disease but rather is a generalized inflammatory biomarker, because serum LRG levels are reported to be increased in patients with bacterial infection and several types of cancers. Nevertheless, serum LRG satisfies the condition of an inflammatory biomarker in the point that its concentration is high at diagnosis, correlated well with disease activity and is a possible predictor of the responsiveness to biological agents. For these reasons, serum LRG is a novel inflammatory biomarker potentially surrogate for CRP. Further studies are in progress in our laboratory to determine the pathophysiological function of LRG and the clinical benefit of LRG measurement.

4. Conclusion

Autoimmune diseases including RA are not only rare but also difficult to treat. In the clinical field, biological agents have emerged as attractive therapeutic options for these diseases, because of their rapid and/or dramatic effectiveness to intractable diseases. However, biological agents are expensive and their usage is occasionally accompanied with severe adverse effects such as immunosuppression and fatal infection. To maximize the therapeutic potential and to minimize the adverse effects of biological agents, novel biomarkers are required for the selection of agents, monitoring of the disease activity and therapeutic efficacy or differential diagnosis of infection. In this respect, LRG we identified from iTRAQ analysis is a candidate of novel biomarkers useful for clinical practice of biological agents since it correlates with disease activity and therapeutic effectiveness of biological agents. In addition, the application of iTRAQ analysis, the novel quantitative proteomic approach, is useful for the identification of new serological biomarkers in patients with autoimmune diseases. Further studies using this approach may lead to the development of additional new biomarkers and may help to clarify the pathogenesis and identify therapeutic targets in autoimmune diseases.

5. References

Ackermann, C., and Kavanaugh, A. (2007). Tumor necrosis factor as a therapeutic target of rheumatologic disease. Expert Opin Ther Targets *11*, 1369-1384.

Aggarwal, K., Choe, L.H., and Lee, K.H. (2006). Shotgun proteomics using the iTRAQ isobaric tags. Brief Funct Genomic Proteomic *5*, 112-120.

Andreakos, E.T., Foxwell, B.M., Brennan, F.M., Maini, R.N., and Feldmann, M. (2002). Cytokines and anti-cytokine biologicals in autoimmunity: present and future. Cytokine Growth Factor Rev *13*, 299-313.

Brennan, F.M., and McInnes, I.B. (2008). Evidence that cytokines play a role in rheumatoid arthritis. J Clin Invest *118*, 3537-3545.

Cohen, S.B., Emery, P., Greenwald, M.W., Dougados, M., Furie, R.A., Genovese, M.C., Keystone, E.C., Loveless, J.E., Burmester, G.R., Cravets, M.W., *et al.* (2006). Rituximab for rheumatoid arthritis refractory to anti-tumor necrosis factor therapy: Results of a multicenter, randomized, double-blind, placebo-controlled, phase III trial evaluating primary efficacy and safety at twenty-four weeks. Arthritis Rheum *54*, 2793-2806.

Cong, Y.S., Fan, E., and Wang, E. (2006). Simultaneous proteomic profiling of four different growth states of human fibroblasts, using amine-reactive isobaric tagging reagents and tandem mass spectrometry. Mech Ageing Dev *127*, 332-343.

DeSouza, L., Diehl, G., Rodrigues, M.J., Guo, J., Romaschin, A.D., Colgan, T.J., and Siu, K.W. (2005). Search for cancer markers from endometrial tissues using differentially labeled tags iTRAQ and cICAT with multidimensional liquid chromatography and tandem mass spectrometry. J Proteome Res *4*, 377-386.

Dwivedi, R.C., Dhindsa, N., Krokhin, O.V., Cortens, J., Wilkins, J.A., and El-Gabalawy, H.S. (2009). The effects of infliximab therapy on the serum proteome of rheumatoid arthritis patients. Arthritis Res Ther *11*, R32.

Efthimiou, P., and Markenson, J.A. (2005). Role of biological agents in immune-mediated inflammatory diseases. South Med J *98*, 192-204.

Emery, P., Keystone, E., Tony, H.P., Cantagrel, A., van Vollenhoven, R., Sanchez, A., Alecock, E., Lee, J., and Kremer, J. (2008). IL-6 receptor inhibition with tocilizumab improves treatment outcomes in patients with rheumatoid arthritis refractory to anti-tumour necrosis factor biologicals: results from a 24-week multicentre randomised placebo-controlled trial. Ann Rheum Dis *67*, 1516-1523.

Feltelius, N., Fored, C.M., Blomqvist, P., Bertilsson, L., Geborek, P., Jacobsson, L.T., Lindblad, S., Lysholm, J., Rantapaa-Dahlqvist, S., Saxne, T., and Klareskog, L. (2005). Results from a nationwide postmarketing cohort study of patients in Sweden treated with etanercept. Ann Rheum Dis *64*, 246-252.

Ferraccioli, G., De Santis, M., Peluso, G., Inzitari, R., Fanali, C., Bosello, S.L., Iavarone, F., and Castagnola, M. (2010). Proteomic approaches to Sjogren's syndrome: a clue to interpret the pathophysiology and organ involvement of the disease. Autoimmun Rev *9*, 622-626.

Fujimoto, M., Serada, S., Mihara, M., Uchiyama, Y., Yoshida, H., Koike, N., Ohsugi, Y., Nishikawa, T., Ripley, B., Kimura, A., *et al.* (2008). Interleukin-6 blockade suppresses autoimmune arthritis in mice by the inhibition of inflammatory Th17 responses. Arthritis Rheum *58*, 3710-3719.

Fujiwara, H., Nishimoto, N., Hamano, Y., Asanuma, N., Miki, S., Kasayama, S., and Suemura, M. (2009). Masked early symptoms of pneumonia in patients with rheumatoid arthritis during tocilizumab treatment: a report of two cases. Mod Rheumatol *19*, 64-68.

Genovese, M.C., Becker, J.C., Schiff, M., Luggen, M., Sherrer, Y., Kremer, J., Birbara, C., Box, J., Natarajan, K., Nuamah, I., *et al.* (2005). Abatacept for rheumatoid arthritis refractory to tumor necrosis factor alpha inhibition. N Engl J Med *353*, 1114-1123.

Gomez-Reino, J.J., and Carmona, L. (2006). Switching TNF antagonists in patients with chronic arthritis: an observational study of 488 patients over a four-year period. Arthritis Res Ther *8*, R29.

Han, C., Smolen, J.S., Kavanaugh, A., van der Heijde, D., Braun, J., Westhovens, R., Zhao, N., Rahman, M.U., Baker, D., and Bala, M. (2007). The impact of infliximab treatment on quality of life in patients with inflammatory rheumatic diseases. Arthritis Res Ther *9*, R103.

Hardt, M., Witkowska, H.E., Webb, S., Thomas, L.R., Dixon, S.E., Hall, S.C., and Fisher, S.J. (2005). Assessing the effects of diurnal variation on the composition of human parotid saliva: quantitative analysis of native peptides using iTRAQ reagents. Anal Chem *77*, 4947-4954.

Haruta, H., Ohguro, N., Fujimoto, M., Hohki, S., Terabe, F., Serada, S., Nomura, S., Nishida, K., Kishimoto, T., and Naka, T. (2011). Blockade of interleukin-6 signaling suppresses not only th17 but also interphotoreceptor retinoid binding protein-specific Th1 by promoting regulatory T cells in experimental autoimmune uveoretinitis. Invest Ophthalmol Vis Sci 52, 3264-3271.

Hirao, M., Hashimoto, J., Tsuboi, H., Nampei, A., Nakahara, H., Yoshio, N., Mima, T., Yoshikawa, H., and Nishimoto, N. (2009). Laboratory and febrile features after joint surgery in patients with rheumatoid arthritis treated with tocilizumab. Ann Rheum Dis *68*, 654-657.

Hohki, S., Ohguro, N., Haruta, H., Nakai, K., Terabe, F., Serada, S., Fujimoto, M., Nomura, S., Kawahata, H., Kishimoto, T., and Naka, T. (2010). Blockade of interleukin-6 signaling suppresses experimental autoimmune uveoretinitis by the inhibition of inflammatory Th17 responses. Exp Eye Res *91*, 162-170.

Hueber, W., and Robinson, W.H. (2006). Proteomic biomarkers for autoimmune disease. Proteomics *6*, 4100-4105.

Hyrich, K.L., Lunt, M., Watson, K.D., Symmons, D.P., and Silman, A.J. (2007). Outcomes after switching from one anti-tumor necrosis factor alpha agent to a second anti-tumor necrosis factor alpha agent in patients with rheumatoid arthritis: results from a large UK national cohort study. Arthritis Rheum *56*, 13-20.

Karlsson, J.A., Kristensen, L.E., Kapetanovic, M.C., Gulfe, A., Saxne, T., and Geborek, P. (2008). Treatment response to a second or third TNF-inhibitor in RA: results from the South Swedish Arthritis Treatment Group Register. Rheumatology (Oxford) *47*, 507-513.

Keystone, E., Burmester, G.R., Furie, R., Loveless, J.E., Emery, P., Kremer, J., Tak, P.P., Broder, M.S., Yu, E., Cravets, M., *et al.* (2008). Improvement in patient-reported outcomes in a rituximab trial in patients with severe rheumatoid arthritis refractory to anti-tumor necrosis factor therapy. Arthritis Rheum *59*, 785-793.

Laas, K., Peltomaa, R., Puolakka, K., Kautiainen, H., and Leirisalo-Repo, M. (2009). Early improvement of health-related quality of life during treatment with etanercept and adalimumab in patients with rheumatoid arthritis in routine practice. Clin Exp Rheumatol *27*, 315-320.

Launois, R., Avouac, B., Berenbaum, F., Blin, O., Bru, I., Fautrel, B., Joubert, J.M., Sibilia, J., and Combe, B. (2011). Comparison of Certolizumab Pegol with Other Anticytokine Agents for Treatment of Rheumatoid Arthritis: A Multiple-treatment Bayesian Metaanalysis. J Rheumatol.

Ling, X.B., Park, J.L., Carroll, T., Nguyen, K.D., Lau, K., Macaubas, C., Chen, E., Lee, T., Sandborg, C., Milojevic, D., *et al.* (2010). Plasma profiles in active systemic juvenile idiopathic arthritis: Biomarkers and biological implications. Proteomics *10*, 4415-4430.

Lovell, D.J., Reiff, A., Ilowite, N.T., Wallace, C.A., Chon, Y., Lin, S.L., Baumgartner, S.W., Giannini, E.H., and Pediatric Rheumatology, C. (2008). Safety and efficacy of up to eight years of continuous etanercept therapy in patients with juvenile rheumatoid arthritis. Arthritis and Rheumatism *58*, 1496-1504.

Maini, R.N., Taylor, P.C., Szechinski, J., Pavelka, K., Broll, J., Balint, G., Emery, P., Raemen, F., Petersen, J., Smolen, J., *et al.* (2006). Double-blind randomized controlled clinical trial of the interleukin-6 receptor antagonist, tocilizumab, in European patients with rheumatoid arthritis who had an incomplete response to methotrexate. Arthritis Rheum *54*, 2817-2829.

Maini, S.R. (2004). Infliximab treatment of rheumatoid arthritis. Rheum Dis Clin North Am *30*, 329-347, vii.

McInnes, I.B., and Schett, G. (2007). Cytokines in the pathogenesis of rheumatoid arthritis. Nat Rev Immunol *7*, 429-442.

Nash, P.T., and Florin, T.H. (2005). Tumour necrosis factor inhibitors. Med J Aust *183*, 205-208.

Nishimoto, N., Miyasaka, N., Yamamoto, K., Kawai, S., Takeuchi, T., and Azuma, J. (2009). Long-term safety and efficacy of tocilizumab, an anti-IL-6 receptor monoclonal antibody, in monotherapy, in patients with rheumatoid arthritis (the STREAM study): evidence of safety and efficacy in a 5-year extension study. Ann Rheum Dis *68*, 1580-1584.

Prieto, S., and Grau, J.M. (2010). The geoepidemiology of autoimmune muscle disease. Autoimmun Rev *9*, A330-334.

Prince, H.E. (2005). Biomarkers for diagnosing and monitoring autoimmune diseases. Biomarkers *10 Suppl 1*, S44-49.

Ramos-Casals, M., Brito-Zeron, P., Soto, M.J., Cuadrado, M.J., and Khamashta, M.A. (2008). Autoimmune diseases induced by TNF-targeted therapies. Best Pract Res Clin Rheumatol *22*, 847-861.

Rubbert-Roth, A., and Finckh, A. (2009). Treatment options in patients with rheumatoid arthritis failing initial TNF inhibitor therapy: a critical review. Arthritis Res Ther *11 Suppl 1*, S1.

Serada, S., Fujimoto, M., Ogata, A., Terabe, F., Hirano, T., Iijima, H., Shinzaki, S., Nishikawa, T., Ohkawara, T., Iwahori, K., *et al.* (2010). iTRAQ-based proteomic identification of leucine-rich alpha-2 glycoprotein as a novel inflammatory biomarker in autoimmune diseases. Ann Rheum Dis *69*, 770-774.

Sfikakis, P.P., Markomichelakis, N., Alpsoy, E., Assaad-Khalil, S., Bodaghi, B., Gul, A., Ohno, S., Pipitone, N., Schirmer, M., Stanford, M., *et al.* (2007). Anti-TNF therapy in the management of Behcet's disease--review and basis for recommendations. Rheumatology (Oxford) *46*, 736-741.

Strand, V., and Singh, J.A. (2007). Improved health-related quality of life with effective disease-modifying antirheumatic drugs: evidence from randomized controlled trials. Am J Manag Care *13 Suppl 9*, S237-251.

Takeuchi, T., Nakanishi, T., Tabushi, Y., Hata, A., Shoda, T., Kotani, T., Shimizu, A., Takubo, T., Makino, S., and Hanafusa, T. (2007). Serum protein profile of rheumatoid arthritis treated with anti-TNF therapy (infliximab). J Chromatogr B Analyt Technol Biomed Life Sci *855*, 66-70.

Terabe, F., Fujimoto, M., Serada, S., Shinzaki, S., Iijima, H., Tsujii, M., Hayashi, N., Nomura, S., Kawahata, H., Jang, M.H., *et al.* (2011). Comparative analysis of the effects of anti-IL-6 receptor mAb and anti-TNF mAb treatment on CD4+ T-cell responses in murine colitis. Inflamm Bowel Dis *17*, 491-502.

Triolo, G., Vadala, M., Accardo-Palumbo, A., Ferrante, A., Ciccia, F., Giardina, E., Citarrella, P., Lodato, G., and Licata, G. (2002). Anti-tumour necrosis factor monoclonal antibody treatment for ocular Behcet's disease. Ann Rheum Dis *61*, 560-561.

Veres, G., Baldassano, R.N., and Mamula, P. (2007). Infliximab therapy for pediatric Crohn's disease. Expert Opin Biol Ther *7*, 1869-1880.

Yazici, Y., Krasnokutsky, S., Barnes, J.P., Hines, P.L., Wang, J., and Rosenblatt, L. (2009). Changing patterns of tumor necrosis factor inhibitor use in 9074 patients with rheumatoid arthritis. J Rheumatol *36*, 907-913.

Yokota, S., Imagawa, T., Mori, M., Miyamae, T., Aihara, Y., Takei, S., Iwata, N., Umebayashi, H., Murata, T., Miyoshi, M., *et al.* (2008). Efficacy and safety of tocilizumab in patients with systemic-onset juvenile idiopathic arthritis: a randomised, double-blind, placebo-controlled, withdrawal phase III trial. Lancet *371*, 998-1006.

Zhang, Y., Wolf-Yadlin, A., Ross, P.L., Pappin, D.J., Rush, J., Lauffenburger, D.A., and White, F.M. (2005). Time-resolved mass spectrometry of tyrosine phosphorylation sites in the epidermal growth factor receptor signaling network reveals dynamic modules. Mol Cell Proteomics *4*, 1240-1250.

6

Application of Monoclonal Antibody Therapies in Autoimmune Diseases

Adrienn Angyal[1], Jozsef Prechl[2], Gyorgy Nagy[3] and Gabriella Sarmay[1]
[1]*Dept. of Immunology, Eotvos Lorand University, Budapest,*
[2]*Immunology Research Group of the Hungarian Academy of Sciences, at Eotvos Lorand University, Budapest,*
[3]*Buda Hospital of Hospitaller Brothers of St. John, Budapest*
Hungary

1. Introduction

A better understanding of the pathogenesis of autoimmunity makes it possible to select more specific therapeutic targets and design biological agents that can replace or enhance the effect of immunosuppressive drugs; these include monoclonal antibodies, soluble receptors and molecular mimetics. This chapter aims to give a brief summary on different protein-based medications: first on the biologicals targeting cytokines that induce inflammatory responses, then on drugs depleting B cells via CD20 and CD22 and finally, on agents that inhibit cell-cell contacts and block cell survival factors. Immunogenicity of these protein preparations causes a significant problem therefore the last section gives an overview of biotechnological approaches aiming to reduce this effect.

2. The blockade of cytokines inducing inflammatory responses

TNFα-blocking agents (Etanercept, Adalimumab, Infliximab)

Currently, there are 3 major TNFα-blockers available for patients who do not react well to standard therapies like methotrexate or other disease modifying anti-rheumatic drugs (DMARDs), these are: etanercept, infliximab and adalimumab. Most common side effects of anti-TNFα therapy are a higher susceptibility for infections and possible flares of TB.

Etanercept, a fusion protein consisting of two extracellular binding domains of the TNF ⟨ receptor 2 and the Fc-part of a human IgG1 molecule is acting like a soluble decoy receptor by inhibiting ligand-binding to TNF-receptors, only with an extended in vivo half-life due to the presence of the Fc-part. It is licensed by the FDA for the treatment of RA, polyarticular juvenile idiopathic arthritis (JIA), psoritic arthritis, ankylosing spondylitis and plaque psoriasis (1).

Infliximab (Remicade) is a chimeric monoclonal antibody specific for TNFα that was approved by the FDA in 1998 for the treatment of Crohn's disease (2). Its use has been extended since then to the treatment of psoriasis, ankylosing spondylitis, psoriatic arthritis, rheumatoid arthritis and ulcerative colitis.

Adalimumab (Humira), another monoclonal antibody of fully human origin was derived by a phage display library and used to treat RA patients first. Since then, clinical trials proved its effectiveness in psoriatic arthritis, ankylosing spondylitis, Crohn's disease, psoriasis and juvenile idiopathic arthritis (3).

Infliximab and adalimumab were shown to neutralize biological activity of TNFα by binding to its soluble, membrane- or receptor-bound forms, while etanercept is unable to neutralize the receptor-bound form of TNFα due to its structural features. Additionally, the anti-TNF monoclonal antibodies can induce Fc-receptor-mediated cell lysis and infliximab has been also shown to induce apoptosis of lamina propria T cells in Crohn's patients in a TNFα-dependent manner.

In a follow-up comparative study Bacquet-Deschryver et al. evaluated the effects of the 3 different anti-TNFα biologics on the re-emerginig of anti-nuclear antibodies (ANA), anti-dsDNA antibodies, RF and anti-CCP in rheumatoid arthritis and spondyloarthropathy patients (3). They found that the response to treatment is independent of the induction of ANA production and anti-dsDNA autoantibody variations regardless of the rheumatism and the anti-TNFα treatment prescribed.

Another study conducted in human TNFα transgenic mice showed that in a strictly TNFα-driven model of RA the number of $CD3^+CD25^+FoxP3^+$ Treg cells is initially lower than in wild-type counterparts, but gets elevated during the course of the disease. This population of regulatory T cells is attenuated in its suppressor activity, which can be restored with either passive (infliximab treatment) or active (TNF-K immunization) TNFα-blocking approaches. Moreover, the differentiation of a $CD62L^-$ regulatory T cell population is induced (4).

Blockade of IL-6 (tocilizumab)

IL-6 is a widely expressed pleiotropic cytokine, best known as main mediator of fever and acute phase reactions alongside IL-1 and TNFα. In hepatocytes it strongly induces production of acute phase proteins e.g. C-reactive protein, mannan-binding lectin, or serum amyloid protein A, and it also causes immobilization of neutrophil granulocytes from the bone marrow. Besides supporting B cell differentiation into antibody plasma cells, it has been shown to be essential in Th17 cell differentiation as well. The IL-6R consists of two chains, the 80-kDa IL-6-binding subunit and the 130-kDa membrane glycoprotein gp130 that is responsible for signal transduction (5). The expression of membrane bound IL6R is restricted to only few cell types including macrophages, neutrophils, some T-cell subpopulations and hepatocytes. On the other hand, gp130 is ubiquitously expressed. IL-6R is either shed from the cell surface by matrix metalloproteases or in human, expressed as a result of alternative splicing. Association of the IL-6/sIL-6R complex to gp130 mediates agonistic signaling events (trans-signaling) (6).

Excessive levels of the IL-6/IL-6R complex can be detected in the synovial fluid of many RA patients, which could highly contribute to osteoclast-like cell formation and therefore, joint destruction (7). Also, IL-6 production of synovial fibroblasts induces excess production of vascular endothelial growth factor (VEGF) resulting in enhanced angiogenesis and increased vascular permeability of synovial tissue. Serum IL-6 levels were found elevated in other autoimmune conditions e.g. in SLE as well (8).

Tocilizumab is a humanized IL6R-specific monoclonal antibody that blocks IL-6 mediated signal transduction via the inhibition of ligand-binding to the IL-6Rs. Phase III clinical studies showed a remarkable inhibition of radiological damage of joints. It has been approved as a therapeutic drug for the treatment of RA and in Japan for Castelman's disease and systemic juvenile idiopathic arthritis. Tocilizumab is a potential candidate drug for the therapy of several other disorders including SLE, Crohn's disease or multiple sclerosis (9).

Inhibition of the IL-1 mediated responses with a recombinant IL-1R antagonist (anakinra)

Like TNFα or IL-6, IL-1α and β also induce a wide spectrum of biological responses that contribute to fight infections: these include the production of acute phase proteins, raising body temperature (hence the term endogenous pyrogens) or mobilization of neutrophils, thus promoting microbe clearance by phagocytosis. The main source for IL-1α and β are macrophages and epithelial cells, whereas IL-1Ra, a naturally occurring IL-1R antagonist is released also by monocytes and hepatocytes (10). The IL-1 receptors CD121a and b are expressed on different subsets of lymphocytes, monocytes and macrophages.
Recombinant IL-1a (anakinra) is an approved therapeutic drug for RA that mimics the effects of endogenous IL-1Ra, thus blocking the IL-1 binding site on the receptor without inducing any further signaling events. The treatment with anakinra is well tolerated, with less occurring opportunistic infections than in case of TNFα blockage, and it was shown to improve joint swelling, pain and inflammation, although with less efficacy (11, 12, 13).

Induction of alterations in IL-21 mediated cellular responses

IL-21 is a type I cytokine expressed by activated $CD4^+$ T cells and NKT cells (14), and induces the differentiation and activation of NK cells, promotes NKT proliferation, enhances the differentiation of Th17 cells and was found to regulate mature B cell responses depending on the type of co-stimulation (within a wide range of inducing proliferation to cell death) (15). $IL21R^{-/-}$mice showed no defects in B cell development, but had severe problems with class-switch to IgG1 and IgG2b, and the down-regulation of the germinal center reaction. As a consequence they experienced a decrease in the number of plasma cells and an increase in memory B cells (16).
Although IL-21 fulfills a complex role in the immune regulation, experimental animal models indicate that its targeting could be of therapeutic benefits. In MRL/lpr mice inhibition of IL-21 improved symptoms of the disease, the mice showing a reduction in proteinuria, skin lesions, circulating dsDNA autoantibodies and lymphadenopathy (17). In collagen-induced arthritis and in adjuvant-induced arthritis, the blockade of IL-21R with an IL-21R-Fc fusion protein reversed clinical disease activity, most probably via the down-regulation of TNFα and production of IL-17 (18). In RA patients, IL-21R is expressed in the synovial macrophages and fibroblasts. In addition, a significantly higher percentage of IL-21R is to be found in the blood and synovial fluid of these individuals, where it might contribute to an increase in TNFα and IFNγ secretion upon T cell activation, thus, in up-regulating the pro-inflammatory response (19, 20).

3. B cell depletion therapies mediated via CD20 and CD22

While initially systemic autoimmunity was considered as a T cell-driven condition, multiple functions of B cells have been described in orchestrating autoimmune disorders, including self-reactive antibody production, auto-antigen presentation and co-stimulation of T lymphocytes, formation of ectopic lymphoid structures (neo-organogenesis) in the end-target organs and pro-inflammatory cytokine production.

CD20-mediated B cell depletion

Due to their central role in the immune pathogenesis of systemic autoimmunity and the observation that patients treated with non-Hodgkin's lymphoma and coexisting RA showed improvements in symptoms of RA after anti-CD20 (Rituximab) treatment, several therapies target B cells.

Physiological autoimmunity, thus the production of auto-antibodies in healthy individuals emerges upon infection and facilitates the clearing of apoptotic cells at the site of inflammation. Defects in down-regulation of this response can lead to the development of pathologic conditions. One of the several criteria by the diagnosis of autoimmunity is the presence of self-reactive antibodies in the circulation that are often present decades before the onset of clinical symptoms. During the course of B cell development, many checkpoints exist to prevent the escape of self-reactive B cells to the periphery these include receptor revision, clonal deletion and anergy (21, 22). Once an auto-reactive B cell is activated though by a self-structure first extra-follicular short-lived plasma cells are formed that produce low-affinity antibodies. Some of these auto-reactive cells also enter the germinal centers where they undergo affinity maturation and class switch, and develop into long-lived auto-reactive memory cells.

Antibodies can contribute to disease pathogenesis in two different ways: direct action by binding to its target e.g. in myasthenia gravis where anti-acetylcholine receptor antibodies bind post-synaptic receptors and compromise motor functions in neurons (23), or in Graves' disease, where the anti-thyroid stimulating hormone (TSH) receptor auto-antibodies can act as receptor agonists (24). The indirect contribution of auto-antibodies to autoimmunity consists of the formation of immune complexes inducing Fc-receptor mediated phagocytosis and/or activation of the complement system and production of pro-inflammatory cytokines, thus leading to tissue damage.

In addition to antibody production B cells also have an important role as antigen presenting cells. B cell deficiency in mice results in a disrupted lymphoid structure in the spleen, lack of follicular dendritic cell network and absence of Peyer's patches (25). B cell depletion studies in mice showed a defect in CD4+ T cell priming in the absence of B cell co-stimulation, especially when the antigen is available only at low concentrations. B cells not only provide support to T cells via direct cell-cell contact, but also shape the immune response by producing either pro-inflammatory cytokines including IL-6, IFNγ and LTα. Certain subsets are also able to produce IL-10 that has a regulatory function and contributes to the attenuation of the disease (26).

Tertiary ectopic lymphoid structures have been described at the end-organ in several autoimmune disorders: in the synovium of RA patients organized zones of B, T and follicular dendritic cells can be found in more than 50% of the cases, while kidneys of SLE patients also often contain such organized structures. B cell depletion or the blockade of B cell-T cell contacts has been proved to disrupt these ectopic lymphoid follicles and attenuate disease severity in several animal models of autoimmunity (27).

One of the most effective disease modifying anti-rheumatic drugs (DMARDs) is rituximab, a human CD20-specific chimeric monoclonal antibody. CD20 is a 35-37kDa tetra-spanning integral membrane protein first expressed on late pre-B cells in the bone marrow, present on naïve and mature B cells, down-regulated on antibody-secreting plasmablasts and extinguishing on plasma cells. It has been shown to regulate early steps of cell cycle progression, B cell proliferation and apoptosis. Upon cell activation, it gets trans-located to membrane lipid rafts, where it can act as a Ca^{2+}-channel (28). CD20 is also expressed on a small subset of basally activated IL1β- and TNF α–producing T cells (0.1-6.8% in healthy individuals) that showed enhanced susceptibility to apoptosis (29). Within an hour Rituximab treatment induces a ~90% reduction of the pre-treatment state in circulating $CD20^{+}$ B cell numbers that lasts for at least 3 months and also mediates a decrease in the number of resident $CD20^+$ B cells in the damaged tissues, although with variable efficacy: 70% of cells residing in the spleen and lymph nodes are depleted after 24 hours, while access to peritoneal B cells is limited (30, 31). Success of the depletion also varies among B cell subpopulations: splenic marginal zone B cells, germinal center B cells and peritoneal B1 cells are significantly more protected.

The reemerging of the B cell population usually occurs in the majority of the patients after 4-6 months and follows a definite pattern by immature $CD5^+$ $CD38^{high}$ transitional B cells and re-circulating plasmablasts appearing first and later circulating naïve B cells.

Monitoring of serum antibody levels in rituximab treated patients revealed that while titers of RF and anti-CCP antibodies significantly dropped, the humoral immune response towards most pathogens remained unaffected (e.g. pneumococcal capsular polysaccharide, tetanus toxoid) (32). Reduction in IgM-RF levels reflected to changes in total serum IgM levels, but the levels of IgA-RF, IgG-RF, and IgG anti-CCP antibodies decreased significantly more than those of their corresponding total serum immunoglobulin classes, which suggests that rituximab induces a selective reduction of short-lived autoantibody-secreting plasma cells. Two independent studies investigating changes in the synovial tissue composition of RA patients before and after rituximab treatment showed a significant decrease in B cell numbers in the synovium indicating that efficacy of the treatment lies in the disruption of extrafollicular lymphoid structures and the inhibition of B-T cell interactions (33).

Data about the efficacy of B cell depletion in SLE are contradictory: several studies involving only a small group of patients reported a significant clinical improvement upon rituximab treatment, while phase II/III trials showed no difference in BILAG scores. In contrast, B cell deficient lupus-prone MRL/lpr mice do not develop nephritis due to the reduced activation of the T cell compartment while transgenic mice expressing only membrane bound BCR on the cell surface (mIgM.MRL/lpr) still develop the disease (34). Another study found that mouse strains prone to develop autoimmunity are a lot more resistant to B cell depletion. These data indicate a more complex role for B cells in SLE than the production of auto-reactive antibodies. CD20-mediated B cell depletion at an early age in pristane-primed NZB/W F1 mice resulted in acceleration of the onset of disease, possibly due to the lack of IL-10 production by regulatory B cells. Treatment following the outbreak of symptoms on the other hand attenuated the intensity of the disease (35).

CD22-mediated B cell depletion

Another B lymphocyte restricted target is the Ig-superfamily member CD22, a 135kDa glycoprotein that is first detected in the cytoplasm of pro- and pre-B cells, becoming present on the cell surface of mature peripheral B cells. It remains expressed on germinal center B cells but is absent on plasmablasts and terminally differentiated plasma cells. Known ligands of CD22 include the tyrosine phosphatase CD45 and the lectin CD33, both binding through α2,6-linked sialic acid motifs. While CD22 was reported to inhibit BCR-mediated cell activation *in vitro* via the recruitment of SHP-1 phosphatase to its cytoplasmic ITIM sequences upon phosphorylation by the tyrosine kinase Lyn (36), its *in vivo* role is less clarified. CD22-deficient mice develop hyper-proliferative B-lymphocytes and in consequence increased levels of auto-antibodies.

Epratuzumab, a humanized monoclonal IgG1 CD22-specific antibody recognizes a non-ligand-binding site of the CD22 molecule. It is predicted to alter BCR-signaling by inducing disruption of cell surface signaling complexes and antibody-mediated depletion of B cells (37). Epratuzumab is shown to cause phosphorylation and internalization of CD22 on peripheral B cells *in vitro*. On a small cohort of SLE-patients, when administered four times every second week it was reported to improve clinical symptoms in all of the patients based on the 6-, 10- or 18-week assessments (38).

4. Inhibition of cell-cell contacts and survival factors

Several other monoclonal antibodies currently under clinical trial target B cell survival factors and cytokines like B-cell activating factor (BAFF), a proliferation inducing ligand (APRIL), IL-6 or IL-10.

Inhibition of the B cell survival factors BAFF and APRIL

BAFF and APRIL are members of the TNF superfamily that maintain peripheral B cell- and plasma cell homeostasis by supporting cell survival. Access to BAFF modifies the stringency of negative selection of naïve B cells, as auto-reactive B cells depend more on BAFF relative to naïve mature cells. BAFF is produced by neutrophil granulocytes, monocytes, macrophages, dendritic cells and T cells as a trans-membrane protein and cleaved from the cell surface by the protease furin (39). In the serum, BAFF and APRIL are found as both homo- and hetero-trimers. The expression of receptors for soluble BAFF (BR3/BAFFR, TACI and BCMA) varies depending on the B-cell developmental stage. Highest levels of BR3/BAFFR are observed on primary and activated follicular and marginal B cells, while expression is decreased but still detectable on germinal center B cells. BR3/BAFFR is reduced or absent on antibody producing plasma cells, whereas TACI and BCMA are abundantly expressed on these cells. Memory B cells express all three BAFF-receptors. Neutralizing antibodies against BAFF cause a loss of transitional-2, marginal zone and follicular B cells *in vivo*, but transitional-1, B1 B cells, and plasma cells are not affected because latter cells receive survival signals by TACI as well (40).

Monoclonal antibody	Type	Target molecule	Autoimmune disease
Adalimumab (Humira)	human	TNFα	RA, psoriatic arthritis, ankylosing spondylitis, Crohn's disease, psoriasis, juvenile idiopathic arthritis
Belimumab (Benlysta)	human	BAFF	SLE
Certolizumab pegol (Cimzia)	humanized	TNFα	RA, Crohn's disease
Epratuzumab	humanized	CD22	SLE
Infliximab (Remicade)	chimeric	TNFα	Crohn's disease, psoriasis, ankylosing spondylitis, psoriatic arthritis, RA, ulcerative colitis
Natalizumab (Tysabri)	humanized	α4 integrin	Multiple sclerosis, Crohn's disease
Rituximab (Rituxan)	chimeric	CD20	RA
Tocilizumab (Actemra)	humanized	IL-6R	RA, Castelman's disease

Table 1. Examples of therapeutic antibodies for the treatment of autoimmune disorders approved by the FDA

In the serum of patients with active SLE and Sjogren's syndrome, the expression levels of soluble BAFF have been found elevated. Therefore, it is a potential target molecule in autoimmune disorders. Belimumab a humanized IgG1 monoclonal antibody blocks BAFF-binding to its receptors, thereby inhibiting the persistence of antibody producing B cells by mediating apoptotic cell death of early plasmablasts, naïve B cells and activated B cells (41) (42). Restriction of BAFF levels might facilitate the function of regulatory B cell populations. Atacicept is a fully human chimeric molecule consisting of the TACI ligand-binding extracellular domain fused to the Fc-portion of a human IgG1. It blocks both TACI- and BAFF-binding to their receptors and resulted to be successful in phase I clinical trials for the treatment of RA (43, 44, 45).

Inhibition of B-T cell interactions

For RA patients who give an inadequate response to anti-TNFα therapy, there is an increasing number of DMARDs that offer improvement of clinical symptoms by the inhibition of T cell-antigen presenting cell (APC) interactions.
Activation of T cells by antigens not only requires TCR-binding to the specific peptide-MHC complex on the APC, but also the ligation of co-stimulatory molecules like CD40, inducible T cell co-stimulator (ICOS) and CD28. Therefore, biologics that block these interactions may interfere with sufficient helper T cell activation and inhibit B cell differentiation into antibody producing plasma cells.
Abatacept is a soluble, fully human fusion protein of the extracellular domain of CTLA-4 and the hinge region, the CH2 and CH3 domains of a human IgG1 molecule. It recognizes B7 (CD80/86) with a high affinity and blocks its interaction with CD28, this way selectively inhibiting T cell activation. Abatacept is approved for the treatment of RA and juvenile idiopathic arthritis, and in a phase I trial it was shown to improve the clinical symptoms of psoriasis patients via the reduction of the size of the intralesional T cell population. Combination of abatacept with TNFα-blockers is not advised as it increases the occurrence of infections and provides no additional benefits (11).
Although the role of ICOS in T cell signaling has not been completely resolved yet, experimental data demonstrate that ICOS/ICOSL is an important regulator of T cell activation. It is expressed on resting T cells only at low amounts, while it gets strongly up-regulated upon activation. Highest level of expression is observed on T follicular helper cells. Blockade of ICOS/ICOSL interactions with monoclonal antibodies has been reported to improve collagen-induced arthritis and murine models of lupus (46). At the early stage of experimental autoimmune encephalomyelitis (EAE), a mouse model of sclerosis multiplex, inhibition of the ICOS/ICOSL interaction seemed to aggravate the disease, while it induced an improvement when administered at later phases (47). In glucose-6-phosphate isomerase (G6PI)-induced arthritis, early ICOSL-specific monoclonal antibody treatment resulted in significant loss of disease severity, but treatment at later stages of arthritis reduced symptoms only marginally. The number of G6PI-specific T helper cells decreased, but there was no difference in the antigen-specific antibody levels in the sera of the animals (48).

5. Biotechnical approaches for the reduction of immunogenicity in monoclonal antibody therapies

By the application of recombinant proteins in human medicine immunogenicity is one of the major concerns as several examples (insulin-, growth hormone-, factor VIII treatment or muronomab itself) had already shown us (49). The immune system may recognize these structures as foreign and develop an antibody response towards them, which may result in reduction of bioactivity. Factors like the sequence of the antibody, the secondary structure, the purity of the product, the dosage and frequency of administration, the diversity in MHC alleles within the population, the site of injection and the physical status of the individual all contribute to the outcome of the immunological response towards the protein-based medication (50, 51).

The clinical effects of the antibodies raised against the therapeutic protein depend on the epitope they recognize, their affinity and titer: some cause no reduction in bioactivity while others induce complications besides affecting the therapeutic benefits. These complications include increased risk of infusion reactions such as fever or rashes, pure red-cell aplasia or even cardiopulmonary and anaphylactic-like adverse events (52). In general, the emerging antibody response can inhibit the binding of the ligand to the receptor, or change the conformation and therefore the affinity and signaling properties of the soluble mediator (e.g. in case of IFNβ treatment). Immunological responses against monoclonal antibodies often enhance clearance by complex formation or block target recognition by binding to the variable region (idiotype). Rituximab, a mouse-human chimeric antibody induces the development of human anti-chimeric antibodies (HACA) in 1-5% of Non Hodgin's lymphoma and RA patients and in 65% of SLE patients, resulting in a reduction of the efficacy of B cell depletion and often in hypersensitivity reactions (53, 54).

Several different techniques exist to attenuate the break-through of tolerance against monoclonal antibodies, these include:

a. The replacement of murine constant regions with human sequences, where the specificity of the antibody remains intact (chimera design)

   The hybridoma technology enabled us to produce monoclonal murine antibodies in large quantities (55). On the other hand, generation of human hybridomas is difficult because they produce only small amounts of IgM and are very unstable. Recombinant DNA techniques make it possible to change the constant regions of murine immunoglobulins to human domains (56). The heavy and light chain genes are clustered into exons that represent the domain structures, which facilitates domain exchanges in antibody molecules. The vector selection is a critical step in the *in vitro* production of these monoclonal antibody constructs, as glycosylation patterns highly vary between species. Mammalian non-immune cells (HeLa or CHO cells) or certain myeloma cell lines are frequently used for this purpose. (57)

   The choice of the heavy chain isotype frequently defines the mechanism of action: IgG1 is binding with high affinity to FcγRs, therefore, the therapeutic antibody of such isotype is more likely to cause additional cell depletion via antibody-dependent cell-mediated cytotoxicity (ADCC). On the other hand IgG2 interacts only weakly with low affinity FcγRs, so the therapeutic effects observed are mainly attributed to the capacity of the antibody for blocking or altering cellular signaling through the targeted receptor.

b. Humanization or reshaping of the variable region, thus partial exchange of framework residues to human sequences

   The antigen specificity of the antibody is defined by only a few amino acids that are exposed to the surface of the antigen-binding pocket (paratope) and interact with the antigen. By transferring this set of residues from a nonhuman origin to a human frame (FR), the specificity of the antibody should remain (58).

The engrafting of the complementary determining regions (CDR) consists of different steps: the determination of the sequences in the nonhuman antibody that participate in the specific recognition of the antigen, the selection of the fitting human frame to engraft it in, and finally, the assembly of the nonhuman CDR and the human FR to a functional antibody via the insertion of back mutations. In order to minimize the presence of nonhuman sequences within the humanized antibody construct, several methods e.g. specificity determining residue (SDR) engrafting or superhumanization had been proposed. While the first is based on the computational analysis of the three-dimensional structure of the antigen-antibody complex, suggesting that only 20-33% of CDR residues are in contact with the antigen, the latter relies on the *in silico* selection of the best matching canonical structures of both the nonhuman and human sequences (59, 60).

For the engraftment, most frequently human germline sequences are used to minimize potential immunogenicity (61). The objective of the back mutations by establishing the functional antibody is to maintain, or if possible, even improve the affinity of the antibody. To obtain this several methods exist, such as e.g. error-prone PCR with low fidelity polymerases under nonstandard conditions or pooling random DNA fragments after digestion of the variable region with DNase I (62, 63).

Despite the fact that humanized antibodies retain less than 5% of the murine sequences, a significant anti-drug response can still be observed in 0.1-9% of the treated patients (64, 65, 66).

c. Selection of human antibody V regions using a phage library screen based on the affinity towards the antigen.

Besides attempts to avoid immunogenicity, antigen display also provides the best method to overcome limitations of the hybridoma technology concerning toxic or highly conserved antigen structures. Several display systems that apply insertion of variable region fragments to the phage genome have been developed for phage T7 (67), phage λ (68, 69, 70) and the Ff class (genus Inovirus) of the filamentous phage f1, fd, and M13 (71). The source for antibody fragments can either be a naive, a semi-synthetic or an entirely synthetic library. Naive libraries are generated by mRNA isolation and cDNA synthesis from B cells (naïve or antigen exposed cells), and the variable region genes are either expressed separately with a two or three step cloning strategy or fused as an scFv in a polymerase chain reaction (PCR). If the assembly PCR is involving randomization of the CDR3 region, namely the usage of oligonucleotide primers encoding various CDR3 and J gene segments (72), a semi-synthetic library is established. Entirely synthetic libraries use various different V_H and V_L germline master frameworks, combined with synthetically created CDR cassettes.

The pIII minor coat protein of the filamentous phage M13 is widely used to fuse the antibody fragment of interest with, thus resulting in the expression of the antibody fragment on the surface of the phage. High affinity binding constructs can be then selected by panning, a method that consists of incubation cycles (2-5) with surface-bound antigen, followed by a restricting washing to remove non-specific clones. Specificity of selected constructs can be evaluated then using enzyme-linked immunosorbent assay (ELISA).

As a final step for the generation of therapeutic antibodies, the selected variable region genes need to be inserted into a human frame sequence.

Clinical data show that despite the fully human sequence, many of the monoclonal antibodies produced by phage display technology e.g. the TNFα-specific adalimumab are still immunogenic (73). An explanation for this could be that *in vitro* affinity maturation lacks several control steps, as there is an additional *in vivo* selection for attributes such as stability and aggregation besides molecular recognition.

d. Human antibody production of transgenic mice expressing human immunoglobulin genes

Strategies to establish mouse strains with germ line modifications in their immunoglobulin genes usually aim for homologous recombination in mouse embryonic stem cells that disrupt endogenous Ig heavy and light chains, and introduce the human transgenes. In the past, different technologies were successfully applied to produce and deliver the human sequence transgenes: Lonberg et al. used pronuclear microinjection to introduce reconstructed minilocus transgenes (74), while Green et al. established transgenes with yeast artificial chromosome (YAC) (75). Initially, mouse heavy and κ light chain sequences were 'replaced' for several different V_H, D_H and J_H regions with γ1, μ or δ heavy chain constant region fragments and V_κ, all five J_κ and the C_κ light chain genes. These transgenic animals were able to mount human antibodies in response to a targeted antigen.

There have been many initiatives undertaken since then to broaden the size of the V-region repertoire, as it has a strong influence on multiple checkpoints in B cell development and therefore the size of the mature B cell population (76). Following selection of the most efficient clones, for large-scale production usually a recombinant expression system is established to reduce costs (77).

In contrast to chimeric, humanized or *in vitro* generated therapeutic monoclonal antibodies, there are no reported cases of the generation of anti-human Ig responses towards transgenic therapeutic antibodies. Table 1 summarizes the currently available monoclonal constructs and their origin.

6. Conclusions

Since the development of the hybridoma technique several monoclonal antibodies have been approved for the treatment of autoimmune diseases. Immunogenicity of murine sequences caused initial complications, which could be attenuated and finally overcome by the production of chimeric and humanized antibodies and with the generation of transgenic mouse strains for human Ig-sequences. One of the crucial steps by the design of a monoclonal antibody for therapeutic applications is the selection of the right target molecule. In autoimmune disorders several options exist: the blockade of the pro-inflammatory cytokines TNFα, IL-1 or IL-6, the inhibition of T cell-B cell interactions, B cell depletion to reduce autoantibody production and the establishment of ectopic lymphoid structures or the blockade of B cell survival factors. Although we still need to face adverse events upon the application of these therapeutic antibodies, targeting specific molecules will help us to reduce the severity of occurring side effects and provide more efficient medications.

7. Acknowledgement

This work was supported by a grant from the Research and Technology Innovation Fund (KTIA-OTKA 80689) and the National Innovation Office (NIH)-ANR bilateral grant.

8. References

Sethi, G., B. Sung, A. B. Kunnumakkara, and B. B. Aggarwal. 2009. Targeting TNF for Treatment of Cancer and Autoimmunity. *Adv Exp Med Biol* 647: 37-51.

Colombel, J. F., E. V. J. Loftus, W. J. Tremaine, L. J. Egan, W. S. Harmsen, C. D. Schleck, R. Zinsmeister, and W. J. Sandborn. 2004. The safety profile of infliximab in patients with Crohn's disease: the Mayo clinic experience in 500 patients. *Gastroenterology* 126: 19-31.

Bacquet-Deschryver, H., F. Jouen, M. Quillard, J. F. Menard, V. Goeb, T. Lequerre, O. Mejjad, A. Daragon, F. Tron, X. Le Loet, and O. Vittecoq. 2008. Impact of three anti- TNFalpha biologics on existing and emergent autoimmunity in rheumatoid arthritis and spondylarthropathy patients. *J Clin Immunol* 28: 445-455.

Biton, J., L. Semerano, L. Delavallee, D. Lemeiter, M. Laborie, G. Grouard-Vogel, M. C. Boissier, and N. Bessis. 2011. Interplay between TNF and Regulatory T Cells in a TNF-Driven Murine Model of Arthritis. *J Immunol*

Hibi, M., M. Murakami, M. Saito, T. Hirano, T. Taga, and T. Kishimoto. 1990. Molecular cloning and expression of an IL-6 signal transducer, gp130. *Cell* 63: 1149-1157.

Kishimoto, T. 2005. Interleukin-6: from basic science to medicine--40 years in immunology. *Annu Rev Immunol* 23: 1-21.

Nishimoto, N., K. Terao, T. Mima, H. Nakahara, N. Takagi, and T. Kakehi. 2008. Mechanisms and pathologic significances in increase in serum interleukin-6 (IL-6) and soluble IL-6 receptor after administration of an anti-IL-6 receptor antibody, tocilizumab, in patients with rheumatoid arthritis and Castleman disease. *Blood* 112: 3959-3964.

Grondal, G., I. Gunnarsson, J. Ronnelid, S. Rogberg, L. Klareskog, and I. Lundberg. 2000. Cytokine production, serum levels and disease activity in systemic lupus erythematosus. *Clin Exp Rheumatol* 18: 565-570.

Tanaka, T., M. Narazaki, and T. Kishimoto. 2011. Anti-interleukin-6 receptor antibody, tocilizumab, for the treatment of autoimmune diseases. *FEBS Lett*

Hannum, C. H., C. J. Wilcox, W. P. Arend, F. G. Joslin, D. J. Dripps, P. L. Heimdal, L. G. Armes, A. Sommer, S. P. Eisenberg, and R. C. Thompson. 1990. Interleukin-1 receptor antagonist activity of a human interleukin-1 inhibitor. *Nature* 343: 336-340.

Smolen, J. S., D. Aletaha, M. Koeller, M. H. Weisman, and P. Emery. 2007. New therapies for treatment of rheumatoid arthritis. *Lancet* 370: 1861-1874.

O'Dell, J. R. 2004. Therapeutic strategies for rheumatoid arthritis. *N Engl J Med* 350: 2591-2602.

Goldbach-Mansky, R. 2009. Blocking interleukin-1 in rheumatic diseases. *Ann N Y Acad Sci* 1182: 111-123.

Coquet, J. M., K. Kyparissoudis, D. G. Pellicci, G. Besra, S. P. Berzins, M. J. Smyth, and D. I. Godfrey. 2007. IL-21 is produced by NKT cells and modulates NKT cell activation and cytokine production. *J Immunol* 178: 2827-2834.

Leonard, W. J., and R. Spolski. 2005. Interleukin-21: a modulator of lymphoid proliferation, apoptosis and differentiation. *Nat Rev Immunol* 5: 688-698.

Ozaki, K., R. Spolski, C. G. Feng, C. F. Qi, J. Cheng, A. Sher, H. C. r. Morse, C. Liu, P. L. Schwartzberg, and W. J. Leonard. 2002. A critical role for IL-21 in regulating immunoglobulin production. *Science* 298: 1630-1634.

Herber, D., T. P. Brown, S. Liang, D. A. Young, M. Collins, and K. Dunussi-

Joannopoulos. 2007. IL-21 has a pathogenic role in a lupus-prone mouse model and its blockade with IL-21R.Fc reduces disease progression. *J Immunol* 178: 3822-3830.

Young, D. A., M. Hegen, H. L. Ma, M. J. Whitters, L. M. Albert, L. Lowe, M. Senices, P. W. Wu, B. Sibley, Y. Leathurby, T. P. Brown, C. Nickerson-Nutter, J. C. J. Keith, and M. Collins. 2007. Blockade of the interleukin-21/interleukin-21 receptor pathway ameliorates disease in animal models of rheumatoid arthritis. *Arthritis Rheum* 56: 1152-1163.

Li, J., W. Shen, K. Kong, and Z. Liu. 2006. Interleukin-21 induces T-cell activation and proinflammatory cytokine secretion in rheumatoid arthritis. *Scand J Immunol* 64: 515-522.

Jungel, A., J. H. Distler, M. Kurowska-Stolarska, C. A. Seemayer, R. Seibl, A. Forster, B. A. Michel, R. E. Gay, F. Emmrich, S. Gay, and O. Distler. 2004. Expression of interleukin-21 receptor, but not interleukin-21, in synovial fibroblasts and synovial macrophages of patients with rheumatoid arthritis. *Arthritis Rheum* 50: 1468-1476.

Monroe, J. G., and K. Dorshkind. 2007. Fate decisions regulating bone marrow and peripheral B lymphocyte development. *Adv Immunol* 95: 1-50.

von Boehmer, H., and F. Melchers. 2010. Checkpoints in lymphocyte development and autoimmune disease. *Nat Immunol* 11: 14-20.

Ruff, R. L., and V. A. Lennon. 2008. How myasthenia gravis alters the safety factor for neuromuscular transmission. *J Neuroimmunol* 201-202: 13-20.

Brown, R. S. 2009. Autoimmune thyroid disease: unlocking a complex puzzle. *Curr Opin Pediatr* 21: 523-528.

Ngo, V. N., R. J. Cornall, and J. G. Cyster. 2001. Splenic T zone development is B cell dependent. *J Exp Med* 194: 1649-1660.

Yanaba, K., J. D. Bouaziz, K. M. Haas, J. C. Poe, M. Fujimoto, and T. F. Tedder. 2008. A regulatory B cell subset with a unique CD1dhiCD5+ phenotype controls T cell- dependent inflammatory responses. *Immunity* 28: 639-650.

Weyand, C. M., Y. M. Kang, P. J. Kurtin, and J. J. Goronzy. 2003. The power of the third dimension: tissue architecture and autoimmunity in rheumatoid arthritis. *Curr Opin Rheumatol* 15: 259-266.

Tedder, T. F., and P. Engel. 1994. CD20: a regulator of cell-cycle progression of B lymphocytes. *Immunol Today* 15: 450-454.

Wilk, E., T. Witte, N. Marquardt, T. Horvath, K. Kalippke, K. Scholz, N. Wilke, R. E. Schmidt, and R. Jacobs. 2009. Depletion of functionally active CD20+ T cells by rituximab treatment. *Arthritis Rheum* 60: 3563-3571.

Hamaguchi, Y., J. Uchida, D. W. Cain, G. M. Venturi, J. C. Poe, K. M. Haas, and T. F. Tedder. 2005. The peritoneal cavity provides a protective niche for B1 and conventional B lymphocytes during anti-CD20 immunotherapy in mice. *J Immunol* 174: 4389-4399.

Uchida, J., Y. Hamaguchi, J. A. Oliver, J. V. Ravetch, J. C. Poe, K. M. Haas, and T. F. Tedder. 2004. The innate mononuclear phagocyte network depletes B lymphocytes through Fc receptor-dependent mechanisms during anti-CD20 antibody immunotherapy. *J Exp Med* 199: 1659-1669.

Bingham, C. O. r., R. J. Looney, A. Deodhar, N. Halsey, M. Greenwald, C. Codding, B. Trzaskoma, F. Martin, S. Agarwal, and A. Kelman. 2010. Immunization responses in rheumatoid arthritis patients treated with rituximab: results from a controlled clinical trial. *Arthritis Rheum* 62: 64-74.

Lund, F. E., and T. D. Randall. 2010. Effector and regulatory B cells: modulators of CD4(+) T cell immunity. *Nat Rev Immunol* 10: 236-247.

Chan, O. T., L. G. Hannum, A. M. Haberman, M. P. Madaio, and M. J. Shlomchik. 1999. A novel mouse with B cells but lacking serum antibody reveals an antibody-independent role for B cells in murine lupus. *J Exp Med* 189: 1639-1648.

Haas, K. M., R. Watanabe, T. Matsushita, H. Nakashima, N. Ishiura, H. Okochi, M. Fujimoto, and T. F. Tedder. 2010. Protective and pathogenic roles for B cells during systemic autoimmunity in NZB/W F1 mice. *J Immunol* 184: 4789-4800.

Carnahan, J., P. Wang, R. Kendall, C. Chen, S. Hu, T. Boone, T. Juan, J. Talvenheimo, S. Montestruque, J. Sun, G. Elliott, J. Thomas, J. Ferbas, B. Kern, R. Briddell, J. P. Leonard, and A. Cesano. 2003. Epratuzumab, a humanized monoclonal antibody targeting CD22: characterization of in vitro properties. *Clin Cancer Res* 9: 3982S- 3990S.

Carnahan, J., R. Stein, Z. Qu, K. Hess, A. Cesano, H. J. Hansen, and D. M. Goldenberg. 2007. Epratuzumab, a CD22-targeting recombinant humanized antibody with a different mode of action from rituximab. *Mol Immunol* 44: 1331-1341.

Dorner, T., J. Kaufmann, W. A. Wegener, N. Teoh, D. M. Goldenberg, and G. R. Burmester. 2006. Initial clinical trial of epratuzumab (humanized anti-CD22 antibody) for immunotherapy of systemic lupus erythematosus. *Arthritis Res Ther* 8: R74.

Bodmer, J. L., P. Schneider, and J. Tschopp. 2002. The molecular architecture of the TNF superfamily. *Trends Biochem Sci* 27: 19-26.

O'Connor, B. P., V. S. Raman, L. D. Erickson, W. J. Cook, L. K. Weaver, C. Ahonen, L. L. Lin, G. T. Mantchev, R. J. Bram, and R. J. Noelle. 2004. BCMA is essential for the survival of long-lived bone marrow plasma cells. *J Exp Med* 199: 91-98.

Furie, R., W. Stohl, E. M. Ginzler, M. Becker, N. Mishra, W. Chatham, J. T. Merrill, A. Weinstein, W. J. McCune, J. Zhong, W. Cai, and W. Freimuth. 2008. Biologic activity and safety of belimumab, a neutralizing anti-B-lymphocyte stimulator (BLyS) monoclonal antibody: a phase I trial in patients with systemic lupus erythematosus. *Arthritis Res Ther* 10: R109.

Stohl, W., J. L. Scholz, and M. P. Cancro. 2011. Targeting BLyS in rheumatic disease: the sometimes-bumpy road from bench to bedside. *Curr Opin Rheumatol* 23: 305-310.

Seyler, T. M., Y. W. Park, S. Takemura, R. J. Bram, P. J. Kurtin, J. J. Goronzy, and C. M. Weyand. 2005. BLyS and APRIL in rheumatoid arthritis. *J Clin Invest* 115: 3083-3092.

Bracewell, C., J. D. Isaacs, P. Emery, and W. F. Ng. 2009. Atacicept, a novel B cell-targeting biological therapy for the treatment of rheumatoid arthritis. *Expert Opin Biol Ther* 9: 909-919.

Nestorov, I., A. Munafo, O. Papasouliotis, and J. Visich. 2008. Pharmacokinetics and biological activity of atacicept in patients with rheumatoid arthritis. *J Clin Pharmacol* 48: 406-417.

Nurieva, R. I., P. Treuting, J. Duong, R. A. Flavell, and C. Dong. 2003. Inducible costimulator is essential for collagen-induced arthritis. *J Clin Invest* 111: 701-706.

Galicia, G., A. Kasran, C. Uyttenhove, K. De Swert, J. Van Snick, and J. L. Ceuppens. 2009. ICOS deficiency results in exacerbated IL-17 mediated experimental autoimmune encephalomyelitis. *J Clin Immunol* 29: 426-433.

Matsumoto, I., H. Zhang, T. Yasukochi, K. Iwanami, Y. Tanaka, A. Inoue, D. Goto, S. Ito, A. Tsutsumi, and T. Sumida. 2008. Therapeutic effects of antibodies to tumor necrosis factor-alpha, interleukin-6 and cytotoxic T-lymphocyte antigen 4 immunoglobulin in mice with glucose-6-phosphate isomerase induced arthritis. *Arthritis Res Ther* 10: R66.

Schellekens, H., and N. Casadevall. 2004. Immunogenicity of recombinant human proteins: causes and consequences. *J Neurol* 251 Suppl 2: II4-9.

Hermeling, S., D. J. Crommelin, H. Schellekens, and W. Jiskoot. 2004. Structure-immunogenicity relationships of therapeutic proteins. *Pharm Res* 21: 897-903.

Cohen, B. A., J. Oger, A. Gagnon, and G. Giovannoni. 2008. The implications of immunogenicity for protein-based multiple sclerosis therapies. *J Neurol Sci* 275: 7- 17.

Edwards, J. C., L. Szczepanski, J. Szechinski, A. Filipowicz-Sosnowska, P. Emery, D. R. Close, R. M. Stevens, and T. Shaw. 2004. Efficacy of B-cell-targeted therapy with rituximab in patients with rheumatoid arthritis. *N Engl J Med* 350: 2572-2581.

Saito, K., M. Nawata, S. Iwata, M. Tokunaga, and Y. Tanaka. 2005. Extremely high titer of anti-human chimeric antibody following re-treatment with rituximab in a patient with active systemic lupus erythematosus. *Rheumatology (Oxford)* 44: 1462-1464.

Sabahi, R., and J. H. Anolik. 2006. B-cell-targeted therapy for systemic lupus erythematosus. *Drugs* 66: 1933-1948.

Kohler, G., and C. Milstein. 1975. Continuous cultures of fused cells secreting antibody of predefined specificity. *Nature* 256: 495-497.

Jones, P. T., P. H. Dear, J. Foote, M. S. Neuberger, and G. Winter. 1986. Replacing the complementarity-determining regions in a human antibody with those from a mouse. *Nature* 321: 522-525.

Whittle, N., J. Adair, C. Lloyd, L. Jenkins, J. Devine, J. Schlom, A. Raubitschek, D. Colcher, and M. Bodmer. 1987. Expression in COS cells of a mouse-human chimaeric B72.3 antibody. *Protein Eng* 1: 499-505.

Studnicka, G. M., S. Soares, M. Better, R. E. Williams, R. Nadell, and A. H. Horwitz. 1994. Human-engineered monoclonal antibodies retain full specific binding activity by preserving non-CDR complementarity-modulating residues. *Protein Eng* 7: 805- 814.

Gonzales, N. R., E. A. Padlan, R. De Pascalis, P. Schuck, J. Schlom, and S. V. Kashmiri. 2003. Minimizing immunogenicity of the SDR-grafted humanized antibody CC49 by genetic manipulation of the framework residues. *Mol Immunol* 40: 337-349.

Tan, P., D. A. Mitchell, T. N. Buss, M. A. Holmes, C. Anasetti, and J. Foote. 2002. "Superhumanized" antibodies: reduction of immunogenic potential by complementarity-determining region grafting with human germline sequences: application to an anti-CD28. *J Immunol* 169: 1119-1125.

Gonzales, N. R., E. A. Padlan, R. De Pascalis, P. Schuck, J. Schlom, and S. V. Kashmiri. 2004. SDR grafting of a murine antibody using multiple human germline templates to minimize its immunogenicity. *Mol Immunol* 41: 863-872.

Neylon, C. 2004. Chemical and biochemical strategies for the randomization of protein encoding DNA sequences: library construction methods for directed evolution. *Nucleic Acids Res* 32: 1448-1459.

Stemmer, W. P. 1994. Rapid evolution of a protein in vitro by DNA shuffling. *Nature* 370: 389-391.

Pendley, C., A. Schantz, and C. Wagner. 2003. Immunogenicity of therapeutic monoclonal antibodies. *Curr Opin Mol Ther* 5: 172-179.

Hwang, W. Y., and J. Foote. 2005. Immunogenicity of engineered antibodies. *Methods* 36: 3-10.

Bartelds, G. M., C. L. Krieckaert, M. T. Nurmohamed, P. A. van Schouwenburg, W. F. Lems, J. W. Twisk, B. A. Dijkmans, L. Aarden, and G. J. Wolbink. 2011. Development of antidrug antibodies against adalimumab and association with disease activity and treatment failure during long-term follow-up. *JAMA* 305: 1460- 1468.

Danner, S., and J. G. Belasco. 2001. T7 phage display: a novel genetic selection system for cloning RNA-binding proteins from cDNA libraries. *Proc Natl Acad Sci U S A* 98: 12954-12959.

Huse, W. D., L. Sastry, S. A. Iverson, A. S. Kang, M. Alting-Mees, D. R. Burton, S. J. Benkovic, and R. A. Lerner. 1989. Generation of a large combinatorial library of the immunoglobulin repertoire in phage lambda. *Science* 246: 1275-1281.

Mullinax, R. L., and J. A. Sorge. 2003. Preparing lambda libraries for expression of proteins in prokaryotes or eukaryotes. *Methods Mol Biol* 221: 271-287.

Kang, A. S., T. M. Jones, and D. R. Burton. 1991. Antibody redesign by chain shuffling from random combinatorial immunoglobulin libraries. *Proc Natl Acad Sci U S A* 88: 11120-11123.

McCafferty, J., A. D. Griffiths, G. Winter, and D. J. Chiswell. 1990. Phage antibodies: filamentous phage displaying antibody variable domains. *Nature* 348: 552-554.

Akamatsu, Y., M. S. Cole, J. Y. Tso, and N. Tsurushita. 1993. Construction of a human Ig combinatorial library from genomic V segments and synthetic CDR3 fragments. *J Immunol* 151: 4651-4659.

Aarden, L., S. R. Ruuls, and G. Wolbink. 2008. Immunogenicity of anti-tumor necrosis factor antibodies-toward improved methods of anti-antibody measurement. *Curr Opin Immunol* 20: 431-435.

Lonberg, N., L. D. Taylor, F. A. Harding, M. Trounstine, K. M. Higgins, S. R. Schramm, C. C. Kuo, R. Mashayekh, K. Wymore, J. G. McCabe, and a. et. 1994. Antigen- specific human antibodies from mice comprising four distinct genetic modifications. *Nature* 368: 856-859.

Green, L. L., M. C. Hardy, C. E. Maynard-Currie, H. Tsuda, D. M. Louie, M. J. Mendez, H. Abderrahim, M. Noguchi, D. H. Smith, Y. Zeng, and a. et. 1994. Antigen-specific human monoclonal antibodies from mice engineered with human Ig heavy and light chain YACs. *Nat Genet* 7: 13-21.

Green, L. L., and A. Jakobovits. 1998. Regulation of B cell development by variable gene complexity in mice reconstituted with human immunoglobulin yeast artificial chromosomes. *J Exp Med* 188: 483-495.

Lonberg, N. 2005. Human antibodies from transgenic animals. *Nat Biotechnol* 23: 1117-1125.

7

Thionamides-Related Vasculitis in Autoimmune Thyroid Disorders

Elisabetta L. Romeo[1], Giuseppina T. Russo[1], Annalisa Giandalia[1], Provvidenza Villari[1], Angela A. Mirto[1], Mariapaola Cucinotta[2], Giuseppa Perdichizzi[1] and Domenico Cucinotta[1]
[1]*Department of Internal Medicine, University of Messina, Messina,*
[2]*Section of Nuclear Medicine, Department of Radiology, University of Messina, Messina, Italy*

1. Introduction

Hyperthyroidism is the consequence of excessive thyroid hormone action (AACE Thyroid Guidelines, 2002). In many cases, it results from excessive activity of the thyroid gland, with a pathologically increased production of thyroid hormones. The causes of hyperthyroidism include several conditions, that are listed in Table 1.

• Toxic diffuse goiter (Graves' disease)
• Toxic adenoma
• Toxic multinodular goiter (Plummer's disease)
• Painful subacute thyroiditis
• Silent thyroiditis, including lymphocytic and postpartum variations
• Iodine-induced hyperthyroidism (for example, related to amiodarone therapy)
• Excessive pituitary TSH or trophoblastic disease
• Excessive ingestion of thyroid hormone

Table 1. Causes of hyperthyroidism (AACE Thyroid Guidelines,2002)

Graves' disease is the most common cause of hyperthyroidism. It is an autoimmune disorder, caused by the presence of autoantibodies directed against the thyroid-stimulating hormone (TSH) receptor (TRAb), chronically stimulating thyroid hormone synthesis and secretion, and resulting in an excessive amount of triiodothyronine (T3) and thyroxine (T4) and gland growth. In iodine sufficient areas, this prototypical autoimmune disease is the most common cause of thyrotoxicosis in young women as well as in children and adolescents, and it is characterized by thyrotoxicosis, goitre and typical manifestations such as ophthalmopathy and pretibial myxedema.
According to the American Association of Clinical Endocrinologists guidelines (AACE, 2002), the diagnosis of hyperthyroidism relates on TSH values. Thus, with the exception of the excess of TSH secretion, hyperthyroidism of any cases results in a lower-than-normal or

suppressed TSH level, together with an increase of free T4 and free T3 in the case of overt disease.

Once hyperthyroidism has been diagnosed, three main therapeutic options are available, including radioactive iodine, surgical intervention (thyroidectomy) and anti-thyroid drug.

In US, radioactive iodine is currently the treatment of choice for adults with Graves' disease, except for pregnant or breast-feeding women, because of its adverse effects on fetal gland and its appearance in the breast milk. Overall, radioactive iodine is a safe and effective therapy, that can be either administered through an ablative or with a smaller doses regimen in order to render the patient euthyroid. In any case, hypothyroidism requiring a lifelong thyroid replacement therapy is an inevitable consequence with radioiodine therapy.

Thyroidectomy was frequently used in the past, but its use is now limited to pregnant women intolerant to antithyroid drugs, or to patients refusing radioactive iodine as a definitive treatment. Possible complications associated with surgical treatment of Graves' disease include laryngeal nerve damage and vocal cord paralysis, hypoparathyroidism and hypothyroidism.

Anti-thyroid drug treatment is still a widely used approach in the treatment of hyperthyroidism. Since the 1940s, thionamides have been used as anti-thyroid drugs in the management of Grave's disease (Laurberg et al., 2006). This class of drugs includes propylthiouracil (PTU), benzylthiouracil, carbimazole and methimazole (MMI), and all of them have been shown to have comparable efficacy in inducing hyperthyroidism remission (Cooper, 2005).

All these compounds act through the inhibition of thyroid peroxidase, the enzyme responsible for the synthesis of thyroid hormones, thus leading to a reduced hormone secretion (Laurberg et al., 2006). Recently, an alternate mechanism of action has been proposed, relating their efficacy in patients with Graves' disease to a direct immunosuppressive effect (Laurberg et al., 2006).

Despite the similar efficacy, the choice of the anti-thyroid drug is conditioned by other drug characteristics and/or by their pharmacokinetics profile. For instance, MMI has a longer half-life than PTU, and thanks to its once-a-day administration, it represents the best choice when addressing patients compliance. On the other hand, PTU is the drug of choice for treating pregnant and breast-feeding women, because of its limited transfer into the placenta and breast milk (Streetman et al., 2003). PTU is often preferred to MMI also for the additional property of inhibiting the peripheral conversion of T4 to T3.

Although widely used, anti-thyroid drugs have been reported to be associated with a wide range of adverse effects, such as skin eruptions, liver dysfunction and agranulocytosis; fever, arthralgias and arthritis are other common clinical manifestation, usually occurring within the first few months of administration.

The occurrence of these side-effects can be influenced by several factors, such as drug starting dose or treatment duration (Nakamura et al., 2003).

In addition, over the past 2 decades, several cases of thionamides-associated autoimmune vasculitis have been reported, with variable clinical presentation and severity.

Vasculitis are a heterogeneous group of inflammatory disorders of the blood vessels, that occur as a part of several autoimmune disorders. In many cases they are largely mediated by the deposition of immune complexes that precipitate and become trapped within vessel

walls, stimulating an immune response that ultimately leads to vascular injury. This mechanism usually occurs in secondary vasculitis, frequently associated with infections or systemic autoimmune diseases, whereas in the primary vasculitis, immune deposits are generally absent (Kallenberg & Heeringa, 1998).
Clinical manifestations of vasculitis largely depend on the type of vessels and the specific disctrict involved, resulting in a wide-range of signs and symptoms.
The Chapel Hill Consensus Conference nomenclature is one of the most widely used to distinguish different forms of vasculitis, based on vessel size (large, medium, and small), as shown in Table 2 (Jennette & Falk, 2007).

Large Vessel Vasculitis
• Giant Cell Arteritis • Takayasu Arteritis
Medium-Sized Vessel Vasculitis
• Polyarteritis Nodosa • Kawasaki Disease
Small Vessel Vasculitis
• Wegener's Granulomatosis • Churg-Strauss Syndrome • Microscopic Polyangiitis • Henoch-Schönlein Purpura • Cryoglobulinemic Vasculitis • Cutaneous leukocytoclastic angiitis

Table 2. Classification of vasculitis according to the Chapel Hill Consensus Conference

2. Thionamides-related vasculitis in autoimmune thyroid disorders

2.1 Autoimmune markers of thionamides-related vasculitis

Overall, vasculitis have been mainly reported in patients treated with PTU, and most of PTU-induced vasculitis are associated with an increase of anti-neutrophil cytoplasmic antibody (ANCA) circulating levels.
ANCA are antibodies directed against myeloid lysosomal enzymes, that can be identified by indirect immunofluorescence (IIF) with human neutrophils. These autoantibodies can have a cytoplasmic (cANCA) or a perinuclear (pANCA) distribution pattern, that can be detected by ELISA (Savige et al., 2000). In particular, cANCA are directed against antiproteinase3 (PR3-ANCA), and they are specific for Wegener's granulomatosis (Van der Wonde et al., 1985), whereas pANCA can be directed against several antigens, the most important being myeloperoxidase (MPO-ANCA). pANCA is a serological marker for microscopic polyangiitis, but it can also be detected in patients with systemic lupus erythematosus, rheumatoid arthritis and drug-induced vasculitis (Jennette & Falk, 1997).
Any of these patterns can occur in patients with drug-induced ANCA-positive vasculitis and atypical ANCA against several antigens, like elastase, azurocin, cathepsine G, lactoferrin and lyzozim have been also reported.
Although the pathogenetic role of these autoantibodies in drug-induced vasculitis has not been fully elucidated yet, several hypotheses have been proposed.

Thus, it has been reported that PTU can selectively accumulate into neutrophils where it can bind to myeloperoxidase, changing or inactivating the heme structure of the enzyme (Lee et al., 1988). It has been suggested that, in susceptible individuals, the enzyme altered by PTU could then stimulate the production of anti-myeloperoxidase antibodies, inducing neutrophils degranulation and vascular damage (D'Cruz et al., 1995). In particular, MPO-ANCA seems to play an important role in the development of tissue damage in vasculitis or glomerulonephritis (Ashizawa et al., 2003; Arimura et al., 1993). It has also been suggested that viral infections could trigger the development of the autoimmune chain reaction.

Overall, ANCA autoantibodies are frequently detected in patients with Graves' disease treated with anti-thyroid drugs, regardless of the presence of clinical manifestations of vasculitis.

Anti-thyroid drugs ANCA-associated vasculitis occurs more frequently in women, consistently with the fact that Graves' disease is more common in female gender.

It has been reported that the prevalence of MPO-ANCA is higher in patients treated with PTU than in those treated with MMI (Wada et al., 2002).

Thus, the prevalence of ANCA positivity has been estimated to average 26% of PTU-treated subjects (Gunton et al., 2000), being even higher in treated children (Hirokazu et al., 2000).

In a study of 117 patients with Graves' disease, Sera et al. reported that MPO-ANCA was negative in all patients treated with MMI as well as in untreated patients, whereas it was detected in 37.5% of patients receiving PTU (Sera et al., 2000). Furthermore, the proportion of patients positive for MPO-ANCA increased with the prolongation of PTU treatment (Sera et al., 2000).

In a retrospective study of 61 patients with Graves' disease, Wada et al. reported that 25% of patients treated with PTU showed positive MPO-ANCA, unlike 3.4% of patients receiving MMI. Moreover, the sole patient MPO-ANCA positive treated with MMI had been taking PTU for six years before starting MMI treatment (Wada et al., 2002).

The annual incidence of MPO-ANCA-associated vasculitis in patients treated with anti-thyroid drugs has been estimated to be between 0.53 and 0.79 patients per 10,000, although several mild cases may not have been reported (Noh et al., 2009).

However, not all ANCA positive patients develop the clinical manifestations of vasculitis, and several factors such as type of drug, ethnicity, timing and dose, treatment duration may concur to the development of overt clinical manifestations.

Overall, the incidence of ANCA positive vasculitis is higher with PTU, being estimated to be 39.2 times the incidence reported with MMI (Noh et al., 2009).

As for ethnicity, the prevalence of ANCA positivity seems to be similar in different ethnical groups, although Gunton et al. suggested that ANCA-positive vasculitis may be more common in patients of Asian origin, being nearly half of the reported cases of PTU-induced ANCA-associated vasculitis from Japan (Gunton et al., 1999).

The timing and doses of thionamides reported in ANCA-associated vasculitis have also been variable. In fact, even if long-term treatment with anti-thyroid drugs seems to have a stronger association with the risk of vasculitis, these complications can also occur within few months after starting the treatment. Furthermore, ANCA-associated vasculitis have been also reported in patients treated with low doses of both MMI and PTU (Noh et al., 2009).

Moreover, it seems that drug dose and duration of anti-thyroid treatment use, together with the titers of antibodies could be related with the clinical course of ANCA-associated vasculitis. Thus, Morita et al. (Morita et al., 2000) reported that anti-thyroid drug-induced ANCA-associated vasculitis was more frequent in patients resistant to drug treatment, who were receiving high doses over a prolonged period of time and with high titers of MPO-ANCA; furthermore, clinical manifestations disappeared according to decreasing values of antibodies. This finding suggests that high titer of MPO-ANCA may be necessary to induce vasculitis.

Beside the role of thionamides in inducing the formation of specific autoantibodies, an alternate hypothesis has to be taken into account.

Thus, given the common autoimmune background, a possible association of ANCA-positivity with the autoimmune disease itself has been suggested.

This hypothesis has been tested in a prospective study, where a group of patients with newly diagnosed Graves' disease were followed up before and during therapy with PTU, and compared to a cross-sectional group of previously diagnosed Graves' patients who had already been treated with PTU, of patients with Hashimoto thyroiditis and those with toxic nodular goiter, as well as to healthy controls. As a result, all untreated newly diagnosed Graves' patients were ANCA negative, but 32.1% became ANCA positive after initiating PTU administration. On the other hand, patients with Hashimoto disease, untreated toxic nodular goiter and euthyroid subjects did not show ANCA positivity. This study suggested that it is PTU treatment, and not hyperthyroidism or autoimmunity, which induces ANCA production (Ozduman Cin et al., 2009). In agreement with this, ANCA prevalence is increased in Graves' disease, but not in patients with other autoimmune thyroid disease, such as Hashimoto thyroiditis (Harper et al., 2004). Furthermore, it has also been demonstrated that PTU administration is associated with ANCA positivity at a similar rate in both patient with Graves' disease and those with toxic multinodular goiter, suggesting that PTU but not Graves' disease itself is the most important factor for ANCA development (Yazisiz et al., 2008).

2.2 Clinical manifestations of thionamides-related vasculitis

Clinical presentation and severity of anti-thyroid drug-induced vasculitis are variable, and largely related to the type of vessels and to the anatomical district involved.

Thus, although not all ANCA positive patients develop a clinical disease, a wide-range of clinical symptoms have been reported in patients with thionamides-related vasculitis.

ANCA-associated vasculitis is usually characterized by small vessel inflammation and necrosis, that may involve any system and organ, being arthralgia and fever the most commonly reported clinical manifestations (Morita et al., 2000).

An ANCA-positive vasculitis in association with anti-thyroid drugs was first reported in 1992 by Stankus and Johnson, who described a patient treated with PTU who developed respiratory failure and MPO-ANCA positive test (Stankus & Johnson, 1992).

Since then, several cases of ANCA-associated vasculitis in patients with Graves' disease treated with anti-thyroid drugs have been described, although ANCA-positive vasculitis have also been reported in patients with toxic multi-nodular goiter treated with PTU. Thus, in 1999 a case report of a PTU-induced vasculitis was described in an elderly women with toxic multi-nodular goiter, presenting with haemoptysis and acute renal failure (Gunton et al., 1999).

Overall, drug-induced vasculitis presenting symptoms may include renal involvement (67%), arthralgia (48%), fever (37%), skin manifestations (30%), respiratory tract involvement (27%), myalgia (22%), scleritis (15%) as well as other manifestations (18%) (Gunton et al., 1999).

As for skin manifestations, leukocytoclastic vasculitis, principally affecting the lower limbs, is the most common cutaneous manifestation (Gunton et al., 1999; Day et al., 2003).

In addition, several cases of pulmonary involvement have been reported, including pulmonary infiltrates associated with respiratory failure, eosinophilic pleuritis, interstitial pneumonitis or respiratory distress syndrome and pulmonary harmorrhage (Stankus & Johnson, 1992; Chevrolet et al., 1991).

Renal involvement in drug-induced vasculitis is also common. In 1995, D'Cruz et al. published the first report of renal biopsy-proven vasculitis in two patients treated with anti-thyroid drugs. Both patients developed a crescentic glomerulonephritis and responded to immunosuppressive therapy and dismission of anti-thyroid drugs (D'Cruz et al., 1995).

Recently, Chen YX et al. published a retrospective study of 19 patients with ANCA-positive vasculitis associated with PTU treatment. In this study, renal injury was the most common manifestation, occurring in 94.74% of cases. At renal biopsy, focal proliferative glomerulonephritis and necrotizing glomerulonephritis with crescent formation, minor glomerular abnormalities, IgA nephropathy, membranous nephropathy, focal proliferative glomerulonephritis, granulomatous interstitial nephritis and focal segmental glomerular sclerosis were all described (Chen YX et al., 2007).

Rare fatalities have been also reported in patients with anti-thyroid drugs-associated vasculitis. Batchelor et al. described the case of a 60-year-old man with a history of Graves' disease, treated with PTU, and presenting with rash, pancytopenia, and lymphadenopathy and subsequently developing acute renal failure and diffuse alveolar hemorrhage, who died despite the discontinuation of PTU and an aggressive therapy including immunosuppressive drugs and plasmapheresis (Batchelor & Holley, 2006).

Thus, even if in the majority of cases vasculitis usually resolve after the discontinuation of anti-thyroid drugs, patients can present with more severe or life-threatening manifestations.

In a study evaluating cutaneous and systemic manifestations following thionamides administration, death occurred in 10% of all published cases, with a predominance in patients with involvement of multiple organ systems (ten Holder et al., 2002).

Until 2005, the main case reports of thionamides induced-vasculitis described above all renal, musculoskeletal and cutaneous manifestations. In that period, the first case of thionamides-induced central nervous system (CNS) vasculitis has been also reported (Vanek et al., 2005): a PTU-treated patients presenting with generalized muscle spasms, amnesia and confusion, who showed a complete resolution of CNS symptoms after cessation of drug administration.

Since most of thionamides-related vasculitis have been associated with PTU, MMI treatment has been advocated as safer for the treatment of Graves' disease; however, several cases of vasculitis following MMI administration have been reported.

In 1995, Kawaki et al. reported the first case of ANCA-associated vasculitis caused by MMI: a 24-year-old woman with Graves' disease treated with MMI for 4 years, who developed recalcitrant ulcers on the lower legs and ANCA positivity, improved after MMI was withdrawn (Kawaki et al., 1995).

Besides skin manifestations, also renal involvement, such as crescentic glomerulonephritis (D'Cruz et al., 1995), and pulmonary involvement, with hemoptysis and hypoxic respiratory failure (Tsai et al., 2001) have been reported in MMI-treated patients.

Furthermore, we recently reported the first case of MMI induced CNS vasculitis in a young woman with Graves' disease, completely recovered after the discontinuation of treatment (Tripodi et al., 2008). CNS vasculitis was suspected on the basis of the clinical features and neurological examination, and confirmed by brain magnetic resonance imaging (RMN) and single-photon emission computed tomography (SPECT). In our patient, ANCA test was negative, supporting the concept that ANCA are not critical for the development of drug-induced vasculitis.

Thus, although less common than with PTU, vasculitis associated with other thionamides-drugs therapy have been also described.

Although more infrequently, carbimazole-associated vasculitis have been reported. Carbimazole has been associated with leukocytoclastic vasculitis and acute renal failure secondary to interstitial nephritis, without any evidence of ANCA positivity (Day et al., 2003), and to ANCA-positive vasculitis with crescentic glomerulonephritis (D'Cruz et al., 1995). Respiratory involvement in carbimazole-treated patients appears to be less common, although a case of MPO-ANCA vasculitis with massive pulmonary hemorrhage and necrotizing glomerulonephritis has been described (Calanas-Continente et al., 2005). Also a case of polyneuropathy, with evidence of microvasculitis in nerve biopsy, was reported as associated to this drug administration (Leger et al., 1984).

In a large cross-sectional study of 407 patients with Graves' disease, Harper et al. reported that both PTU and carbimazole therapy were associated with an increases rate of ANCA-positivity, although the risk in carbimazole-treated patients was smaller than in PTU-treated ones (15.9% and 33.3% respectively vs 4,6% of controls) (Harper et al., 2004). Its administration has also been related to the development of rare side effects, such as those described by Sève et al., who reported the first case of eosinophilic granulomatous vasculitis localized to the stomach in a patient with Graves' disease treated for five months with carbimazole, with complete resolution of clinical manifestations after drug dismission (Sève et al., 2005).

Since there are no evidence that carbimazole can accumulate in neutrophils or to act as a hapten as PTU, the underlying mechanism associated to the development of vasculitis related with other thionamides-drugs has not been yet elucidated.

2.3 Anti-thyroid-induced ANCA-associated vasculitis and idiophatic ANCA vasculitis: Comparison of clinical manifestations and outcomes

Clinical and serological characteristics of drug-induced and idiophatic systemic vasculitis are similar; however, the appropriate diagnosis is of great importance since they may have a different treatment and prognosis.

Thus, the removal of anti-thyroid drugs is usually associated with the resolution of the clinical symptoms of vasculitis, whereas patients with idiophatic vasculitis always need to be treated more aggressively with immunosuppressive and anti-inflammatory drugs, or plasmapheresis.

Clinical and serological data from idiophatic and anti-thyroid drug-induced ANCA positive vasculitis were compared in a 11-year retrospective study. In this cohort (Bonaci-Nikolic et al., 2005), both groups of patients showed a similar high frequency of arthralgia and myalgia, whereas skin involvement, especially represented by urticaria and urticaria-like vasculitis, was more common in patients treated with anti-thyroid drugs, with histological evidence of leucocytoclastic vasculitis. Furthermore, patients with idiophatic systemic vasculitis showed more frequently fever, weight loss, renal and respiratory manifestations, pulmonary-renal syndrome, ear/nose and nervous system manifestations.

As for serological profile, patients with drug-induced vasculitis, showed positivity for ANAs and antihistone antibodies, and had high levels of IgM anticardiolipin antibodies cryoglobulinemia and low C4 values (Wiik et al., 2005; Bonaci-Nikolic et al., 2005).

Hence, drug-induced vasculitis seem to have a milder course and a better long-term prognosis, since the withdrawal of anti-thyroid drugs usually leads to the resolution of clinical manifestations in the vast majority of cases.

Thus, the prognosis of anti-thyroid-induced ANCA-associated vasculitis is usually good as long as the drug is discontinued. However, early recognition of clinical symptoms is very important because of the potential risk of life-threatening injury, such as pulmonary-renal syndrome, with pulmonary hemorrhage and renal failure. In these patients, additional treatment with steroids and/or immunosuppressive agents should be recommended.

In a retrospective study of fifteen patients with PTU-induced ANCA-associated vasculitis, Gao et al. investigated treatment protocols and outcomes of patients, suggesting that immunosuppressive therapy should be administrated only in those patients with vital organ involvement, such as lung and kidney vasculitis, in order to prevent progression to irreversible disease.

Interestingly, unlike what is normally found in patients with primary ANCA-associated vasculitis (Hogan et al., 2005), none of the patients with drug-induced vasculitis experienced relapse after the discontinuation of immunosuppressive therapy at follow-up (Gao et al.,2008).

Moreover, immunosuppressive therapy may be administered only for a shorter period of time, usually 6-12 months, than in primary ANCA-associated vasculitis, without any further maintenance therapy (Gao et al., 2008).

3. Conclusion

Anti-thyroid drugs are a common and widespread treatment for Graves' disease and the other forms of hyperthyroidism. It is a safe and efficacy treatment, and it is the treatment of choice in patients refusing radioactive iodine as definitive treatment or during pregnancy and breast-feeding.

However, this treatment has been associated with several side effects and among them, vasculitis, with a wide-range of severity and clinical presentations.

Vasculitis are more commonly reported in PTU-treated patients, with a long duration of treatment, and with positivity for ANCA autoantibodies.

Thionamides-related vasculitis usually recover after discontinuation of therapy, although rare cases of fatalities have been also reported.

4. References

AACE Thyroid Guidelines. (2002). *Endocrine Practice*, Vol. 8, No. 6, pp. 457-69.

Arimura, Y.; Minoshima, S.; Kamiya, Y.; Tanaka, U.; Nakabayashi, K.; Kitamoto, K.; Nagasawa, T.; Sasaki, T. & Suzuki, K. (1993). Serum myeloperoxidase and serum cytokines in anti-myeloperoxidase antibody-associated glomerulonephritis. *Clinical Nephrology*, Vol. 40, No. 5, pp. 256-2641

Ashizawa, K. & Eguchi, K. (2003). Serum anti-myeloperoxidase antineutrophil cytoplasmic antibodies (MPO-ANCA) in patients with Graves' disease receiving anti-thyroid medication. *Internal Medicine*, Vol. 42, No. 6, pp.463-464

Batchelor, N. & Holley, A. (2006). A fatal case of propylthiouracil-induced ANCA-positive vasculitis. *Medscape General Medicine*, Vol. 8, No.4, p. 10

Bonaci-Nikolic, B.; Nikolic, M.M.; Andrejevic, S.; Zoric, S. & Bukilica, M. (2005). Antineutrophil cytoplasmic antibody (ANCA)-associated autoimmune disease induced by antithyroid drugs: comparison with idiopathic ANCA vasculitides. *Arthritis Research & Therapy*, Vol. 7, No. 5, pp. R1072-1081

Calanas-Continente, A.; Espinosa, M.; Manzano-Garcìa, G.; Santamarìa, R.; Lopez-Rubio, F. & Aljama, P. (2005). Necrotizing glomerulonephritis and pulmonary hemorrhage associated with carbimazole therapy. *Thyroid*, Vol. 15, No. 3

Chen, Y.X.; Yu, H.J.; Ni, L.Y.; Zhang, W.; Xu, Y.W.; Ren, H.; Chen, X.N.; Wang, X.L.; Li, X.; Pan, X.X.; Wang, W.M. & Chen, N. (2007). Propylthiouracil-associated antineutrophil cytoplasmic autoantibody-positive vasculitis: retrospective study of 19 cases. *The Journal of Rheumatology*, Vol. 34, No. 12, pp. 2451-2456

Chevrolet, J.C.; Guelpa, G. & Schifferli, J.A. (1991). Recurrent adult respiratory distress-like syndrome associated with propylthiouracil therapy. *European Respiratory Journal*, Vol. 4, No. 7, pp. 899-901

Cooper, D.S. (2005). Antithyroid drugs. *New England Journal of Medicine*, Vol. 352, No. 9, (March 3), pp. 905-17

D'Cruz, D.; Chesser, A.M.S.; Lightowler, C.; Comer, M.; Hurst, M.J.; Baker, L.R.I. & Raine, A.E.G. (1995). Antineutrophil cytoplasmic antibody-positive crescentic glomerulonephritis associated with anti-thyroid drug treatment. *British Journal of Rheumatology*, Vol. 34, No. 11, pp.1090-1091

Day, C.; Bridger, J.; Rylance, P.; Jackson, M.; Nicholas, J. & Odum, J. (2003). Leukocytoclastic vasculitis and interstitial nephritis with carbimazole treatment. *Nephrology Dialysis Transplantion*, Vol. 18, No. 2, pp. 429-431

Gao, Y.; Chen, M.; Ye, H.; Yu, F.; Guo, X.H. & Zhao, M.H. (2008). Long-term outcomes of patients with propylthiouracil-induced anti-neutrophil cytoplasmic auto-antibody-associated vasculitis. *Rheumatology*, Vol. 47, No. 10 , pp. 1515-1520

Gunton, J.E.; Stiel, J.; Caterson, R.J. & McElduff, A. (1999). Anti-thyroid drugs and antineutrophil cytoplasmic antibody positive vasculitis. A case report and review of the literature. *Journal of Clinical Endocrinology and Metabolism*, Vol. 84, No. 1, pp. 13-16, ISSN 0021-972X

Gunton, J.E.; Stiel, J.; Clifton-Bligh, P.; Wilmshurst, E. & McElduff, A. (2000). Prevalence of positive anti-neutrophil cytoplasmic antibody (ANCA) in patients receiving anti-thyroid medication. *European Journal of Endocrinology*, Vol. 142, No. 6, pp. 587-590, ISSN 0804-4643

Harper, L.; Chin, L.; Daykin, J.; Allahabadia, A.; Heward, J.; Gough, S.C.; Savage, C.O. & Franklyn, J.A. (2004). Propylthiouracil and carbimazole associated-antineutrophil cytoplasmic antibodies (ANCA) in patients with Graves' disease. *Clinical Endocrinology*, Vol. 60, No. 6, pp. 671-675

Hogan, S.L.; Falk, R.J.; Chin, H.; Cai, J.; Jennette, C.E.; Jennette, J.C. & Nachman, P.H. (2005). Predictors of releapse and treatment resistance in antineutrophil cytoplasmic antibody-associated small-vessel vasculitis. *Annals of Internal Medicine*, Vol. 143, No. 9, pp. 621-631

Jennette, J.C. & Falk, R.J. (1997). Small vessel vasculitis. *New England Journal of Medicine*, Vol.337, No. 21, pp. 1512-1523

Jennette, J.C. & Falk, R.J. (2007). The role of pathology in the diagnosis of systemic vasculitis. *Clinical and Experimental Rheumatology*, Vol. 25, No. 1 supp 44, pp. S52-56

Kallenberg, C.G. & Heeringa, P. (1998). Pathogenesis of vasculitis. *Lupus*, Vol. 7, No. 4, pp. 280-284

Kawaki, Y.; Nukaga, H.; Hoshito, M.; Iwata, M. & Otsuka, F. (1995). ANCA associated vasculitis and lupus like syndrome caused by methimazole. *Clinical and Experimental Dermatology*, Vol. 20, No. 4, pp. 345-347

Laurberg, P. (2006). Remission of Graves' disease during anti-thyroid drug therapy. Time to reconsider the mechanism? *European Journal of Endocrinology*, Vol. 155, No. 6, pp. 783-786, ISSN 0804-4643

Laurberg, P.; Andersen, S. & Karmisholt, J. (2006). Antithyroid drug therapy of Graves' hyperthyroidism: realistic goals and focus on evidence. *Expert Review of Endocrinology & Metabolism*, Vol.1, pp. 91-102

Lee, E.; Hirouchi M.; Hosokawa, M.; Sayo, H.; Kohno, M. & Kariya, K. (1988). Inactivation of peroxidase of rat bone marrow by repeated administration of propylthiouracil is accompanied by a change in the heme structure. *Biochemical Pharmacology*, Vol. 37, No. 11, pp.2151-2153

Leger, J.M.; Dancea, S.; Brunet, P. & Hauw, JJ. (1984). Polyneuropathy during treatment with carbimazole. *Revue Neurologique (Paris)*, Vol. 140, No. 11, 652-656

Morita, S.; Ueda, Y. & Eguchi, K. (2000). Anti-thyroid drug-induced ANCA-associated vasculitis: a case report and review of the literature. *Endocrine Journal*, Vol. 47, No. 4, pp. 467-470

Nakamura, H.; Noh, J.Y.; Itoh, K.; Fukata, S.; Miyauchi, A. & Hamada, N. (2007). Comparison of methimazole and propylthiouracil in patients with hyperthyroidism caused by Graves' disease. *Journal of Clinical Endocrinology and Metabolism*, Vol. 92, No. 6, pp. 2157-2162

Ozduman Cin, M.; Morris, Y.; Tiryaki Aydintug, O.; Kamel, N. & Gullu, S. (2007). Prevalence and clinical significance of antineutrophil cytoplasmic antibody in Graves' patients treated with propylthiouracil. *International Journal of Clinical Practice*, Vol. 63, No. 2, pp. 299-302

Sato, H.; Hattori, M.; Fujieda, M.; Sugihara, S.; Inomata, H.; Hoshi, M. & Miyamoto, S. (2000). High prevalence of antineutrophil cytoplasmic antibody positivity in childhood onset Graves' disease treated with propylthiouracil. *Journal of Clinical Endocrinology and Metabolism*, Vol. 85, No. 11, pp. 4270-4273, ISSN 0021-972X

Savige, J.; Davies, D.; Falk, R.J.; Jennette, J.C. & Wiik, A. (2000). Antineutrophil cytoplasmic antibodies and associated disease: a review of the clinical and laboratory features. *Kidney International*, Vol. 57, No. 3, pp. 846-862

Sève, P.; Stankovic, K.; Michalet, V.; Vial, T.; Scoazec, J.Y. & Broussolle, C. (2005). Carbimazole induced eosinophilic granulomatous vasculitis localized to the stomach. *Journal of Internal Medicine*, Vol. 258, No. 2, pp. 191-195

Sera, N.; Ashizawa, K.; Ando, T.; Abe, Y.; Ide, A.; Usa, T.; Tominaga, T.; Ejima, E.; Yokoyama, N. & Eguchi, K. (2000). Treatment with propylthiouracil is associated with appearance of antineutrophil cytoplasmic antibodies in some patients with Graves' disease. *Thyroid*, Vol. 10, No. 7, pp. 595-599

Stankus, S.J. & Johnson, N.T. (1992). Propylthiouracil-induced hypersensitivity vasculitis presenting as respiratory failure. *Chest*, Vol. 102, No. 5, pp. 1595-1596

Streetman, D.D. & Khanderia, U. (2003). Diagnosis and treatment of Graves disease. *Annals of Pharmacotherapy*, Vol. 37, No.7-8, pp. 1100-1109

Ten Holder, S.M.; Joy, M.S. & Falk, R.J. (2002). Cutaneous and systemic manifestation of drug-induced vasculitis. *Annals of Pharmacotherapy*, Vol. 36, No. 1, pp. 130-147

Tripodi, P.F.; Ruggeri, R.M.; Campennì, A.; Cucinotta, M.; Mirto, A.; Lo Gullo, R.; Baldari, S.; Trimarchi, F.; Cucinotta, D. & Russo, G.T. (2008). Central nervous system after starting methimazole in a woman with Graves' disease. *Thyroid*, Vol. 18, No. 9, pp. 1011-1013

Tsai, M.H.; Chang, Y.L.; Wu, V.C.; Chang, C.C. & Huang, T.S. (2001). Methimazole-induced pulmonary haemorrhage associated with antimyeloperoxidase-antineutrophil cytoplasmic antibody: a case report. *Journal of the Formosan Medical Association*, Vol. 100, No. 11, pp. 772-775

Van der Wonde, F.J.; Rasmussen, N.; Lobatto, S.; Wiik, A.; Permin, H.; van Es, L.A.; van der Giessen, M.; van der Hem, G.K. & The, T.H. (1985). Autoantibodies against neutrophils and monocytes: tool for diagnosis and marker of disease activity in Wegener's granulomatosis. *Lancet*, Vol. 1, No. 8426, pp. 425-429

Vanek, C. & Samuels, M.H. (2005). Central nervous system vasculitis caused by propylthiouracil therapy: a case report and literature review. *Thyroid*, Vol. 15, No. 1, pp. 80-84

Wada, N.; Mukai, M.; Kohno, M.; Notoya, A.; Ito, T. & Yoshioka, N. (2002). Prevalence of serum anti-myeloperoxidase antineutrophil cytoplasmic antibodies (MPO-ANCA) in patients with Graves' disease treated with propylthiouracil and thiamazole. *Endocrine Journal*, Vol. 49, No. 3, pp.329-334

Wiik, A. (2005). Clinical and laboratory characteristics of drug-induced vasculitic syndromes. *Arthritis Research & Therapy*, Vol. 7, No. 5, pp. 191-192

Yazisiz, V.; Ongut, G.; Terzioglu, E. & Karayalcin, U. (2010). Clinical importance of antineutrophil cytoplasmic antibody positivity during propylthiouracil treatment. *International Journal of Clinical Practice*, Vol. 41, No. 1, pp. 19-24

8

The Emerging Role of Monoclonal Antibodies in the Treatment of Systemic Lupus Erythematosus

Ewa Robak and Tadeusz Robak
Medical University of Lodz
Poland

1. Introduction

Systemic lupus erythematosus (SLE) is an autoimmune disease characterized by B cell hyperactivity and defective T-cell function, with production of high titer autoantibodies and clinical involvement in multiple organ systems. Patients with mild SLE can generally be maintained on a combination of non-steroidal anti-inflammatory drugs and antimalarials. Corticosteroids, azathioprine and cyclophosphamide remain important for long term management of most patients with active disease and even those in clinical remission. However, these agents have considerable side effects and are not effective in all patients with SLE. Novel immunological therapies include both B and T cell directed treatments, anticytokine and complement directed therapies. These modalities enable more specific immunosuppression, and include cyclosporin, high-dose intravenous immunoglobulin, mycophenolate mofetil, tacrolimus and new purine nucleoside analogs (Schröder and Zeunerorts 2009).

In recent years, clinical studies have been undertaken with selected monoclonal antibodies (mAbs) in the treatment of several hematological diseases, especially in malignant disorders. However, some clinical observations indicate that mAbs may be an important alternative for the conventional therapy of some autoimmune disorders (Robak 2004).

B-lymphocytes are an essential component of the acquired immune response (La Cava 2010). They randomly express cell-surface receptors which are often autoreactive and must be controlled by the process of B-cell tolerance. In SLE, the number of B-cells in the peripheral blood is often decreased, and those that are present have abnormal phenotypes indicative of activation. The important role of B cells in the pathogenesis of SLE has provided a strong rationale to target B cells in SLE. Selective therapeutic depletion of B-cells became possible with the availability of the anti-CD20 antibody rituximab.

2. Anti-CD20 monoclonal antibodies

The CD20 (B1) antigen is a 33–35 kDa integral membrane protein expressed on the surfaces of non-malignant and most malignant B cells (Cragg, Walshe et al. 2005). The CD20 protein consists of cytoplasmic N- and C-termini and four hydrophobic regions for anchoring the molecule in the membrane (Robak 2008). The characteristics that make CD20 a good target antigen include its relatively high level of expression and close location of the extracellular epitopes to the cell surface. The intensity of antigen expression or the number of receptor sites on the cell surface appears to correlate with the clinical response. The cytotoxic activity of mAbs directed against CD20+ cells is thought to be based on antibody-dependent cellular cytotoxicity (ADCC) via natural killer (NK) cell responses, complement-dependent cytotoxicity (CDC), or by the induction of cell signaling followed by apoptosis. At present, rituximab is the most important mAb of clinical value in patients with autoimmune disorders and B-cell lymphoid malignancies. Over the last few years, new generations of anti-CD20 mAbs have been developed for potential benefits over rituximab (Robak and Robak 2011; Lim, Beers et al. 2010). They were engineered to have augmented antitumor activity by increasing CDC or ADCC activity and increased Fc binding affinity for the low-affinity variants of the FcγRIIIa receptor (CD16) on immune effector cells. The second-generation mAbs are humanized or fully human to reduce immunogenicity, but with an unmodified Fc region. They include ofatumumab, veltuzumab, and ocrelizumab. The third-generation mAbs are also humanized but in comparison with the second-generation mAbs they also have an engineered Fc region designed to increase their effector functions by increasing binding affinity for the FcγRIIIa receptor (Ruuls, Lammerts et al. 2008). Both polymorphisms in FcγRIIIa and structure of mAb Fc can impact on the affinity between FcγRIIIa and mAb. The third-generation mAbs include AME133v, Pro13192, and GA-101.

2.1 Rituximab

Rituximab is an IgG-1κ immunoglobulin, containing murine light- and heavy-chain variable-region sequences and human constant region sequences. Rituximab is known as the first-generation mAb. Since approval in 1997, rituximab has become the standard of care in follicular B-cell lymphomas (FL), CLL, and aggressive lymphomas when combined with chemotherapy (Hauptrock and Hess 2008). Rituximab is administered as an intravenous infusion with a recommended dosage of 375 mg/m^2 given once weekly for 4 weeks. Treatment with this agent is usually well tolerated. However, infusion-related reactions occur in the majority of patients. These adverse events are typically fever, chills, rigors and rare hypotension and bronchospasm, although the incidence of these side effects decreases with subsequent rituximab infusion. Moreover, prolonged impairment of antibody production causes the increased risk of viral and bacterial infections. It should be also remembered that rituximab is a human mouse chimeric antibody and hence treated patients may be susceptible to the development of human antichimeric antibodies, which can impact on responsiveness.

A recent study has shown that treatment with rituximab affects both the cellular and humoral arm of the immune system in patients with SLE (Lu, Ng et al. 2009).

A number of prospective studies and several retrospective cohort studies of rituximab in the treatment of SLE have been reported (Cambridge, Isenbergetal. 2008). In 2005 Leonardo et al. (Leandro, Cambridge et al. 2005) described female patients with SLE who were treated with combination of rituximab, CY and prednisolone. Each patient received two infusions of rituximab (500 mg/dose), two infusions of cyclophosphamide (750 mg/dose) and 60 mg prednisolone per day for five days. Five patients were analyzed and one patient was lost to follow up after 3 months. All five patients showed an improvement in British Isles Lupus Assessment Group (BILAG) scores from a median of 14 at baseline to a median of 6 at six months. Recently, the same group reported the results of 46 patients with active SLE were treated with a 1 gm of rituximab, 750 mg of cyclophosphamide, and 100-250 mg of methylprednisolone, administered on 2 occasions 2 weeks apart (Lu, Ng et al. 2009). Twenty one patients (47%) reached partial remission after one cycle (mean followup 39.6 months). Treatment resulted in a decrease in median global BILAG scores from 12 to 5 ($P < 0.0001$) and median anti-double-stranded DNA antibody titers from 106 to 42 IU/ml ($P < 0.0001$). In addition an increase in the median C3 level from 0.81 to 0.95 mg/liter ($P < 0.02$) at 6 months was observed. Five serious adverse events were noted.

Willems et al. (Willems, Haddad et al. 2006) described the safety and efficacy of rituximab in 11 girls (mean age 13.9 years) with severe SLE including 8 girls with class IV or V lupus nephritis, 2 girls with severe autoimmune cytopenia and 1 girl with an antiprothrombin antibody. Patients received 2 to 12 intravenous infusions of rituximab (350-450 mg/m^2/ infusion) with corticosteroids. Remission was achieved in 6 of 8 patients with lupus nephritis and in two patients with autoimmune cytopenia. However, severe adverse events occurred in 45% of the patients in this study.

Looney et al. reported the results of the first dose escalation study of rituximab for the treatment of SLE (Looney, Anolik et al. 2004). The drug was added to ongoing therapy in 18 patients with moderately active SLE. Six patients received a single infusion of 100 mg/m^2, six received one infusion of 375 mg/m^2 and six patients received four weekly doses of 375 mg/m^2. In this study, rituximab-induced B cell depletion was translated into a significant improvement in SLE disease activity even in the absence of substantial serologic responses. Most patients were able to decrease corticosteroid dose from 13 to 10 mg by the end of the study and three patients were able to discontinue concomitant immunosuppressives. The clinical response was most notable for rashes and arthritis.

Terrier et al. analyzed recently prospective data from the French AutoImmunity and Rituximab (AIR) registry, which includes data on patients with autoimmune disorders treated with rituximb (Terrier, Amoura et al. 2010). Overall response was observed in 80 of 113 patients (71%) by the SELENA-SLEDAI (SLE Disease Activity Index Score assessment). Efficacy was similar between patients receiving rituximab monotherapy and those receiving concomitant immunosuppressive agents. Articular, cutaneous, renal, and hematologic improvements were noted in 72%, 70%, 74%, and 88% of patients, respectively. In relapsed patients response was observed in 91% after retreatment with rituximab. Severe infections were observed in 12 patients (9%), corresponding to a rate of 6.6/100 patient-years. Most severe infections occurred within the first 3 months after the last rituximab infusion. Five patients died, due to severe infection ($n = 3$) or refractory autoimmune disease ($n = 2$).

Merrill et al reported the results of the Exploratory Phase II/III SLE Evaluation of Rituximab (EXPLORER) trial, a placebo-controlled, double-blind, multicenter study of rituximab in patients with moderately-to-severely active extrarenal SLE (Merrill, Neuwelt et al. 2010). Patients were randomized at a 2:1 ratio to receive intravenous rituximab (1,000-mg) or placebo on days 1, 15, 168, and 182, which was added to prednisone. Of the 257 patients, 88 were assigned to receive placebo, and 169 were randomized to the rituximab arm. At week 52, no difference was observed in major clinical responses or partial clinical responses between the placebo group. Decreases in the level of anti-dsDNA autoantibodies and increases in complement C3 and C4 levels were greater in the rituximab group than in the placebo group. The overall response rate was 28.4% and 29.6%, respectively. The proportion of patients in whom serious infection developed was 17% in the placebo group and 9.5% in the rituximab group.

Rituximab is also an active treatment agent in patients with lupus nephritis and central nervous system (CNS) involvement. Sfikakis et al. reported clinical response in 80% and sustained complete response in 40% of patients with class III and IV nephritis treated with rituximab and moderate doses of corticosteroids (Sfikakis, Boletis et al. 2005). In the study of Ng et al. 21 patients with renal involvement were treated with rituximab and cyclophosphamide (Ng, Cambridge et al. 2007). They had a decrease in median urinary protein creatinine ratio (PCR) from 446 to 190 mg/mmol 6 months. More recently, Pepper et al. treated 18 patients with class III/IV/V lupus nephritis with rituximab. All patients were on steroids prior to the development of lupus nephritis (Pepper, Griffith et al. 2009). The patients received mycophenolate mofetil maintenance therapy. Fourteen of 18 patients achieved complete or partial remission with a sustained response of 67% at 1 year. In addition, serum albumin increased from a mean of 29 g/L at presentation to 34 g/L at 1 year (P = 0.001). Importantly, following treatment with rituximab, 6 patients stopped prednisolone, 6 patients reduced their maintenance dose and 6 patients remained on the same dose (maximum 10 mg). No severe infections were observed.

The study performed by Tokunaga et al. showed marked improvement following rituximab therapy in patients with neuropsychiatric SLE (Tokunaga, Saito et al. 2007). A monoclonal antibody was administered at doses of 375 mg/m^2 once weekly for four weeks or 1000 mg once weekly for two weeks in 10 patients with refractory neuropsychiatric SLE. Treatment resulted in rapid improvement of CNS-related manifestations, particularly acute confusional state. Rituximab also improved cognitive dysfunction psychosis and seizure and reduced the SLEDAI on day 28 in all 10 patients. These effects lasted for more than a year in 5 patients. In another study, Smith et al. (Smith, Jones et al. 2006) evaluated prospectively the effects of rituximab treatment for refractory SLE and vasculitis. Patients received four weekly infusions of rituximab at a dose of 375 mg/m^2. Intravenous cyclophosphamide (500 mg) was administered along with the first infusion in an effort to achieve early disease control. Remission followeing rapid B cell depletion was achieved in all 11 patients including 6 complete responses and 5 partial responses. Moreover, a renal response occurred in all 6 patients with lupus nephritis. Clinical improvement was accompanied by a significant reduction in the daily dose of prednisone. Seven of 11 patients experienced a relapse, a median of 12 months after treatment. After relapse, six patients with SLE were re-treated with rituximab and all achieved remission and did so more quickly than after the primary treatment.

Rituximab is generally well tolerated. Even fewer adverse events have been observed in patients treated for SLE than in the lymphoma patients (Tokunaga, Saito et al. 2007). The most common adverse events during or following rituximab therapy are infusion related symptoms, typically fever, chills, rigors and hypotension. In patients who receive premedication consisting of antipyretic and antihistaminic drugs together with corticosteroids, infusion-related side effects are usually only mild or moderate and do not require discontinuation of rituximab administration. Occasionally, serious infections were also reported. However, these may have been related to the underlying disease and/or concomitant therapy with other immunosuppressive agents. In 2006, an FDA alert was reported after two SLE patients treated with rituximab had died from progressive multifocal leukoencephalopathy (PML) (Ermann and Bermas 2007). However, both patients had received additional treatment with cyclophosphamide. At present, it is difficult to estimate the risk of this complication in SLE patients treated with rituximab. In recent analysis, among the rheumatic diseases, 43 cases of PML (0.44%) were associated with SLE, 24 (0.25%)

with rheumatoid arthritis (RA), and 25 (0.26%) with other connective tissue diseases (CTDs) (Molloy and Calabrese 2009). Additional controlled studies with new designs are needed to define the place of rituximab in the therapeutic arsenal for SLE.

2.2 New generations of Anti-CD20 monoclonal antibodies

Over the last few years, new generations of anti-CD20 monoclonal antibodies have been developed for potential benefits over the classical, first-generation mAb rituximab. Compared with rituximab, new mAbs have enhanced antitumor activity resulting from increased CDC and ADCC, and increased Fc binding affinity for the low-affinity variants of the FcγRIIIa receptor (CD16) on immune effector cells (Czuczman & Gregory 2010).

2.2.1 Ofatumumab

Ofatumumab (HuMax-CD20; Arzerra™, GlaxoSmithKline plc/Genmab A/S) is a second-generation, fully human, anti-CD20, IgG1 mAb in phase I, II and III trials for hematological malignancies and autoimmune diseases such as rheumatoid arthritis (RA) and multiple sclerosis. Ofatumumab specifically recognizes an epitope encompassing both the small and large extracellular loops of CD20 molecule, and is more effective than rituximab at CDC induction and killing target cells. In April 2010, the European Medicines Agency granted a conditional marketing authorization for ofatumumab, for the treatment of fludarabine-refractory CLL patients. It has been reported recently that ofatumumab, administered as 2 i.v. infusions at doses 300 mg, 700 mg, or 1,000 mg is clinically effective in patients with active RA (Østergaard , Baslund et al. 2010). Rapid and sustained peripheral B cell depletion was noted in all dose groups. Overall, 70% of patients receiving ofatumumab had a moderate or good response according to the European League Against Rheumatism (EULAR) criteria at week 24.

2.2.2 Veltuzumab

Veltuzumab (IMMU-106, hA20; Immunomedics Inc., Morris Plains, NJ) is a second-generation, type 1, humanized, anti-CD20, IgG1 mAb with complementarity-determining regions (CDRs) similar to rituximab (Goldenberg, Rossi et al. 2009). This mAb is generated using the same human immunoglobulin as epratuzumab and has a >90% humanized framework. It is also very similar to rituximab in terms of antigen binding, specificity binding, and dissociation constant. Veltuzumab differs from rituximab by one amino acid (Asp101 instead of Asn101) in the CDR 3 of the variable heavy chain. Smaller murine regions may reduce infusion reactions, infusion times, and immunogenicity. This antibody has enhanced binding avidities and a stronger effect on CDC compared with rituximab in selected cell lines. Veltuzumab is safe and active agent in NHL. B cells were depleted after the first infusion of all tested doses, including dose levels less than those typically used with rituximab (Morschhauser, Leonard et al. 2009).

2.2.3 Ocrelizumab

Ocrelizumab (Genentech Inc/Biogen Idec Inc/Chugai Pharmaceutical Co Ltd/Roche Holding Ag) is a second-generation, type 1, humanized, anti-CD20, IgG1 mAb with modifications of the Fc region that lead to enhanced ADCC and reduced CDC activities compared with rituximab (Kausar, Mustafa et al. 2009).This agent has the potential for enhanced efficacy compared with rituximab due to increased binding affinity for the low-affinity variants of the FcγRIIIa receptor on immune effector cells (Genovese, Kaine et al. 2008). Ocrelizumab binds to a different, but overlapping, epitope of the extracellular domain of CD20 as compared with rituximab. Ocrelizumab is a humanized mAb with the potential for enhanced efficacy in lymphoid malignancies compared with rituximab due to increased binding affinity for the low-affinity variants of the FcγRIIIa receptor (Faria & Isenberg 2010).

2.2.4 GA-101

GA-101 (RO5072759) is a fully humanized, type II, IgG1 mAb derived from humanization of the parental B-Ly1 mouse antibody and subsequent glycoengineering using GlycoMab® technology. GA-101 was designed for enhanced ADCC and superior direct cell-killing properties, in comparison with currently available type I antibodies (Robak 2009). In contrast to rituximab GA101, mediated significant NK cell degranulation in whole blood samples. Thus, CDC and ADCC are believed to be the major effector mechanisms of GA101 in whole blood assays (Bologna, Gotti et al. 2011).

2.2.5 TRU-015

TRU-015 (CytoxB20G, Trubion Pharmaceuticals Inc and Pfizer Inc) is a small modular immunopharmaceutical (SMIP) derived from key domains of an anti-CD20 antibody. TRU-015 represents a novel biological compound that retains Fc-mediated effector functions and is smaller than mAbs (Rubbert-Roth 2010). SMIPs belong to a novel proprietary biologic compound class that retain Fc-mediated effector functions and are smaller than mAbs (Robak, Robak et al. 2009). A SMIP molecule is a single-chain polypeptide consisting of one binding domain, one hinge domain, and one effector domain. The TRU-015 SMIP molecule is the homogeneous single-chain immunotherapeutic derived from key domains of an anti-CD20 antibody, for the potential intravenous infusion treatment of RA, SLE and B-cell lymphoid malignancies (Hayden-Ledbetter, Cerveny et al. 2009). This molecule is a compact dimer of 104 kDa that co-migrates with albumin in size exclusion chromatography and retains a long half-life *in vivo*. It is effective in mediating target cell killing in the mechanism of ADCC but has reduced CDC activity compared with rituximab. TRU-015 could represent a novel therapy for the treatment of SLE, although the efficacy, safety profile, and advantages of this compound compared with existing therapeutic options would need to be established in clinical trials (Burge, Bookbinder et al. 2008). TRU-015 has shown clinical efficacy and tolerability in phase IIa and IIb studies in patients with rheumatoid arthritis, and clinical development efforts for the treatment of lymphoma and inflammatory disease are ongoing. In the ongoing trial pharmacokinetics of TRU-015 after a single administration in subjects with membranous nephropathy secondary SLE is investigated (ClinicalTrials.gov Identifier: NCT00479622).

All new anti-CD20 mAbs are potentially useful in the treatment of SLE. However, the advantage of these new drugs over rituximab should be proven by well-designed clinical trials in rituximab-refractory patients or through head-to-head comparison.

3. Other B cell targeting monoclonal antibodies

3.1 Anti-CD22 antibody epratuzumab

Epratuzumab (Immunomedics, Inc.) is a humanized monoclonal IgG antibody that specifically targets the CD22 antigen on B cells (Leonard & Goldenberg 2007). This monoclonal antibody is 90% to 95% of human origin thus greatly reducing the potential for immunogenicity. Unconjugated anti-CD22 antibodies only partially deplete B cells, but might deliver a negative signal by binding CD22 to the cell surface (Daridon, Blassfeld et al. 2010). Treatment of SLE patients with epratuzumab leads to a reduction of circulating CD27 negative B-cells, although epratuzumab is weakly cytotoxic to B-cells *in vitro*. Epratuzumab binding was higher on B-cells relative to T-cells. In addition, weak non-specific binding of epratuzumab on monocytes was noted. On B-cells, binding of epratuzumab was enhanced on CD27negative B-cells compared to CD27 positive B-cells, primarily related to a higher expression of CD22 on CD27negative B-cells. Epratuzumab also enhanced the migration of CD27negative B-cells towards the chemokine CXCL12.

Recently, Dorner et al. reported the results of an open-label, single-center study of 14 patients with moderately active SLE (Dörner, Kaufmann et al. 2006). Patients received 360 mg/m^2 of epratuzumab intravenously every 2 weeks for 4 doses with analgesic antihistamine premedication prior to each dose. Total BILAG scores decreased by ≥50% in all 14 patients at some point during the study with 92% having decrease in various amounts continuing to at least 18 weeks.

Epratuzumab toxicity consisted primarily of mild to moderate transient infusion-related events during the first infusion. These results support conducting multicenter controlled studies to examine the effects of epratuzumab in broader patient populations. A U.S. patent has been issued to Immunomedics, Inc. for epratuzumab as a potential new treatment for lupus.

3.2 Anti-BlyS monoclonal antibodies

The B-lymphocyte Stimulator (BLyS) and A Proliferatiave Inducing Ligand (APRIL) are ligands for receptors BAFF-R (B Cell Activation Factor), BCMA (B Cell Maturation Associate) and TACI (Transmembrane Activator and Calcium Reproducing Initiator). BLyS also known as BAFF, THANK, TALL-1 or zTNF4, is a member of TNF super-family, which stimulates immunoglobulin (Ig) production by binding to specific receptors (King and Hahn 2007). In patients with SLE, the serum levels of BLyS are elevated and its neutralization has suggested that higher levels of BLyS contribute to the generation of autoantibodies and is important in SLE pathogenesis (Toubi, Kessel et al. 2006). In consequence, neutralization of BLyS may play a role in the therapy of this disease.

3.2.1 Belimumab

Belimumab (Human Genome Sciences, (Rockville, MD, USA)/Glaxo Smith Kline, (Uxbridge, UK)) is a fully human IgG1 mAb that specifically binds and inhibits the biological activity of BLyS (Wiglesworth, Ennis et al. 2010). The antibody exerts its biological activity by preventing the binding of BLyS to its receptors, resulting in autoreactive B cell apoptosis (Baker, Edwards et al. 2003). It also inhibits soluble BLyS activity at subnanomolar concentrations in a murine model. Belimumab inhibits also BLyS- induced proliferation of B-cells *in vitro* and prevents human BLyS-induced increases in splenic B-cell numbers and serum IgA titers in mice.

The safety, tolerability, immunogenicity, and pharmacology of belimumab were investigated in a phase I, randomized, placebo controlled, double-blind study in patients with SLE (Furie, Stohl et al. 2008). Seventy patients with mild to moderate disease were enrolled in this trial. Fifty-seven patients were treated with mAb and 13 with placebo. The drug was administered at 4 different doses (1.0, 4.0, 10 and 20 mg/kg) as single infusions, 21 days apart. The incidence of adverse events and laboratory abnormalities was similar among the belimumab and placebo groups. A significant reduction in the median percentage of CD20+ B-cells was noted with a one and two doses of belimumab versus placebo. However, SLE activity did not change after treatment with this mAb.

Wallace et al. assessed the safety, tolerability, biological activity, and efficacy of belimumab in combination with standard of care therapy in patients with active SLE (Wallace, Stohl et al. 2009). In this phase II, randomized trial 449 patients with SELENA-SLEDAI score ≥ 4 were randomly assigned to belimumab (1, 4, 10 mg/kg) or placebo in a 52-week study. In this study, belimumab treatment did not result in significant improvement compared with placebo. Percentage change in the SELENA-SLEDAI score at week 24, the primary endpoint of the study, was similar in both arms (19.5% in the belimumab group versus 17.2% in the placebo group). There was no significant difference in time to first SFI-defined flare over 52 weeks between the belimumab and placebo groups (67 versus 83 days, respectively). However, the median time to first SLE flare during weeks 24–52 was significantly longer with belimumab treatment (154 versus 108 days; P=0.0361). During the 52-week study and 8-week follow-up period, the incidence of AEs were similar in all treatment groups, including placebo. Only urticaria was statistically more frequent in belimumab-treated patients (4% versus 0%).

The efficacy and safety of belimumab in patients with active SLE was also assessed in a large, randomized, multicenter study recently reported by Navarra et al 2011 (Navarra, Guzmán et al. 2011). In this trial, 865 patients with scores of at least 6 on the Safety of Estrogens in Lupus Erythematosus National Assessment-Systemic Lupus Erythematosus Disease Activity Index (SELENA-SLEDAI) were randomly assigned to belimumab 1 mg/kg or 10 mg/kg, or placebo by intravenous infusion in 1 h on days 0, 14, and 28, and then every 28 days until 48 weeks, with standard of care. Significantly higher Systemic Lupus Erythematosus Responder Index (SRI) rates were noted with belimumab 1 mg/kg (51%, P=0.0129) and 10 mg/kg (58%, p=0.006) than with placebo (44%) at week 52. In addition, more patients had SELENA-SLEDAI score reduced by at least 4 points during 52 weeks with belimumab 1 mg/kg (53%, P=0.0189) and 10 mg/kg (58%, P=0.0024) than with placebo (46%). Moreover, more patients receiving belimumab 1 mg/kg (78%, P=0.1064) and 10 mg/kg (81%, P=0.0181) had no new BILAG A or no more than 1 new B flare than did those receiving placebo (73%). There was no difference in rates of adverse events in patients given belimumab 1 mg/kg and 10 mg/kg, and placebo. Serious infection was noted in 8%, 4%, and 6% patients, respectively. Severe or serious hypersensitivity reactions on an infusion day were reported in four patients.

3.2.2 LY2127399

Anti-BAFF monoclonal antibody LY2127399 (Eli Lilly & Company Limited) is a fully human IgG4 antibody with neutralizing activity against both membrane-bound and soluble BAFF. This may reduce the activity, proliferation and survival of B-cells. The ongoing study evaluates the efficacy, safety and tolerability of two different doses of LY2127399 administered in addition to standard of care therapy in patients with active SLE (ClinicalTrials.gov Identifier: NCT01205438).

4. Monoclonal antibodies inhibiting T cell costimulation

Cytotoxic lymphocyte-associated antigen-4 (CTLA-4) is a potent inhibitor of the costimulation pathway necessary to activate T cells. Abatacept (CTLA-4 immunoglobulin; CTLA4-Ig,

Orencia) is a recombinant fully humanized fusion protein, composed of the extracellular domain of human CTLA-4 and a modified Fc part of IgG-1that was engineered to prevent complement fixation (St Clair 2009). It targets T cell activation by interfering with one of the costimulatory mechanisms that are essential for cell activation. CTLA4-Ig binds to B7-1 and B7-2 on antigen presenting cells and downregulates T cell activation by disrupting CD28-B7 costimulatory interaction. Abatacept blocks the interaction between CD28 expressed on the surface of T cells and CD80/CD86 on the surface of antigen-presenting cells. The drug was approved for RA by the FDA US (Food and Drug Administration) in 2005. Abatacept was compared to placebo in a randomized, placebo controlled, phase II trial of patients with active SLE characterized by arthritis, serositis, or rash (Merrill, Burgos-Vargas et al. 2010). SLE patients were randomized at a ratio of 2:1 to receive abatacept (10 mg/kg of body weight) or placebo. Prednisone (30 mg/day or equivalent) was given for 1 month, and then the dosage was tapered. There was no difference in the percentage of patients who experienced the primary endpoint of SLE flare, as defined by BILAG, over the course of 52 weeks. However, the investigators discerned a difference in flare rates between the abatacept group (64%) and placebo group (83%). This difference was especially pronounced in the subgroup of patients with arthritis. The frequency of adverse events was comparable in the abatacept and placebo groups (90.9% versus 91.5%), but serious adverse events were higher in the abatacept group (19.8 versus 6.8%). Most serious adverse events were single, disease-related events occurring during the first 6 months. Improvements in certain exploratory measures suggest that abatacept has some efficacy in patients with non-life-threatening manifestations of SLE.

5. Anticytokine monoclonal antibodies

In the course of SLE, a wide variety of cytokines is dysregulated, many of which are likely to influence autoimmunity and lupus tissue inflammation (La Cava. 2010; Robak, Kulczycka et al. 2007). They are not only involved in the immune dysregulation of SLE, but also in the local inflammatory response which ultimately leads to tissue injury. Proinflammatory cytokines such as tumor necrosis factor α (TNFα), iterleukin-6 (IL-6), IL-1 and interferon-γ (IFN-γ) may play an important role in propagating the inflammatory process responsible for tissue damage. IL-12, IL-15 and IL-18 are probably also involved in pathogenesis of SLE. The possibility of blocking the proinflammatory cascade by selective inactivation of cytokines can be a successful therapy for patients with SLE.

5.1 Anti-IL-6 monoclonal antibodies

Data from several studies suggests that IL-6 plays an important role in the B-cell hyperactivity and immunopathology of SLE (Klashman, Martin et al. 1991). One of the most important effects of IL-6 is to induce the maturation of B lymphocytes into plasma cells and augment the imunoglobulin secretion. IL-6 binds to the IL-6 receptors which belong to the type 1 cytokine receptor superfamily that consists of two subunits, namely the IL-6 R and the gp 130. This cytokine may have a direct influence in mediating tissue damage. Elevated levels of IL-6 were detected in the serum, urine and renal glomerulli of patients with active SLE and in murine models of SLE (Grondal, Gunnarsson et al. 2000).
Tocilizumab (ACTEMRA, MRA, Roche Pharmaceuticals) is a humanized anti-human IL-6R mAb considered as a therapeutic option for patients with SLE. It is an antibody which inhibits the interleukin-6 receptor. It binds to both soluble IL-6R and transmembrane IL-6R

and inhibit IL-6 binding to its receptors, leading to the blockade of IL-6 signaling through both receptors (Jones and Ding 2010). Tocilizumab suppresses the biological activity of IL-6 and is now being used in clinical trials for RA and SLE (ClinicalTrials.gov Identifier: NCT00046774). An intraperitoneal administration of an anti-IL-6 mAb decreased the production of anti-ds DNA antibodiess in murine model of SLE and prevented the development of severe kidney disease. These results suggest that treatment with anti-IL-6 mAb has a beneficial effect on autoimmunity in murine SLE and that autoreactive B cells may be the primary target for anti-IL-6 antibody treatment (Liang, Gardner et al. 2006).
Tocilizumab is an effective agent in all the stages of RA (Jones, Sebba et al. 2010). Tocilizumab is the first agent that has been shown to be superior to methotrexate (MTX) as monotherapy for the signs and symptoms of this disease. It is also an active drug in SLE patients. Tocilizumab when used in mild to moderate lupus patient has demonstrated preliminary success and good tolerability in an open-label phase I dosage-escalation study (Illei, Shirota et al. 2010). In this trial 16 patients with mild-to-moderate disease activity were assigned to receive 1 of 3 doses of tocilizumab given intravenously every other week for total of 7 infusions: 2 mg/kg in 4 patients, 4 mg/kg in 6 patients, or 8 mg/kg in 6 patients. Patients were then monitored for an additional 8 weeks. The median decrease in anti-dsDNA antibody levels at week 14 was −9 IU/ml ($P = 0.03$). There was improvement in overall disease activity over the course of treatment. Mean SLAM scores decreased from 7.1 at baseline to 5.0 at week 14 ($P = 0.002$), and mean mSELENA-SLEDAI scores decreased from 9.5 to 5.5 ($P = 0.001$). In addition, there was no SLE flare during the treatment period. The infusions were well tolerated, without any clinically significant infusion reactions. However, the treatment induced dosage-related decreases in the absolute neutrophil count, with a median decrease of 38% in the 4 mg/kg dosage group and 56% in the 8 mg/kg dosage group. Infections were observed in 11 patients between the start of study treatment and the end of the follow up period. This study provides the first evidence that treatment with tocilizumab has an acceptable safety profile and suggests a possible immunologic and clinical benefit in SLE.

5.2 Anti-IL 10 monoclonal antibody

Interleukin-10 (IL-10) is a cytokine produced mainly by monocytes and lymphocytes. It impedes the activation of antigen presenting cells, down-regulates the expression of co-stimulatory molecules and blunts T cell activation and TNF-α secretion. IL-10 boosts B cell proliferation and immunoglobulin class switching resulting in enhanced antibody secretion with the capacity to enter extravascular compartments and promote inflammation in SLE (Yap & Lai 2010). The levels of IL-10 increase in the serum of patients with active SLE and correlates with disease activity. Alteration in IL-10 regulation may result in accelerated T-cell apoptosis and aberrant T-cell dependent B-cell function. In animal models of lupus nephritis, anti-IL 10 blockade offered some benefits in limiting renal damage (Ravirajan, Wang et al. 2004). The beneficial effect of a combined therapy using both anti-IL-10 and anti-C5 mAb to prevent or reduce the effect of the humoral immune response in lupus disease was also suggested. Preliminary data has shown that anti-IL-10 monoclonal antibody improved cutaneous lesions, joint symptoms, and SLEDAI in lupus patients (Llorente, Richaud-Patin et al. 2000). The anti-IL-10 monoclonal antibody was administered to six patients with steroid resistant SLE in an open label pilot study. Treatment consisted of an 20 mg/day intravenous administration of an anti-IL-10 murine mAb (B-N10) for 21 consecutive days, with a follow-up period of 6 months. Therapy was well tolerated and marked improvement in skin lesions and joint symptoms was observed in all patients over the next 6 months. Furthermore, three times lower doses of prednisone were used. The study indicates that the use of IL-10 antagonists may be beneficial in the management of refractory SLE.

6. Anti-CD40 and anti-CD40L monoclonal antibodies

CD40, a member of the tumor necrosis factor receptor super family, is highly expressed in normal B-cells and a variety of B-cell malignancies. CD40 ligand, also called CD154 or gp39, is a protein expressed on activated CD4+ T cells as well as on platelets, mast cells, macrophages, basophils, NK cells and B lymphocytes. An increased expression of CD40L has been found in the peripheral lymphocytes of patients with active SLE (Devi, Van Noordin et al. 1998). Moreover, serum levels of CD154 (CD40L) are higher in lupus patients than in normal persons (van Kooten & Banchereau 2000). The high expression of CD154 on T and B cells may increase production of potentially harmful auto-antibodies. The results of preclinical studies indicate that lupus-prone mice treated with anti-CD40L Abs had diminished inflammation, reduced anti-DNA autoantibody production and prolonged survival. Prolonged administration was particularly helpful in preventing fibrosis in severely nephritic mice (Kalled, Cutler et al. 2001). These results prompted the testing of anti-CD40L mAbs in human SLE.

6.1 Anti-CD40 monoclonal antibodies

Two mAbs directed against CD40 have been developed and investigated in preclinical studies and clinical trials, lucatumumab (HCD122) and dacetuzumab (SGN-40) (Kelley, Gelzleichter et al. 2006).

6.1.1 Lucatumumab

Lucatumumab ((HCD122, CHIR-0.12.12; Novartis Pharmaceuticals) is a fully human anti-CD40 mAb directed against the B-cell surface antigen CD40. It blocks CD40/CD40L interactions *in vitro* and inhibits CD40L-induced proliferation of human peripheral blood lymphocytes without disturbing baseline lymphocyte proliferation. Lucatumumab triggers cell lysis via ADCC in cells overexpressing CD40 (Luqman, Klabunde et al. 2008).

6.1.2 Dacetuzumab

Dacetuzumab (Seattle Genetics, Inc), is another humanized anti-CD40 IgG1 mAb, which induces ADCC and apoptosis of normal and malignant B-cells (Kelley, Gelzleichter et al. 2006). Dacetuzumab is able to initiate multiple signalling cascades upon ligation of CD40 on NHL cell lines. Dacetuzumab-mediated cytotoxicity is associated with up-regulation of cytotoxic ligands of the tumor necrosis factor (TNF) family including Fas/FasL, TNF-related apoptosis-inducing ligand, and TNFalpha.

6.2 Anti-CD40L monoclonal antibodies

6.2.1 IDEC-131

IDEC-131/E6040 (Idec Pharmaceuticals Corp. San Diego) is a humanized mAb against human CD154, comprising human $\gamma 1$ heavy chains and human κ light chains with complementarity-determining regions of murine mAb clone 24-31. In Phase I clinical trial, IDEC-131 was administered in a single intravenous infusion at doses of 0.05-15.0 mg/kg in patients with SLE. Patients were followed for 3 months to evaluate toxicity and pharmacokinetics (Davis, Totoritis et al. 2001). All patients experienced at least one adverse event. However, no infusion related cytokine-release syndrome was observed and all patients completed treatment. In a phase II, double blind, placebo-controlled, multiple-center, multiple-dose study, 85 patients with mild-to-moderately active SLE were randomized to receive 6 infusions of IDEC-131, ranging from 2.5 mg/kg to 10.0 mg/kg, or placebo over 16 weeks (Kalunian, Davis et al. 2002). At week 20, the mean change from baseline total SLEDAI scores indicated improvement in disease activity within each treatment group. In addition, the median global BILAG scores at week 20 indicated a reduction in SLE activity. However, results did not differ among the IDEC-131 treatment and placebo groups, and no dose-response relationship was noted at week 20. Moreover, the changes in levels of anti-dsDNA antibody and serum complement were not statistically significant in any group or between treatment groups and placebo. In addition, the changes in levels of anti-dsDNA antibody and serum complement were not different between treatment groups and placebo. The adverse events were also similar between the IDEC-131 and placebo groups.

6.2.2 BG9588

BG9588 (Biogen, Inc., Cambridge, MA) is a recombinant humanized anti-human CD40L monoclonal antibody that specifically binds to the CD40 ligand expressed on the surface of activated T lymphocytes. It blocks the CD40L/CD40 interaction between T and B cells that is required for the initiation for certain antibody responses. A short course of BG9588 treatment in patients with proliferative lupus nephritis reduced anti-dsDNA antibodies, increased C3 concentrations, and decreased hematuria (Boumpas, Furie et al. 2003). These results indicate that the drug has immunomodulatory action. Additional studies will be needed to evaluate its long-term effects.

7. Anticomplement antibody

Patients with SLE have widespread activation and deposition of the complement fragment in affected tissues. In murine models of SLE, the administration of the anti-C5 monoclonal antibody delayed the onset of proteinuria and prolonged survival. Moreover, pharmacological blockade of C5 receptor with a specific receptor antagonist reduces disease manifestation in experimental lupus nephritis (Cordeiro & Isenberg 2008). Furthermore, in mice with renal disease induced by a human anti-dsDNA antibody, RH-14 anti-C5 monoclonal antibody significantly reduced proteinuria.

Eculizumab (Soliris; Alexion Pharmaceuticals, Inc., Cheshire, CT) is a recombinant humanized monoclonal antibody that works by binding to complement protein C5, inhibiting its enzymatic cleavage, blocking formation of the terminal complement complex, and thus preventing red cell lysis (Parker , Kar et al. 2007). It has a molecular weight of 148 kD. Eculizumab is approved for the treatment of paroxysmal nocturnal hemoglobinuria (PNH) (Hillmen, Young et al. 2006). This antibody is potentially useful for treating patients with lupus nephritis. In this disease, the terminal components of the complement C5b-C9 play an important role in mediating the inflammation and the damage of podocytes and glomerular basement membrane (Robak & Robak 2009). Eculizumab has been recently developed and investigated in a phase I single dose study in SLE.

MoAb	Target	Antibody characteristics
Rituximab	CD20	Type I, 1st generation $IgG_{1-\kappa}$, mAb, containing murine light- and heavy-chain variable-region sequences and human constant region sequences
Ocrelizumab	CD20	Type I, 2nd generation, humanized fusion IgG_1, binding to different CD20 epitope than rituximab, enhanced ADCC, reduced CDC, enhanced affinity for FcγRIIIa RIIIa
Veltuzumab (IMMU-106, hA20)	CD20	Type I, 2nd generation, humanized IgG_1, binding to different CD20 epitope than rituximab, enhanced ADCC, reduced CDC, enhanced affinity for FcγRIIIa RIIIa
Ofatumumab (HuMax-CD20, (Arzerra)	CD20	Type I, 2nd generation, Human IgG_1, binding to different CD20 epitope, more effective at CDC than rituximab
GA-101 (RO5072759)	CD20	Type II, 3rdgeneration, humanized IgG_1, superior ADCC than rituximab and superior direct cell-killing ability
AME-133v (LY2469298)	CD20	Type I, 3rd generation, humanized fusion IgG_1, enhanced affinity for FcγRIIIa, superior ADCC
PRO131921	CD20	Type I, 3rd generation, humanized fusion IgG1, improved binding to FcγRIIIa, better ADCC, superior anti-tumor efficacy
TRU-015	CD20	SMIP derived humanized fusion protein, ADCC and apoptosis induction
Epratuzumab (hLL2)	CD22	Humanized $IgG_{1-\kappa}$, 90% to 95% of human origin , acting as an immunomodulatory agent, stimulating the CD22 molecule
Belimumab	BLyS	Fully human IgG_1 mAb that specifically binds and inhibits the biological activity of BLyS
Abatacept	B7-1 and B7-2	Recombinant fully humanized fusion protein, composed of the Extracellular domain of human CTLA-4 and a modified Fc part of IgG_1
Tocilizumab (ACTEMRA, MRA)	IL-6R	Recombinant, humanised monoclonal IgG_1 antihuman interleukin 6-receptor antibody
IDEC-131	CD40L	IDEC-131/E6040, humanized mAb against human CD154, comprising human γ_1 heavy chains and human κ light chains with complementarity-determining regions of murine mAb clone 24-31
BG9588	CD40L	Recombinant humanized anti-human CD40L mAb consists of the complementarity-determining regions of the murine monoclonal antibody 5c8 (anti-human CD40L antibody) with human variable-region framework residues and IgG_1 constant region

MoAb	Target	Antibody characteristics
Lucatumumab (HCD122, CHIR-0.12.12)	CD40	Human IgG_1 mAb that blocks CD40/CD40L interactions and inducesADCC
Dacetuzumab (SGN-40)	CD40	Humanized anti-CD40 IgG_1 mAb, which induces ADCC and apoptosis of B-cells
Eculizumab	Complementprotein C5	Recombinant humanized mAb binding to complement protein C5, inhibiting its enzymatic cleavage, blocking formation of the terminal complement complex

ADCC=antibody-dependent cellular cytotoxicity; BLyS=B-lymphocyte Stimulator; CDC=complement-dependent cytotoxicity; mAb= monoclonal antibody; SMIP=small modular immunopharmaceutical

Table 1. Monoclonal antibodies potentially useful in systemic lupus erythematosus

8. Conclusions

In recent years, clinical studies have been undertaken with selected mAbs in the treatment of SLE. The most frequently used mAb is rituximab, which is directed against CD20, a membrane protein expressed on B lymphocytes. Rituximab is effective in depleting B cells from peripheral blood, lymph nodes and bone marrow. Recent clinical studies confirm the high activity of rituximab in SLE patients, especially with lupus nephritis and neuropsychiatric involvement. Rituximab was generally well tolerated. However, occasionaly serious infections were reported. Over the last few years new generations of anti-CD20 mAbs have been developed for potential benefits over rituximab. They were engineered to have augmented antitumor activity by increasing CDC or ADCC activity and increased Fc binding affinity for the low-affinity variants of the FcγRIIIa receptor (CD16) on immune effector cells. This mAbs are are highly cytotoxic against B-cell lymphoid cells and are now being evaluated in clinical trials.

More recently, several newer mAbs have been developed and are being evaluated in phase I/II clinical trials. These include anti-cytokine therapies anti-CD40L mAbs, anti-CD-22 mAb, anti-BLys mAbs and anti- C5 mAbs. Belimumab is a fully human monoclonal antibody that binds to BLyS and inhibits its biological activity. Significantly positive results in both phase 3 studies have raised hopes that belimumab may be the long-awaited new effective therapy for SLE. Proinflammatory cytokines such as tumor necrosis factor (TNF) and interleukin- 6 (IL-6) play an important role in propagating the inflammatory process responsible for tissue damage. Blocking of these cytokines by mAbs can be also a successful therapy for patients with SLE. Finally, mAb eculizumab that specifically inhibits terminal complement activation has been recently developed and investigated in a phase I single dose study in SLE. These potentially useful agents should be further evaluated in well designed controlled trials.

9. Acknowledgements

This work was supported in part by the grants from the Medical University of Lodz (No 503-1093-1 and No No 503-1019-1). The authors have no conflicts of interest that are directly relevant to the content of this chapter.

10. References

Baker, K.P.; Edwards, B.M.; Main, S.H. et al. (2003) Generation and characterization of LymphoStat-B, a human monoclonal antibody that antagonizes the bioactivities of B lymphocyte stimulator. *Arthritis Rheum.,* Vol.48. No 11, pp. 3253-3265, ISSN 1044-2626

Bologna, L.; Gotti, E.; Manganini, M. et al. (2011). Mechanism of Action of Type II, Glycoengineered, Anti- CD20 Monoclonal Antibody GA101 in B-Chronic Lymphocytic Leukemia Whole Blood Assays in Comparison with Rituximab and Alemtuzumab. *J Immunol.,* Vol. 186, No. 6, pp. 3762-3769, ISSN 0022-1767

Boumpas, D.T.; Furie, R.; Manzi, S. et al. (2003). BG9588 Lupus Nephritis Trial Group. A short course of BG9588 (anti-CD40 ligand antibody) improves serologic activity and decreases hematuria in patients with proliferative lupus glomerulonephritis. *Arthritis Rheum.,* Vol. 48, No 3, pp. 719–727, ISSN 1044-2626

Burge, D.J.; Bookbinder, S.A.; Kivitz, A.J. et al. (2008). Pharmacokinetic and pharmacodynamic properties of TRU-015, a CD20-directed small modular immunopharmaceutical protein therapeutic, in patients with rheumatoid arthritis: a phase I, open-label, dose-escalation clinical study. *Clin Ther,* Vol. 30, No 10, pp. 1806-1816, ISSN 0149-2918

Cambridge, G.; Isenberg, D.A.; Edwards, J.C. et al. B cell depletion therapy in systemic lupus erythematosus: relationships among serum B lymphocyte stimulator levels, autoantibody profile and clinical response. *Ann Rheum Dis,.* Vol. 67, No. 7, pp. 1011-1016, ISSN 0003-4967

Cordeiro, A.C. & Isenberg, D.A. (2008). Novel therapies in lupus - focus on nephritis. *Acta Reumatol Port.,* Vol. 33, No. 2, pp. 157-169, ISSN 0303-464X

Czuczman, M.S. & Gregory SA. (2010). The future of CD20 monoclonal antibody therapy in B-cell malignancies. *Leuk Lymphoma.,* Vol. 51, No. 6, pp. 983-994, ISSN 1042-8194

Daridon, C.; Blassfeld, D. Reiter, K. et al. (2010). Epratuzumab targeting of CD22 affects adhesion molecule expression and migration of B-cells in systemic lupus erythematosus. *Arthritis Res Ther.,* Vol. 12, No. 6, pp. R204, ISSN 1478-6362

Davis, J.C. Jr.; Totoritis, MC.; Rosenberg, J. et al. (2001). Phase I clinical trial of a monoclonal antibody against CD40-ligand (IDEC-131) in patients with systemic lupus erythematosus.*J Rheumatol,* Vol. 28, No. 1, pp. 95-101, ISSN 0315-162X

Devi, B.S.; Van Noordin, S.; Krausz, T. & Davies, K.A. (1998). Peripheral blood lymphocytes in SLE—hyperexpression of CD154 on T and B lymphocytes and increased number of double negative T cells. *J Autoimmun.,* Vol. 11, No 5, pp. 471–475, ISSN 0896-8411

Dörner, T.; Kaufmann, J.; Wegener, W.A. et al. (2006). Initial clinical trial of epratuzumab (humanized anti-CD22 antibody) for immunotherapy of systemic lupus erythematosus. *Arthritis Res Ther.,* Vol. 8, No. 3, pp. R74, ISSN 1478-6362

Ermann, J.; Bermas, B.L. (2007). The biology behind the new therapies for SLE. *Int. J. Clin. Pract.,* Vol. 61, No. 12, pp. 2113-2119, ISSN 1368-5031

Faria, R.M. & Isenberg, DA. (2010). Three different B-cell depletion (anti-CD20 monoclonal antibodies) treatments for severe resistant systemic lupus erythematosus. *Lupus.,* Vol. 19, No. 10, pp. 1256-1257, ISSN 0961-2033

Furie, R.; Stohl, W.; Ginzler, E.M.; Becker, M.; Mishra, N.; Chatham, W.W, Merrill, J.T.; Weinstein, A.; McCune, W.J.; Zhong, J.; Cai, W.; Freimuth, W. (2008). Biologic activity and safety of belimumab, a neutralizing anti-B-lymphocyte stimulator (BLyS) monoclonal antibody: a phase I trial in patients with systemic lupus erythematosus. Study Group B. *Arthritis Res Ther.*, Vol 110, No 5, R109, ISSN 1478-6362

Genovese, M.C.; Kaine, J.L.; Lowenstein, M.B. et al. (2008). Ocrelizumab, a humanized anti-CD20 monoclonal antibody, in the treatment of patients with rheumatoid arthritis: a phase I/II randomized, blinded, placebo-controlled, dose-ranging study. *Arthritis Rheum*, Vol. 58, No 9, pp. 2652-2661, ISSN 1044-2626

Goldenberg, D.M.; Rossi, E.A., Stein, R. et al. (2009). Properties and structure-function relationships of veltuzumab (hA20), a humanized anti-CD20 monoclonal antibody. *Blood*, Vol. 113, No 5, pp. 1062-1070, ISSN 0006-4971

Grondal, G.; Gunnarsson, I.; Ronnelid, J. et al. (2000). Cytokine production, serum levels and disease activity in systemic lupus erythematosus. *Clin Exp Rheumatol,* Vol. 18, No 5, pp. 565–570, ISSN 0392-856X

Hayden-Ledbetter, M.S.; Cerveny, C.G.; Espling, E. et al. (2009). CD20-directed small modular immunopharmaceutical, TRU-015, depletes normal and malignant B cells. *Clin Cancer Res,* Vol. 15, No 8, pp. 2739-2746 , ISSN 1557-3265

Hauptrock, B.& Hess, G. (2009). Rituximab in the treatment of non-Hodgkin's lymphoma. *Biologics,* Vol. 2, No. 4, pp.619-633 , ISSN 1177-5491

Hillmen, P, Young NS, Schubert J, et al. (2006). The complement inhibitor eculizumab in paroxysmal nocturnal hemoglobinuria. *N Engl J Med.*, Vol. 355, No 12, pp. 1233-1243, ISSN 0028-4793

Illei, G.G; Shirota, Y.; Yarboro, C.H. et al. (2010). Tocilizumab in systemic lupus erythematosus: data on safety, preliminary efficacy, and impact on circulating plasma cells from an open-label phase I dosage-escalation study. *Arthritis Rheum.* Vol. 62, No. 2, pp. 542-552, ISSN 1044-2626

Jones, G. & Ding, C. (2010). Tocilizumab: a review of its safety and efficacy in rheumatoid arthritis. *Clin Med Insights Arthritis Musculoskelet Disord.,* Vol. 19, No. 3, pp. 81-89, ISSN 1179-5441

Jones, G.; Sebba, A.; Gu, J. et al. (2010). Comparison of TCZ monotherapy versus methotrexate monotherapy in patients with moderate to severe rheumatoid arthritis: The AMBITION study. *Ann Rheum Dis.* Vol. 69, No 1, pp. 88–96, ISSN 0003-4967

Kalled, S.L.; Cutler, A.H.; Ferrant, J.L. (2001). Long-term anti-CD154 dosing in nephritic mice is required to maintain survival and inhibit mediators of renal fibrosis. *Lupus,* Vol. 10, No 1, pp. 9–22, ISSN 0961-2033

Kalunian, K.C.; Davis, J.C. Jr.; Merrill, J.T. et al. (2002). IDEC-131 Lupus Study Group. Treatment of systemic lupus erythematosus by inhibition of T cell costimulation with anti-CD154: a randomized, double-blind, placebo-controlled trial. *Arthritis Rheum.,* Vol. 46, No 12, pp. 3251–3258, ISSN 1044-2626

Kausar, F.; Mustafa, K.; Sweis, G. et al. (2009). Ocrelizumab: a step forward in the evolution of B-cell therapy. *Expert Opin Biol Ther,* Vol. 9, No pp. 889-895, ISSN 1471-2598

Kelley, S.K.; Gelzleichter, T.; Xie, D. et al (2006). Preclinical pharmacokinetics, pharmacodynamics, and activity of a humanized anti-CD40 antibody (SGN-40) in rodents and non-human primates. *Br J Pharmacol* Vol. 148, No 8, pp. 1116-1123, ISSN 1476-5381

King, J.K. & Hahn, B.H. (2007). Systemic lupus erythematosus: modern strategies for management: a moving target. *Best Pract Res Clin Rheumatol,*. Vol. 21, No. 6, pp. 971-987, ISSN 1521-6942

Klashman, D.J.; Martin, R.A.; Martinez-Maza, O. & Stevens R.H. (1991). In vitro regulation of B cell differentiation by interleukin-6 and soluble CD23 in systemic lupus erythematosus B cell subpopulations and antigen-induced normal B cells. *Arthritis Rheum.*, Vol. 34, No. 3, pp. 276–286, ISSN 1044-2626

La Cava, A. (2010). Anticytokine therapies in systemic lupus erythematosus. *Immunotherapy,*. Vol. 2, No. 4, pp. 575-582.

La Cava, A. (2010). Targeting B cells with biologics in systemic lupus erythematosus. Expert Opinion *on Biological Therapy*, Vol. 10, No. 11, pp. 1555-1561, ISSN 1471-2598

Liang, B.; Gardner, D.B.; Griswold, D.E. et al. (2006). Anti-interleukin-6 monoclonal antibody inhibits autoimmune responses in a murine model of systemic lupus erythematosus. *Immunology,* Vol. 119, No 3, pp. 296–305, ISSN 0022-1767

Lim, S.H.; Beers, S.A.; French R.R. et al. (2010). Anti-CD20 monoclonal antibodies: historical and future perspectives. *Haematologica.,* Vol. 95, No 1, pp. 135-43, ISSN 0390-6078

Leandro, M.J.; Cambridge, G.; Edwards, J.C. et al. (2005). B-cell depletion in the treatment of patients with systemic lupus erythematosus: a longitudinal analysis of 24 patients. *Rheumatology,* Vol. 44, No. 12, pp. 1542-1545, ISSN 0315-162X

Leonard, J.P. & Goldenberg, D.M. (2007). Preclinical and clinical evaluation of epratuzumab (anti-CD22 IgG) in B-cell malignancies. *Oncogene,* Vol. 26, No. 25, pp. 3704-13, ISSN 0950-9232

Llorente, L.; Richaud-Patin, Y.; Garcia-Padilla, C. et al. (2000). Clinical and biologic effects of anti-interleukin-10 monoclonal antibody administration in systemic Lupus erythematosus. *Arthritis Rheum.* Vol. 43, No. 8, pp. 1790 - 1800, ISSN 1044-2626

Lu, T.Y.; Ng, K.P.; Cambridge, G. et al. (2009). A retrospective seven-year analysis of the use of B cell depletion therapy in systemic lupus erythematosus at University College London Hospital: the first fifty patients. *Arthritis Rheum,* Vol. 61, No.4, pp. 482-487, ISSN 1044-2626

Luqman, M.; Klabunde, S. Lin, K. et al (2008).The antileukemia activity of a human anti-CD40 antagonist antibody, HCD122, on human chronic lymphocytic leukemia cells. *Blood* , Vol. 112, No 3, pp. 711-720, ISSN 0006-4971

Merrill, J.T.; Burgos-Vargas, R., Westhovens, R. et al. (2010). The efficacy and safety of abatacept in patients with non-life-threatening manifestations of systemic lupus erythematosus: results of a twelve-month, multicenter, exploratory, phase IIb, randomized, double-blind, placebo-controlled trial. *Arthritis Rheum.* Vol.62, No.10, pp. 3077-3087, ISSN 1044-2626

Merrill, J.T.; Neuwelt, C.M.; Wallace, D.J. et al. (2010). Efficacy and safety of rituximab in moderately-to-severely active systemic lupus erythematosus: the randomized, double-blind, phase II/III systemic lupus erythematosus evaluation of rituximab trial. *Arthritis Rheum.*, Vol. 62, No. 1, pp. 222-233, ISSN 1044-2626

Molloy, E.S.& Calabrese, LH. (2008). Progressive multifocal leukoencephalopathy: a national estimate of frequency in systemic lupus erythematosus and other rheumatic diseases. *Arthritis Rheum.*, Vol. 60, No. 12, pp. 3761-5, ISSN 1044-2626

Morschhauser, F.; Leonard, J.P.; Fayad, L. et al. (2009). Humanized anti-CD20 antibody, veltuzumab, in refractory/recurrent non-Hodgkin's lymphoma: phase I/II results. *J Clin Oncol.* Vol. 27, No. 20, pp. 3346-3353, ISSN 0732-183X

Navarra, S.V.; Guzmán, R.M.; Gallacher, A.E. et al. BLISS-52 Study Group. (2011). Efficacy and safety of belimumab in patients with active systemic lupus erythematosus: a randomised, placebo-controlled, phase 3 trial. *Lancet.*, Vol. 377, No. 9767, pp. 721-731, ISSN 0140-6736

Ng, K.P.; Cambridge, G., Leandro, M.J. et al. (2007). B cell depletion therapy in systemic lupus erythematosus: long-term follow-up and predictors of response. *Ann Rheum Dis,.* Vol. 66, No. 9, pp. 1259-62, ISSN 0003-4967

Østergaard, M.; Baslund, B.; Rigby, W. et al. (2010). Ofatumumab, a human anti-CD20 monoclonal antibody, for treatment of rheumatoid arthritis with an inadequate response to one or more disease-modifying antirheumatic drugs: results of a randomized, double-blind, placebo-controlled, phase I/II study. *Arthritis Rheum.*, Vol. 62, No. 8, pp. 2227-2238, ISSN 1044-2626

Parker, C.J.; Kar, S. & Kirkpatrick, P. (2007). Eculizumab. *Nat. Rev. Drug Discov.* Vol. 6, No 7, pp. 515–625, ISSN 1474-1776

Pepper, R.; Griffith, M.; Kirwan, C. et al. (2009). Rituximab is an effective treatment for lupus nephritis and allows a reduction in maintenance steroids. *Nephrol Dial Transplant.*, Vol. 24, No. 12, pp. 3717-3723, ISSN 0931-0509

Ravirajan, C.T.; Wang, Y.; Matis, L.A. et al. (2004) Effect of neutralizing antibodies to IL-10 and C5 on the renal damage caused by a pathogenic human anti-ds DNA antibody. *Rheumatology.* Vol. 43, No 4, pp. 442–447. , ISSN 0315-162X

Robak, T. (2004). Monoclonal antibodies in the treatment of autoimmune cytopenias. *Eur J f Haematol.*, Vol. 72, No. 2, pp.79-88, ISSN 0902-4441

Robak, E.; Kulczycka, L.; Sysa-Jedrzejowska, A. et al. (2007). Circulating proangiogenic molecules PIGF, SDF-1 and sVCAM-1 in patients with systemic lupus erythematosus. *Eur Cytokine Netw.*, Vol. 18, No. 4, pp. 181-7, ISSN 1148-5493

Robak, T. (2008). Ofatumumab, a human monoclonal antibody for lymphoid malignancies and autoimmune disorders. *Curr Opin Mol Ther.*, Vol. 10, No. 3, pp. 294-309, ISSN 1355-6568

Robak, T. (2009). GA-101, a third-generation, humanized and glyco-engineered anti-CD20 mAb for the treatment of B-cell lymphoid malignancies. *Curr Opin Investig Drugs.*, Vol. 10, No. 6, pp. 588-596, ISSN 1472-4472

Robak, T.; Robak, P. & Smolewski P. (2009). TRU-016, a humanized anti-CD37 IgG fusion protein for the potential treatment of B-cell malignancies. *Curr Opin Investig Drugs*, Vol. 10, No pp. 1383-1390, ISSN 1472-4472

Robak, E. & Robak, T. (2009). Monoclonal antibodies in the treatment of systemic lupus erythematosus. *Curr Drug Targets,*, Vol. 10, No 1, pp. 26–37, ISSN 1389-4501

Robak, T & Robak, E. (2011). New anti-CD20 monoclonal antibodies for the treatment of B-cell lymphoid malignancies. *BioDrugs*, 2011 Vol. 25, No. 1, pp.13-25, ISSN 1173-8804

Rubbert-Roth, A. (2010). TRU-015, a fusion protein derived from an anti-CD20 antibody, for the treatment of rheumatoid arthritis. *Curr Opin Mol Ther.*, Vol. 12, No. 1, pp. 115-123, ISSN 1355-6568

Ruuls, S.R.; Lammerts van Bueren J.J.; van de Winkel J.G. et al. (2008). Novel human antibody therapeutics: the age of the Umabs. *Biotechnol J*, Vol. 3, No pp. 1157-1171, ISSN 0268-2575

Schröder, J.O. & Zeuner, R.A. (2009). Biologics as treatment for systemic lupus: great efforts, sobering results, new challenges. *Current Drug Discovery Technologies* , Vol.6, No. 4, pp. 252-255, ISSN 1570-1638

Sfikakis, P.P.; Boletis, J.N.; Lionaki, S. et al. (2005). Remission of proliferative lupus nephritis following B cell depletion therapy is preceded by down-regulation of the T cell costimulatory molecule CD40 ligand: an open-label trial. *Arthritis Rheum,*. Vol. 52, No. 2, pp. 501-513, ISSN 1044-2626

Smith, K.G.; Jones, R.B.; Burns, S.M. & Jayne, D.R. (2006). Long-term comparison of rituximab treatment for refractory systemic lupus erythematosus and vasculitis: Remission, relapse, and re-treatment. *Arthritis Rheum.*, Vol. 54, No. 9, pp. 2970-82, ISSN 1044-2626

St Clair, E.W. (2009). Novel targeted therapies for autoimmunity. *Curr Opin Immunol.* Vol. 21, No. 6, pp.648-657, ISSN 0952-7915

Terrier, B.; Amoura, Z.; Ravaud, P. et al. Club Rhumatismes et Inflammation. (2010). Safety and efficacy of rituximab in systemic lupus erythematosus: results from 136 patients from the French AutoImmunity and Rituximab registry. *Arthritis Rheum.*, Vol. 62, No. 8, pp. 2458-66 , ISSN 1044-2626

Tokunaga, M.; Saito, K.; Kawabata, D. et al. (2007). Efficacy of rituximab (anti-CD20) for refractory systemic lupus erythematosus involving the central nervous system. *Ann Rheum Dis.*, Vol. 66, No. 4, pp. 470-5, ISSN 0003- 4967

Toubi, E.; Kessel, A.; Rosner, I. et al. (2006). The reduction of serum B-lymphocyte activating factor levels following quinacrine add-on therapy in systemic lupus erythematosus. *Scand J Immunol.*, Vol. 63, No. 4, pp. 299-303, ISSN 0301-6323

van Kooten, C.; Banchereau, J. (2000). CD40-CD40 ligand. *J Leukoc Biol* ,Vol. 6, pp. 2-17, ISSN 0741-5400

Wallace, D.J.; Stohl, W.; Furie, R.A. et al. (2009). A phase II, randomized, double-blind, placebo-controlled, dose-ranging study of belimumab in patients with active systemic lupus erythematosus. *Arthritis Rheum.*, Vol. 61, No 9, pp. 1168–1178, ISSN 1044-2626

Wiglesworth, A.K.; Ennis, K.M. & Kockler, D.R. (2010). Belimumab: a BLyS-specific inhibitor for systemic lupus erythematosus. *Ann Pharmacother.*, Vol. 44, No.12, pp. 1955-61, ISSN 1060-0280

Willems, M.; Haddad, E.; Niaudet, P.; Koné-Paut, I. et al. French Pediatric-Onset SLE Study Group. (2006). Rituximab therapy for childhood-onset systemic lupus erythematosus. *J Pediatr.*, Vol. 148, No. 5, pp. 623-627, ISSN 0271-6798

Yap, DY.; Lai, KN. (2010). Cytokines and their roles in the pathogenesis of systemic lupus erythematosus: from basics to recent advances. *J Biomed Biotechnol,* 2010:365083. Epub 2010 May 6. ISSN 1110-7243.

9

Role of Fatty Acids in the Resolution of Autoimmune and Inflammatory Diseases

Elena Puertollano, María A. Puertollano,
Gerardo Álvarez de Cienfuegos and Manuel A. de Pablo
University of Jaén, Faculty of Experimental Sciences, Div. of Microbiology Jaén
Spain

1. Introduction

The main role of fatty acids is focused on serving as major substrates for energy production; however, fatty acids are also involved in the formation of cellular structures as well as in the transmission of cellular signals. Among the multiple functions attributed to fatty acids are their anti-inflammatory properties. This important characteristic has been applied in the prevention, attenuation or treatment of inflammatory disorders. Based on the previous argument is obvious that several fatty acids (mainly *n*-3 polyunsaturated or *n*-9 monounsaturated fatty acids) are capable of modulating immune system functions. These fatty acids may alter immune response through different mechanisms such as alteration of membrane fluidity, eicosanoid synthesis, oxidative stress, regulation of gene expression, apoptosis or modulation of gastrointestinal microbiota.

Early studies in Greenland Eskimos determined the low prevalence of inflammatory disorders in this population (Kromann et al., 1980). Despite their beneficial effects in the reduction of inflammatory diseases, other studies have demonstrated that the administration of diets containing long-chain *n*-3 polyunsaturated fatty acids may contribute, at least in part, to the reduction of host resistance against infectious agents. In fact, epidemiological investigations described a high incidence of tuberculosis in native Eskimos (Kaplan et al., 1972), who consume a great amount of *n*-3 polyunsaturated fatty acids. These data are clearly illustrative of the potential action of certain fatty acids on the inflammatory response, and of the consequences derived from an excessive immunosuppression.

It is obvious that these fatty acids contained in the diets produce an immune status able to ameliorate inflammatory conditions. Indeed, a growing number of studies using healthy human subjects as well as animal disease models have undoubtedly demonstrated dietary fish oil or olive oil to possess anti-inflammatory properties. For this reason, polyunsaturated or monounsaturated fatty acids have showed beneficial effects in numerous inflammatory diseases characterized by a overactivation of immune system such as asthma (childhood and adult), multiple sclerosis, glomerulonephritis, inflammatory bowel disease (Crohn's disease, ulcerative colitis) and rheumatoid arthritis . Here, we summarize the involvement of fatty acids as anti-inflammatory agents and the action that these fatty acids contained in the human or animal diets exert on the prevention or treatment of autoimmune diseases.

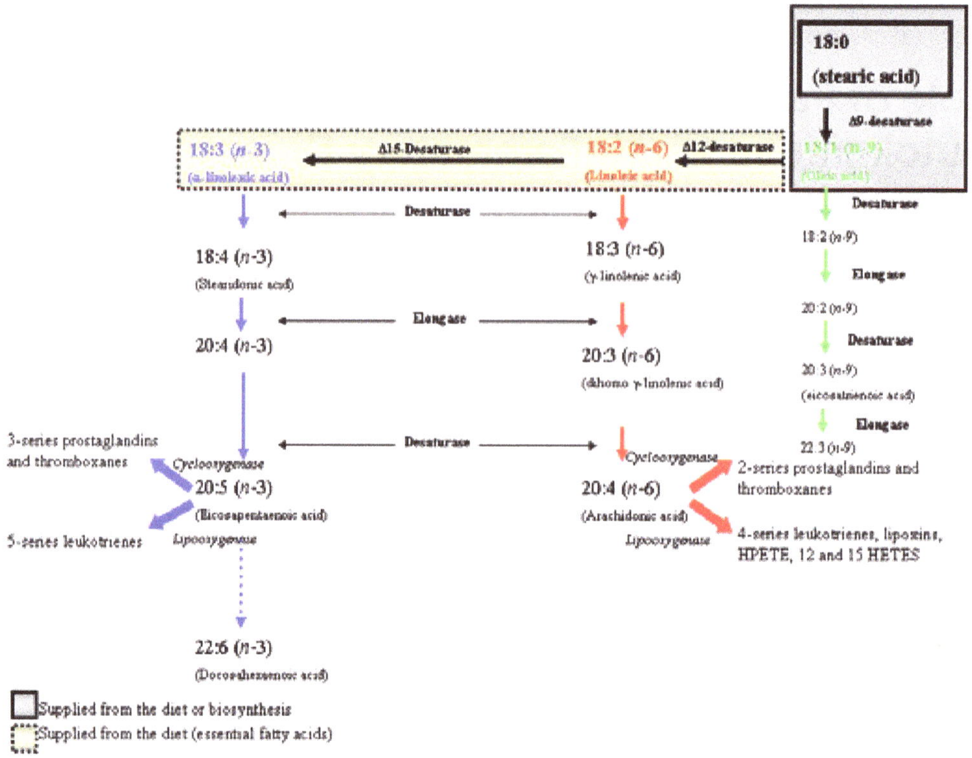

Fig. 1. Different pathways of n-3, n-6 and n-9 fatty acids synthesis. HETEs, hydroxyl-eicosatetraenoic acid; HPETE, hydroperoxy-eicosatetraenoic acids. (Puertollano *et al.*)

2. Fatty acids, inflammation and immune system

Polyunsaturated fatty acids (PUFA) are considered essentials to mammalian cells and should be administered in the diet. These essential fatty acids are divided into two great families: *n-3* series derived from linolenic acid (LNA), and *n-6* series derived from linoleic (LA) acid. Different biochemical processes lead to the production of eicosapentanoic acid (EPA) or docohexaenoic acid (DHA) from LNA, as well as arachidonic acid (AA) from linoleic acid. Likewise, another family of non essential fatty acids such as *n-9* series derived from oleic acid, a monounsaturated fatty acid (MUFA), also seems to play an important role in the immunomodulatory process (Yaqoob, 2002) [Figure 1].

In recent years numerous investigations have examined the mechanisms of action responsible for the modulation of immune system by fatty acids and most of them are in agreement that unsaturated fatty acids are potent immunosupressor especially *n-3* PUFA (reviewed in Puertollano et al., 2008). The main mechanisms of action of fatty acids are schematized in figure 2 and include alterations of immune cells membrane fluidity, eicosanoids synthesis modifications, oxidative alteration, regulation of gene expression and apoptosis mechanisms inducement. Table 1 summarized these mechanisms of actions and others recently proposed such as modulation of gastrointestinal microbiota.

All of these mechanisms of action deal to explain the numerous effects of fatty acids on immune system. It is well known that unsaturated fatty acids are involved on the alteration of lymphocyte proliferation. In general, administration of high level of fatty acids, and especially *n-3* series, are related with a reduction on lymphocyte proliferation in both animals and human studies (Meydani et al., 1991; Yaqoob et al., 1994; Moussa et al., 2000). This fact can be especially interesting in the amelioration of diseases characterized by overactivation of immune response like autoimmune disorder. In addition fatty acids can modify another lymphocyte functions like cytokine production.

- Eicosanoids production
- Membrane fluidity and lipid rafts
- Oxidative stress
- Signaling transduction
- Gene expression
- Apoptosis
- Ability in antigen presentation
- Modulation of gastrointestinal microbiota

Table 1. Hypothetical mechanisms of dietary lipids on immune functions: factors determining the modulation of immune system.

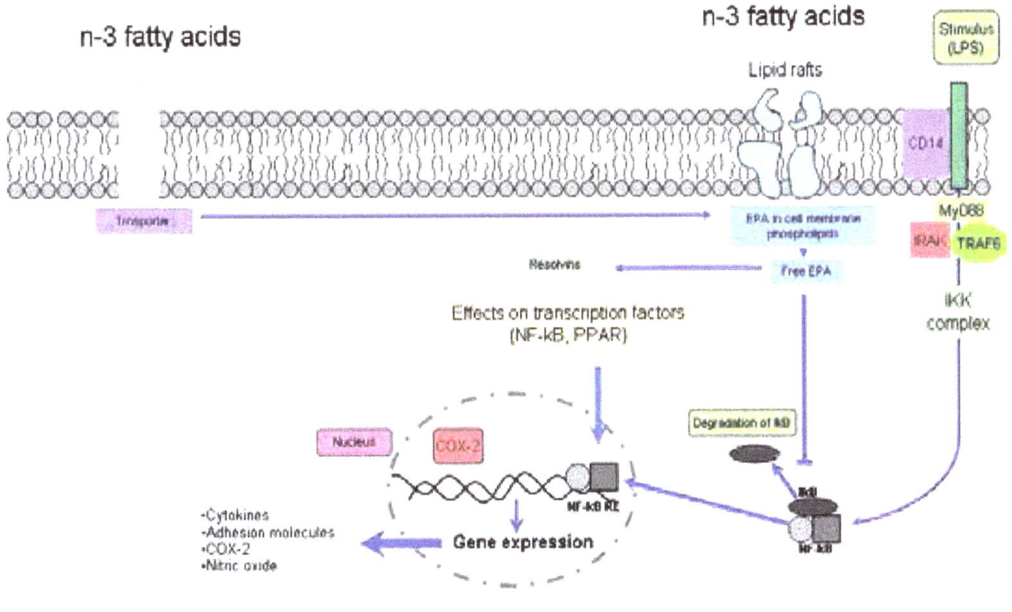

Fig. 2. Schematic diagram of proposed mechanisms of action of *n-3* polyunsaturated fatty acids whereby these fatty acids are involved in the modulation of immune system functions. Abbreviations: CD14, CD14 surface receptor; COX, cyclooxygenase; EPA, eicosapentaenoic acid, IκB, NF-κB inhibitory protein; LPS, lipopolysaccharide; NF-κB, nuclear factor-κB; PPAR, peroxisome proliferator-activated receptor; TLR, Toll-like receptors. (Puertollano *et al.*)

Several studies have demonstrated the immunomodulatory properties of polyunsaturated and monounsaturated fatty acids over reduction of pro and anti-inflammatory cytokines.

In this context interesting investigations indicates that *n-3* PUFA exert a significant inhibition of Th1-type cytokines, whereas they have little effects on Th2-type cytokines (Wallace et al., 2001). In spite of olive oil diets are involved in the reduction of cytokine secretion, their immunosupressant effects are not as potent as those exerted by the administration of a fish oil diet (Puertollano et al., 2004). Fatty acids are able to modify the natural killer (NK) cells activity too. Finally recent studies have proved the action of fatty acids in the expression of adhesion molecules like lymphocyte function antigen-1 (LFA-1) and intercellular adhesion molecule-1 (ICAM-1) (Sanderson et al., 1995; Miles et al., 2001). These facts have been shown in preliminary studies in animal models but it is necessary to confirm it in human studies.

2.1 Dietary lipids and inflammatory response

Inflammation is part of immune response and is a complex process affected by different factors, included mediators generated from fatty acids. Eicosanoids from *n-6* series fatty acids (like prostaglandine E_2 (PGE_2) and leukotriene B_4 (LTB_4) among others) are considered pro-inflammatory mediators while molecules from *n-3* series (like PGE_3 and LTB_5) generally are endowed with lower bioactivity. It is necessary to keep an optimal *n-6*/*n-3* balance to achieve a healthy inflammatory state.

Numerous researches have demonstrated that fish oil rich diet promotes a decrease on inflammatory ecoisanoids production from *n-6* PUFA because of the competition between the two metabolic pathways. In this way *n-3* PUFA supplementation of the human diet is able to decrease production of inflammatory eicosanoids like PGE_2, LTB_4 and thromboxane B_2 (TXB_2) by inflammatory cells (Meydani et al., 1991; Kelley et al., 1999; Trebble et al., 2003; Rees et al., 2006). In addition *n-3* PUFA have other effects over inflammatory response. One of the most important is the generation of resolvins, a group of mediators derived from EPA and DHA that appear to exert potent anti-inflammatory actions (Calder, 2008a). Decreasing antigen presentation via major histocompatibility complex class II (MHC II), inhibiting T-cell reactivity and diminishing inflammatory cytokine production (Calder et al., 2002; Akhtar Khan, 2010; Kim et al., 2010) are others of the anti-inflammatory effects of *n-3* fatty acids. Autoimmunity can be considered as an exacerbated inflammatory response against self structures; therefore *n-3* long chain fatty acids can be useful in the treatment of these diseases.

Oleic acid is the main fatty acid contained in olive oil. Olive oil has traditionally been used as a placebo in the studies investigating the potential action of other dietary lipids on the modulation of immune functions. Thus, MUFA that constitute olive oil were initially considered as neutral fatty acids. Nevertheless different studies demonstrated that olive oil is clearly involved in anti-inflammatory activities and in the modulation of immune response (reviewed in Puertollano et al., 2010). The anti-inflammatory activity of olive oil appears to be associated with the production of the metabolite eicosatrienoic acid from oleic acid (20:3 *n-9*), which is a potent inhibitor of LTB_4 (James et al., 1993). In addition it is possible that beneficial effects of olive oil may be in part due to the presence of natural antioxidants, contributing to an increase in the stability of oil (Linos et al., 1999).

Taken together there is evidence that both *n-3* PUFA and *n-9* MUFA can be useful in treatment of inflammatory disorders associated with autoimmune disease. Table 2 summarizes a list of some of the diseases and conditions with an inflammatory component that could be beneficially affected by *n- 3* and *n-9* series fatty acids.

- Acute cardiovascular events
- Acute respiratory distress syndrome
- Allergic disease
- Asthma (childhood and adult)
- Atherosclerosis
- Cancer cachexia
- Chronic obstructive pulmonary disease
- Cystic fibrosis
- Inflammatory bowel disease (Crohn's disease, ulcerative colitis)
- Lupus
- Multiple sclerosis
- Neurodegenerative disease of ageing
- Obesity
- Psoriasis
- Rheumatoid arthritis
- Systemic inflammatory response to surgery, trauma and critical illness
- Type 1 diabetes
- Type 2 diabetes

Table 2. Inflammatory disorder where fatty acids could be useful. Diseases are listed in an alphabetical order (Adapted from Calder, 2006).

3. Fatty acids and autoimmune disorders

Autoimmunity is the failure of an organism to recognize its own constituent parts as self, which results in immune responses against its own cells and tissues. Autoimmunity involves an inflammatory response against own tissues which are implicated different mechanisms like autoantibodies production, immunocomplex formation and lymphocytes T reactivity. Recently, an important investigation about the implication of fatty acids and dietary lipids in the amelioration of autoimmune diseases has been carried out because of their anti-inflammatory properties (Linos et al., 1999). Below we will summarize the main autoimmune disorder where fatty acids have shown to exert beneficial effects.

3.1 Fatty acids and inflammatory bowel disease

Inflammatory bowel disease (IBD) includes Cronh´s disease and ulcerative colitis which are autoimmune disorders characterized by an exacerbated inflammatory response against innocuous stimulus in gastrointestinal tract. Their pathogenesis is considered to include disorders of the immunomodulation of the bowel mucosa which results in lesions of the epithelium tissue layer caused by activated T cells, mononuclear cells and macrophages. In Crohn's disease the mucosa of the whole alimentary tract from the mouth to the anus can be affected, with maximal manifestation in the ileum and colon, while in ulcerative colitis the mucosa of the colon is mainly affected. In both diseases inflammatory cytokines and eicosanoids like LTB_4 are actively produced in situ (Sharon et al., 1984).

The gastrointestinal system is subjected to sustained exposure to ingested foods throughout the whole life, and this gives rise to interactions between food components and gastrointestinal mucosal cells. Interactions with transporters and transcription factors contribute to the modulation of various responses, including those of cells involved in inflammatory processes. There are, however, specific chronic diseases of the alimentary tract that are based on inflammatory processes and hence are bound to be susceptible to modulation by dietary FA.

3.1.1 Role of dietary lipids on animal models of IBD

Several studies with animal models of IBD, especially chemical induced colitis, have been developed after the recognition of anti-inflammatory properties of *n*-3 PUFA. Generally researches show that fish oil rich diet are involved in the amelioration of the disease comparing with *n-6* fatty acid oil rich diet. In this way different studies have demonstrated convincingly the reduction on colonic damage and ulceration (Vilaseca et al., 1990; Yuceyar et al., 1999), reduction in cell recruitment and activation (Andoh et al., 2003; Whiting et al., 2005) decreasing levels of LTB_4 and PGE_2 on plasma and gut mucosa (Shoda et al., 1995; Nieto et al., 2002; Hudert et al., 2006) and reduction of pro-inflammatory cytokines (Andoh et al., 2003) in animals fed with *n-3* PUFA rich diet.
The effects of fatty acids on an animal model of Cronh's disease have been proved too. Lately Matsunaga et al. have reported for the first time that *n-3* fatty acids ameliorate the ileum inflammation in a murine model of spontaneous and chronic ileitis that closely resembles human Cronh's disease. Specifically these authors have shown that *n-3* fatty acids diets are capable to decrease the ileum inflammation markers, cells recruitment and infiltration and pro-inflammatory mediators like monocyte chemoattractant protein-1(MCP-1) and IL-6 (Matsunaga et al., 2009).
A number of investigators have studied the effect of olive oil rich diet on animals models of IBD too. In this way Camuesco et al. have reported a lower colonic inflammatory response in rats fed with olive oil-based diet and this anti-inflammatory effect is increased when the olive oil diet is supplemented with a 4% of fish oil (Camuesco et al., 2005). Another study has described a beneficial effect of extra virgin olive oil in colitis associated colon carcinogenesis. A reduction on colonic inflammation, proinflammatory cytokines and less incident and multiplicity of tumours have been reported in rats fed with extra virgin olive oil versus sunflower oil (Sanchez-Fidalgo et al., 2010).
Generally animal models have shown a beneficial effect of *n-3* and *n-9* fatty acids in the development of IBD.

3.1.2 Trials in human patients

The established role of AA derived eicsanoids in pathophysiology of inflammatory bowel diet, and especially and inadequate *n*-6/*n*-3 balance, may play an important role in establishing and perpetuating of the disease. Indeed, multivariate analysis suggested that the recently increased consumption of *n*–6 FA in Japan, resulting in an increased ratio of *n*–6 to *n*–3 PUFA and possibly also elevated AA levels, may be responsible for the increased incidence of Crohn's disease in this country (Shoda et al., 1996).
In recent years some pilot studies have been carried out to analyze the effects of fish oil on IBD patients (reviewed by Calder, 2008a). A number of several randomized, placebo-controlled, double-blind studies on the effects of fish oil (2.7–5.6 g/d) in IBD have reported benefits, including improved clinical scores, mucosal histology, sigmoidoscopic score and lower rates of relapse. In this way an interesting study reported a decreased incidence of relapses in patients with Crohn's disease in remission who received a supplemented of enterically coated fish oil for 1 year; there was a significant reduction in the proportion of

relapse on fish oil group, 28%, compared with placebo group, 69%, over 12 months. In addition this difference was maintained at 12 months, with an incidence of remission of 59% in fish oil group versus 26% in placebo group (Belluzzi et al., 1996). However another studies have not found beneficial effects of *n-3* fatty acids supplementation in IBD patients (Loeschke et al., 1996; Lorenz-Meyer et al., 1996).

Studies about the effect of olive oil in IBD patients are limited and most of them used the olive oil as a placebo because *n-9* MUFA was considered as a neutral fat. Although preliminary studies of Dr. Gassull research group had demonstrated that *n-9* MUFA might be beneficial inducing remission of Crohn's disease (Gonzalez-Huix et al., 1993; Fernandez-Banares et al., 1994). The first multicentre, randomized and double-blind trial to evaluate the influence of fat composition in enteral nutrition have not been successful. Nevertheless the results are not conclusive because of the small sample size (smaller than was initially estimated). The study was prematurely finished and the source of oleic acid used in this trial was synthetic trioleate and not olive oil as in the other studies (Gonzalez-Huix et al., 1993). Olive oil contains polyphenols, another components with a potent antioxidant activity and this fact may contribute to different effects of vegetables oil and even though olive oil and *n-9* MUFA (Owen et al., 2000).

Studies in which olive oil have been used as a placebo have reported contradictory results. Lorenz et al. have shown an increased activity of disease in patients of ulcerative colitis and Crohn's disease supplemented with olive oil as a placebo versus fish oil group (Lorenz et al., 1989; Romano et al., 2005). However others authors have not founds differences between both groups of supplementation (Greenfield et al., 1993; Trebble et al., 2005).

In spite of several favourable studies about the use of fatty acids, and specially fish oil, in the treatment of IBD the evidence of clinical benefits are limited. The soundest result was the potential of *n-3* PUFA to maintain the patients of Crohn's disease in remission (Belluzzi et al., 1996). However, this observation was not confirmed in a recent larger study using a similar protocol (Feagan et al., 2008). One reason why dietary lipids might be more effective in animal models than in human patients is the different dose of assay. In human trials the dose of fatty acids are lower compared with the dose in animals studies (higher compared with habitual human consumption doses).

3.2 Fatty acids and rheumatoid arthritis

Rheumatoid arthritis is a chronic inflammatory autoimmune disease that affects about 1% of adult population and is more frequent in women than men. Rheumatoid arthritis is characterized by joint inflammation, swelling, pain, impaired function, stiffness, osteoporosis, muscle wasting, and the participation of inflammatory cells (macrophages, T lymphocytes, plasma cells infiltrating the synovium). All the mediators of inflammation (cytokines, interleukins and typical pro-inflammatory factors and proteins) are actively produced by synovial cells. COX-2 is over-expressed in the synovium of patients, and its eicosanoid products, in addition to those of the 5-LOX, are found in the synovial fluids (Sano et al., 1992; Sperling, 1995). In addition rheumatoid arthritis is also characterised by signs of systemic inflammation, such as elevated plasma concentrations of some cytokines (e.g. IL-6), acute-phase proteins and rheumatoid factors. The relevance of the pro-inflammatory COX pathway is also underlined by the efficacy of the pharmacological inhibition of this pathway (e.g. by non steroidal anti-inflammatory drugs).

There is evidence that rheumatoid arthritis is less severe in Mediterranean countries where consume of fish oil, fruits and vegetables and olive oil are higher than in other countries (Pattison et al., 2004). This report, joint to the special relevance of COX pathway on the development of the disease, has brought about a great number of studies where the role of dietary lipids in the management of rheumatoid arthritis has been evaluated.

3.2.1 Some studies with animal models

Interest in the use of *n-3* fatty acids in rheumatoid arthritis began in the mid-eighties, following the demonstration in several autoimmune strains of mice that *n-3* fatty acids reduced the severity of diffuse proliferative glomerulonephritis (Simopoulos, 2002). Further studies have shown the efficacy of fish oil in the development of the animal disease. For instance in an early study Leslie et al. shown that fish oil increased the time of onset of arthritis and decreased the incidence and severity of this disease in a murine model of type II collagen-induced arthritis(Leslie et al., 1985). Another researchers have reported a mouse model of rheumatoid arthritis fed with fish oil and have shown a significantly lower serum levels of interleukins IL-6, IL-10, IL-12 and in tumour necrosis factor-α (TNF-α), PGE_2, TXB_2 and LTB_4 compared with levels in mice fed corn oil (Venkatraman et al., 1999). Similarly, EPA and DHA incorporation into macrophage phospholipids via oral administration resulted in a reduction of streptococcal cell wall arthritis in Lew/SSN rats (Volker et al., 2000).

On the other hand it is well known that rheumatoid arthritis is characterized by joint and tissue damage and this damage occurs by a variety of mechanisms, many of which involve reactive oxygen species (ROS). ROS can cause destruction of hyaluronic acid and disruption to collagen, proteoglycans, protease inhibitors, and membrane function, the latter via oxidation of membrane fatty acids. The initiation of rheumatoid arthritis is believed to result in an increase in the concentration of macrophages and neutrophils in the synovial fluid and free-radical-producing enzymes. This leads to high levels of ROS in the joints, which increases and prolongs inflammation and damage (Darlington et al., 2001). Olive oil, and especially extra virgin olive oil, is rich in antioxidants compounds. Taking account the role of ROS in joint and tissue damage on development of rheumatoid arthritis, the effect of olive oil can be especially useful in this kind of disease. Indeed Martinez-Dominguez et al. have shown the efficacy of an olive oil supplemented with polyphenols in animal models of arthritis (Martinez-Dominguez et al., 2001).

3.2.2 Efficacy of fatty acids on human disease

During the 80s and 90s several studies in patients with rheumatoid arthritis showed the beneficial effects of *n-3* PUFA on the development of the disease. Several authors reported that fish oils reduces the production of inflammatory mediators like LTB 4 by neutrophils and monocytes (Kremer et al., 1985; Kremer et al., 1987; Cleland et al., 1988; Tulleken et al., 1990; van der Tempel et al., 1990) and IL-1β by monocytes (Kremer et al., 1990). There is also evidence of reduction in the plasma concentrations of IL-1 (Espersen et al., 1992)and C-reactive protein (Kremer et al., 1985), and normalized neutrophil function (Sperling et al., 1987).

A number of randomized, placebo-controlled, double-blind studies of fish oil treatments have been reported. In different reviews Calder have summarized the results of studies with a dose of fatty acids between 1.6 and 7.1 g/d (average of 3.5 g/day EPA + DHA) and almost of them reported some benefit (Calder, 2006; Calder, 2008b; Galli et al., 2009). Clinical symptoms were improved, including reduced duration of morning stiffness, number of tender or swollen joints, joint pain, time of fatigue and increased grip strength. Particular relevance has the reduction of the use of anti-inflammatory drugs.

n-3 PUFA may act as anti-inflammatory agents by competition whit AA for incorporation in the eicosanoid pathway. This efficacy of *n-3* PUFA may be achieved in rheumatoid arthritis by simultaneously decreasing of *n*-6 PUFA intake, especially AA. Indeed Adam et al. have shown that a diet supplemented with *n*-3-PUFA and AA restricted is able to ameliorate clinical signs of inflammation like tenders and swollen joints and to decrease the formation of eicosanoids such as leukotrienes and prostaglandins (Adam et al., 2003). This study shows also that intakes of preformed AA, in addition to formation from the precursor LA, may be a factor in the modulation of AA levels in the body, and since LA and AA are provided by quite different sources (seed oils vs. lean meat), this should be taken into consideration in the evaluation of strategies for optimal *n-3* FA intakes.

Several reviews about the role of fish oil in rheumatoid arthritis patients have been carried out and most of them conclude that there was strong evidence about benefits of *n-3* PUFA on the management of this disease (Cleland et al., 2000). These reviews have shown that fish oil is able to improve the signs of the disease like number and severity of tender joint, number of swollen joints, physician and patients´ global assessment and use of anti-inflammatory drugs among others effect (Simopoulos, 2002; Stulnig, 2003; Calder, 2006; Calder, 2008a; Galli et al., 2009). Indeed an editorial comment about the use of fish oil in this disease concluded that dietary fish oil supplements should be regarded as part of a standard therapy for rheumatoid arthritis (Cleland et al., 2000).

With reference to olive oil a study by Linos et al. (Linos et al., 1991) has suggested that a beneficial anti-inflammatory effect of olive oil consumption on rheumatoid arthritis may be possible. In fact, this study compared the relative risk of development of rheumatoid arthritis in relation to lifelong consumption of olive oil in a Greek population and demonstrated that high consumers of olive oil (almost every day throughout life) had four times less risk than those who consumed olive oil less than six times per month on average throughout their lives; by contrast the effect of fish consumption was also tested without statistically significant findings (Linos et al., 1991).

A number of studies that examined the benefits of fish oil in rheumatoid arthritis used an olive oil placebo for the control groups. Kremer et al. evaluated the effect of fish oil supplementation on the progression and severity of the disease using olive oil as a placebo. Unexpectedly clinical evaluation and immunologic test showed similar results in both groups. No explanation of the improvements showed by the olive oil groups was given, although changes in immune function may be responsible (Kremer et al., 1990). A more recent research has reported an improvement in beneficial effect of fish oil when is mixed together olive oil versus a supplementation with only fish oil , suggesting a positive action of olive oil in signs and symptoms of rheumatoid arthritis (Berbert et al., 2005).

Taking together all these results and facts revised in this section, it can be concluded that there are strong evidences to justify the positive effects of fish oil in the management of rheumatoid arthritis. On the other hand, although the results are still preliminary, combination of olive oil and fish oil may be more favorable because of the antioxidant effect of olive oil joint to the anti-inflammatory potential of both oils.

3.3 Fatty acids in systemic lupus erythematosus

Systemic lupus erythematosus (SLE) is a complex autoimmune disease with heterogeneous clinical manifestations and disease course and most of cases occurring in women of childrenbering age. It is characterized by the deregulated innate and adaptive immune pathways and the development of anti-nuclear antibodies (ANA). Mortality of patients with SLE is significatly correlated wiht development of glomerulonephritis. Binding of autoantibodies, specially IgG anti-DNA, and immunecomplex depositions within the kidneys recruits leukocytes and this infiltration results in an inflammatory response that can lead to irreparale renal parenchymal damage (Pestka, 2010).

3.3.1 Studies with animal models

Several studies with animal models of SLE have been carried out about the role of dietary lipids in the development of the disease and generally most of them concluded a beneficial effect of fish oil (reviewed in Pestka, 2010).

Early studies of Prickett and his research group showed that administration of fish oil to young mice induced a reduction on severity and incidence of renal disease and increased the lifespan of NZB/NZW mice (Prickett et al., 1981; Prickett et al., 1982; Prickett et al., 1983), even fish oil was able to reduce the progression of established renal damage in another mouse model of lupus (Robinson et al., 1986). Other studies have reported a link between increased lifespan and reduced renal damage and reductions of anti-DNA autoantibodies and circulating immunocomplexes in NZB/NZW (Alexander et al., 1987).

Subsequently several studies have demonstrated that the amelioration of disease in these animal models were linked with the action of fish oil over eicosanoids metabolism (Kelley et al., 1985; Spurney et al., 1994; Venkatraman et al., 1999).

Results from Fernandes laboratory have reported that DHA, but not EPA, is the most potent *n-3* fatty acid that suppresses glomerulonephritis and extends life span of systemic lupus erythematosus-prone NZB/NZW mice (Halade et al., 2010). In addition the same authors have proved that the beneficial action of fish oil in lupus animal models is increased by caloric restriction (Jolly et al., 1999; Jolly et al., 2001).

3.3.2 Clinical trials

Numerous studies have evaluated the possible beneficial action of fish oil in lupus patients although the results are not so conclusive like animal studies. Indeed two early clinical trials suggested that fish oil supplementation has little value in management of lupus nephritis when it is compared with olive oil (Westberg et al., 1990; Clark et al., 1993). However two double blind studies have reported a benefit in disease criteria and lupus score (Walton et al., 1991; Duffy et al., 2004). More recently investigations have shown that fish oil, and more specifically EPA, may be useful in the amelioration of lupus disease because of the decreasing oxidative stress, improving endothelial functions and conferring cardiovascular benefits (Nakamura et al., 2005; Wright et al., 2008).

In view of the previous reports we can conclude that, in spite of fish oil supplementation may be useful in the amelioration of lupus and prevention of renal disease, new and larger investigations must be carried out to clarify the role of fatty acids in development of this disease.

3.4 Fatty acids and multiple sclerosis

Multiple sclerosis (MS) is a Central Nervous System-specific demyelinating disease and is the most common neurological disorder that occurs in young adults. Although the aetiology of MS remains unknown there is strong evidence for the presence of autoimmune mechanisms in the disease pathogenesis. Pro-inflammatory cytokines from activated T cells and macrophages have been strongly implicated in the pathogenesis of MS, like the up-regulation of adhesion molecules on endothelial cells and the subsequent infiltration of activated T cells into the Central Nervous System.

An association between dietary fat intake and the incidence of multiple sclerosis was first proposed by Swank in 1950 (Swank, 1950). Some epidemiological studies have been carried out later and the most of them indicate that diets rich in saturated fatty acids are detrimentally associated with MS, while PUFA acid rich diets are beneficially associated with MS. Studies from Harbige laboratory have shown that the relationship between linoleic acid (*n-6*) and dihomo-g-linoleic acid (DGLA), and also between DGLA (*n-6*) and AA is clearly disturbed in MS compared with healthy controls. This may indicate a problem with δ6 and δ5 desaturation and / or a greater requirement for these *n-6* fatty acids in many of the MS patients (Harbige et al., 2007).

3.4.1 Fatty acids in animal models of multiple sclerosis

Experimental autoimmune encephalomyelitis (EAE) is an experimentally induced CD4+ T cell mediated autoimmune inflammatory and demyelinating disease in rodents often used as a useful animal model of MS.

Administration of PUFA can reduce the clinical severity of EAE. Indeed LA supplementation has been shown to reduce the severity of EAE in guinea pigs when it is administered before EAE induction (Meade et al., 1978; Hughes et al., 1980). Harbige et al. also demonstrated that gamma linoleic acid (GLA) supplementation could reduce the severity of both acute EAE and the relapsing phases of chronic. Further analysis revealed an increase in production of transforming growth factor β-1 and PGE_2, both associated with a reduction in the inflammatory response in EAE models (Harbige et al., 1995; Harbige et al., 1997; Harbige et al., 2000).

3.4.2 Clinical trials in human patients

Following the preliminary epidemiological studies by Swank, several researches have attempted the role of PUFA in the development of MS. In this way Millar et al. carried out a double-blind study with LA and olive oil during 24 months. These authors reported an improvement in relapse severity and nonsignificant trends towards lower relapse rates but no difference in disability (Millar et al., 1973). Later, Paty et al. did not find such effects in a similar trial with higher doses of oleic acid as a placebo (Paty et al., 1978). No conclusive data have been found in other trials realized with GLA in combination with LNA (Bates et al., 1977).

However more recently Harbige et al. have reported a randomised double-blind placebo controlled trial to determine the effects of supplementation with selected GLA rich borage oil. Data proved that high dose of this oil reduced the relapse rate and disability progression as measured by EDSS (Expanded Disability Status Scale) and compared with a placebo of polyethylene glycol and with low dose of the same oil (Harbige et al., 2007). Although these data are very positive, the number of patients enrolled in the trial is limited (n=36) and no conclusive statements can be made.

The fish oil action in MS has been investigated too but some studies have not been successful. Two double blind controlled clinical trials have been carried out to evaluate the effect of fish oil in the disease without significant findings. In these trials olive oil was used as a placebo again and although nonsignificant trends, toward less disability and certain improvements in quality of life, have been found the results are inconclusive (Bates et al., 1989; Weinstock-Guttman et al., 2005). However others researchers have found beneficial effects of fish oil in MS patients. Shinto et al. have reported that *n-3* fatty acids supplementation significantly decreased matrix metalloproteinase-9 (MMP-9) levels in relapsing-remitting MS. This enzyme is thought to have a significant role in the transmigration of inflammatory cells into the central nervous system by aiding in the disruption of the blood brain barrier. In this way the ability of *n-3* fatty acids to decrease the levels secreted by immune cells may be a significant observation in spite of significant changes in quality of life have not been found (Shinto et al., 2009).

Taken over all epidemiological data, animal data and clinical trial we can confirm that PUFA, particularly *n-6* fatty acids, have a role in the pathogenesis and treatment of multiple sclerosis. However different factors must be better controlled in the clinical trials to achieve convincing results, like trials design, sample size and the choice of an appropriate placebo. This last item is of a great important because of olive oil has been used as a placebo in most of the reviewed clinical trials, however experience of our laboratory and others clearly proved the great immunomodulator potential of this fat, usually considered relatively inert (Puertollano et al., 2004; Puertollano et al., 2010). In this way olive oil may be acting in immune system of MS patients and no significant different with *n-3* and *n-6* PUFA can be found.

3.5 Action of dietary lipids in type 1 diabetes mellitus

Type 1 diabetes mellitus (T1DM) is an autoimmune disease characterized by the destruction of insulin-producing beta cells in the pancreatic islets. Dietary factors have been implicated in the aetiology of type 1 diabetes as well as in initiating the autoimmune process that leads to clinical disease. Macrophages and T cells, attracted to the islets, secrete soluble mediators such as oxygen free radicals, nitric oxide (NO), and the cytokines IL-1ß, interferon (IFN)-γ and TNF-α. Increasing evidence suggests that these mediators induce apoptosis, the main mode of ß-cell death in the development of T1DM. Fatty acids, because of their properties as anti-inflamatory compounds as well as cell apoptosis modulators, may be useful in the management of T1DM.

3.5.1 Findings from studies in animal models of type 1 diabetes

Earlier investigations suggested that deficiency of essential fatty acids, including *n-6* and *n-3* PUFA, caused a resistance in development of the diabetes in certain animal models (Lefkowith et al., 1990; Wright et al., 1995).

However, in 2001 Krishna Mohan & Das carried out a study to evaluate the effect of supplementation of various PUFA-rich oils on the incidence of alloxan-induced diabetes in experimental animals (Krishna Mohan et al., 2001). These authors have reported that *n-3* and *n-6* fatty acids may prevent alloxan-induced diabetes in experimental animals administered before of the diabetogenic agent and this preventive action may reside in their ability to enhance antioxidant status, suppress cytokine production, and activate PPARs. These researchers have evaluated also the effect of estearic saturated FA, oleic MUFA and *n-6* AA PUFA in the same model finding that only AA was effective (Suresh et al., 2006).

Recently others authors have evaluated the efficacy of a right balance *n-6/n-3* PUFA in diet of T1DM model NOD mice finding that low *n-6/n-3* ratio delays the onset of diabetes

(Kagohashi et al., 2010b). Other studies from the same laboratory have shown that the most effective strategy in prevention of the disease in the offspring is an adequate dose of *n-6/n-3* PUFA in maternal diet during gestation and lactation (Kagohashi et al., 2010a).

3.5.2 Trials with type 1 diabetes mellitus patients

In 2003 an interesting pilot case-study was carried out in Norway to the attempt to test the hypothesis that cod liver oil, taken either by the mother during pregnancy or by the child during the first year of life, is associated with a lower risk of type 1 diabetes among children. A significant association between the use of cod liver oil during the first year of life and a lower risk of type 1 diabetes was found (Stene et al., 2003). In a similar way, an observational longitudinal study was carried out in U.S.A., the Diabetes Autoimmunity Study in the Young (DAISY). During 13 years a total of 1770 children at increased risk for type 1 diabetes were sudied. Th results revealed that dietary intake of *n-3* fatty acids is associated with reduced risk of islet autoimmunity in children at increased genetic risk for type 1 diabetes. This association is further substantiated by the pilot observation of a higher proportion of *n*-3 PUFA in the erythrocyte membranes (Norris et al., 2007). However the same authors later reported that there was a lack of association between *n-3* PUFA intake and conversion to type 1 diabetes in children with islet autoimmunity (Miller et al., 2011).

In spite of certain positive data in animal models and human patients nowadays we can not confirm a justification for the use of fatty acids in preventing the development of type 1 diabetes mellitus.

4. Conclusions

In the recent years the immunonutrition area has advanced significantly to elucidate the role of the diet in development and function of immune system and to prevent or ameliorate numerous diseases in which immune system is implicated like infections, cancer, inflammatory disease, allergies and autoimmune disorders. Among the diet components, fatty acids (PUFA in particular), are especially interesting by their immunomodulator and anti-inflammatory role.

Autoimmune disorders are a complex group of disease characterized by an exacerbated immune response against self structures and an elevated inflammatory state. Several investigations have shown that fatty acids and especially *n-3* PUFA act as potent anti-inflammatory molecules and even induce a strong immunosupression. For this reason, the use of fatty acids has been considered a good a therapeutic strategy in prevention and treatment of these diseases.

In spite of convincing data from the several studies with animal model, clinical trials have not achieved similar results. Only clear evidence in management of rheumatoid arthritis and in remission maintenance in Crohn's disease patients justifies the use of fish oil, and perhaps in combination with olive oil. However results from studies with other diseases like ulcerative colitis, lupus and multiple sclerosis are promising. Future studies with a better control of placebo, number of enrolled patients and design are necessary to justify of use of fatty acids in this type of immune disorders.

Finally epidemiological studies report that Mediterranean countries with a traditionall diet rich in fruits and vegetables, fish oil and olive oil and poor in saturated fats, have lower levels of inflammatory disease than countries with other type of diet. In the same way countries like Japan with changes in the habitual diet to "western diet" have increased rates of inflammatory disease. In our opinion the best strategy recommending to population in general, and autoimmune disease patients in particular, is the maintenance of a healthy diet rich in naturals antioxidants (fruit, vegetables, olive oil), moderate consumption of fats and a well balanced of *n-6/n-3* fatty acids.

5. Acknowledgements

To Dr. José Manuel Martínez Martos and Dr. Mª Jesús Ramírez Expósito , from University of Jaén, Div. of Phisiology, for their assistance with the manuscript.

6. References

Adam, O., Beringer, C., Kless, T., Lemmen, C., Adam, A., Wiseman, M., Adam, P., Klimmek, R. & Forth, W. (2003). Anti-inflammatory effects of a low arachidonic acid diet and fish oil in patients with rheumatoid arthritis. *Rheumatology international,* Vol 23, No.1, pp 27-36, ISSN/ISBN 0172-8172; 0172-8172.

Akhtar Khan, N. (2010). Polyunsaturated fatty acids in the modulation of T-cell signalling. *Prostaglandins, leukotrienes, and essential fatty acids,* Vol 82, No.4-6, pp 179-187, ISSN/ISBN 1532-2823; 0952-3278.

Alexander, N.J., Smythe, N.L. & Jokinen, M.P. (1987). The type of dietary fat affects the severity of autoimmune disease in NZB/NZW mice. *The American journal of pathology,* Vol 127, No.1, pp 106-121, ISSN/ISBN 0002-9440; 0002-9440.

Andoh, A., Tsujikawa, T., Ishizuka, I., Araki, Y., Sasaki, M., Koyama, S. & Fujiyama, Y. (2003). N-3 fatty acid-rich diet prevents early response of interleukin-6 elevation in trinitrobenzene sulfonic acid-induced enteritis. *International journal of molecular medicine,* Vol 12, No.5, pp 721-725, ISSN/ISBN 1107-3756; 1107-3756.

Bates, D., Cartlidge, N.E., French, J.M., Jackson, M.J., Nightingale, S., Shaw, D.A., Smith, S., Woo, E., Hawkins, S.A. & Millar, J.H. (1989). A double-blind controlled trial of long chain n-3 polyunsaturated fatty acids in the treatment of multiple sclerosis. *Journal of neurology, neurosurgery, and psychiatry,* Vol 52, No.1, pp 18-22, ISSN/ISBN 0022-3050; 0022-3050.

Bates, D., Fawcett, P.R., Shaw, D.A. & Weightman, D. (1977). Trail of polyunsaturated fatty acids in non-relapsing multiple sclerosis. *British medical journal,* Vol 2, No.6092, pp 932-933, ISSN/ISBN 0007-1447; 0007-1447.

Belluzzi, A., Brignola, C., Campieri, M., Pera, A., Boschi, S. & Miglioli, M. (1996). Effect of an enteric-coated fish-oil preparation on relapses in Crohn's disease. *The New England journal of medicine,* Vol 334, No.24, pp 1557-1560, ISSN/ISBN 0028-4793; 0028-4793.

Berbert, A.A., Kondo, C.R., Almendra, C.L., Matsuo, T. & Dichi, I. (2005). Supplementation of fish oil and olive oil in patients with rheumatoid arthritis. *Nutrition (Burbank, Los Angeles County, Calif.),* Vol 21, No.2, pp 131-136, ISSN/ISBN 0899-9007; 0899-9007.

Calder, P.C. (2008a). Polyunsaturated fatty acids, inflammatory processes and inflammatory bowel diseases. *Molecular nutrition & food research,* Vol 52, No.8, pp 885-897, ISSN/ISBN 1613-4133; 1613-4125.

Calder, P.C. (2008b). Session 3: Joint Nutrition Society and Irish Nutrition and Dietetic Institute Symposium on 'Nutrition and autoimmune disease' PUFA, inflammatory processes and rheumatoid arthritis. *The Proceedings of the Nutrition Society,* Vol 67, No.4, pp 409-418, ISSN/ISBN 0029-6651; 0029-6651.

Calder, P.C. (2006). N-3 Polyunsaturated Fatty Acids, Inflammation, and Inflammatory Diseases. *The American Journal of Clinical Nutrition,* Vol 83, No.6 Suppl, pp 1505S-1519S, ISSN/ISBN 0002-9165; 0002-9165.

Calder, P.C., Yaqoob, P., Thies, F., Wallace, F.A. & Miles, E.A. (2002). Fatty acids and lymphocyte functions. *The British journal of nutrition,* Vol 87 Suppl 1, pp S31-48, ISSN/ISBN 0007-1145; 0007-1145.

Camuesco, D., Galvez, J., Nieto, A., Comalada, M., Rodriguez-Cabezas, M.E., Concha, A., Xaus, J. & Zarzuelo, A. (2005). Dietary olive oil supplemented with fish oil, rich in EPA and DHA (n-3) polyunsaturated fatty acids, attenuates colonic inflammation in rats with DSS-induced colitis. *The Journal of nutrition,* Vol 135, No.4, pp 687-694, ISSN/ISBN 0022-3166; 0022-3166.

Clark, W.F., Parbtani, A., Naylor, C.D., Levinton, C.M., Muirhead, N., Spanner, E., Huff, M.W., Philbrick, D.J. & Holub, B.J. (1993). Fish oil in lupus nephritis: clinical findings and methodological implications. *Kidney international,* Vol 44, No.1, pp 75-86, ISSN/ISBN 0085-2538; 0085-2538.

Cleland, L.G. & James, M.J. (2000). Fish oil and rheumatoid arthritis: antiinflammatory and collateral health benefits. *The Journal of rheumatology,* Vol 27, No.10, pp 2305-2307, ISSN/ISBN 0315-162X; 0315-162X.

Cleland, L.G., French, J.K., Betts, W.H., Murphy, G.A. & Elliott, M.J. (1988). Clinical and biochemical effects of dietary fish oil supplements in rheumatoid arthritis. *The Journal of rheumatology,* Vol 15, No.10, pp 1471-1475, ISSN/ISBN 0315-162X; 0315-162X.

Darlington, L.G. & Stone, T.W. (2001). Antioxidants and fatty acids in the amelioration of rheumatoid arthritis and related disorders. *The British journal of nutrition,* Vol 85, No.3, pp 251-269, ISSN/ISBN 0007-1145; 0007-1145.

Duffy, E.M., Meenagh, G.K., McMillan, S.A., Strain, J.J., Hannigan, B.M. & Bell, A.L. (2004). The clinical effect of dietary supplementation with omega-3 fish oils and/or copper in systemic lupus erythematosus. *The Journal of rheumatology,* Vol 31, No.8, pp 1551-1556, ISSN/ISBN 0315-162X; 0315-162X.

Espersen, G.T., Grunnet, N., Lervang, H.H., Nielsen, G.L., Thomsen, B.S., Faarvang, K.L., Dyerberg, J. & Ernst, E. (1992). Decreased interleukin-1 beta levels in plasma from rheumatoid arthritis patients after dietary supplementation with n-3 polyunsaturated fatty acids. *Clinical rheumatology,* Vol 11, No.3, pp 393-395, ISSN/ISBN 0770-3198; 0770-3198.

Feagan, B.G., Sandborn, W.J., Mittmann, U., Bar-Meir, S., D'Haens, G., Bradette, M., Cohen, A., Dallaire, C., Ponich, T.P., McDonald, J.W., Hebuterne, X., Pare, P., Klvana, P., Niv, Y., Ardizzone, S., Alexeeva, O., Rostom, A., Kiudelis, G., Spleiss, J., Gilgen, D., Vandervoort, M.K., Wong, C.J., Zou, G.Y., Donner, A. & Rutgeerts, P. (2008). Omega-3 free fatty acids for the maintenance of remission in Crohn disease: the EPIC Randomized Controlled Trials. *JAMA : the journal of the American Medical Association,* Vol 299, No.14, pp 1690-1697, ISSN/ISBN 1538-3598; 0098-7484.

Fernandez-Banares, F., Cabre, E., Gonzalez-Huix, F. & Gassull, M.A. (1994). Enteral nutrition as primary therapy in Crohn's disease. *Gut,* Vol 35, No.1 Suppl, pp S55-9, ISSN/ISBN 0017-5749; 0017-5749.

Galli, C. & Calder, P.C. (2009). Effects of fat and fatty acid intake on inflammatory and immune responses: a critical review. *Annals of Nutrition & Metabolism,* Vol 55, No.1-3, pp 123-139, ISSN/ISBN 1421-9697; 0250-6807.

Gonzalez-Huix, F., de Leon, R., Fernandez-Banares, F., Esteve, M., Cabre, E., Acero, D., Abad-Lacruz, A., Figa, M., Guilera, M. & Planas, R. (1993). Polymeric enteral diets as primary treatment of active Crohn's disease: a prospective steroid controlled trial. *Gut,* Vol 34, No.6, pp 778-782, ISSN/ISBN 0017-5749; 0017-5749.

Greenfield, S.M., Green, A.T., Teare, J.P., Jenkins, A.P., Punchard, N.A., Ainley, C.C. & Thompson, R.P. (1993). A randomized controlled study of evening primrose oil and fish oil in ulcerative colitis. *Alimentary Pharmacology & Therapeutics,* Vol 7, No.2, pp 159-166, ISSN/ISBN 0269-2813; 0269-2813.

Halade, G.V., Rahman, M.M., Bhattacharya, A., Barnes, J.L., Chandrasekar, B. & Fernandes, G. (2010). Docosahexaenoic acid-enriched fish oil attenuates kidney disease and prolongs median and maximal life span of autoimmune lupus-prone mice. *Journal of immunology (Baltimore, Md.: 1950),* Vol 184, No.9, pp 5280-5286, ISSN/ISBN 1550-6606; 0022-1767.

Harbige, L.S. & Sharief, M.K. (2007). Polyunsaturated fatty acids in the pathogenesis and treatment of multiple sclerosis. *The British journal of nutrition,* Vol 98 Suppl 1, pp S46-53, ISSN/ISBN 0007-1145; 0007-1145.

Harbige, L.S., Layward, L., Morris-Downes, M.M., Dumonde, D.C. & Amor, S. (2000). The protective effects of omega-6 fatty acids in experimental autoimmune encephalomyelitis (EAE) in relation to transforming growth factor-beta 1 (TGF-beta1) up-regulation and increased prostaglandin E2 (PGE2) production. *Clinical and experimental immunology,* Vol 122, No.3, pp 445-452, ISSN/ISBN 0009-9104; 0009-9104.

Harbige, L.S., Layward, L., Morris, M. & Amor, S. (1997). Protective mechanisms by omega-6 lipids in experimental autoimmune encephalomyelitis (EAE) are associated with cytokines and eicosanoids. *Biochemical Society transactions,* Vol 25, No.2, pp 342S, ISSN/ISBN 0300-5127; 0300-5127.

Harbige, L.S., Yeatman, N., Amor, S. & Crawford, M.A. (1995). Prevention of experimental autoimmune encephalomyelitis in Lewis rats by a novel fungal source of gamma-linolenic acid. *The British journal of nutrition,* Vol 74, No.5, pp 701-715, ISSN/ISBN 0007-1145; 0007-1145.

Hudert, C.A., Weylandt, K.H., Lu, Y., Wang, J., Hong, S., Dignass, A., Serhan, C.N. & Kang, J.X. (2006). Transgenic mice rich in endogenous omega-3 fatty acids are protected from colitis. *Proceedings of the National Academy of Sciences of the United States of America,* Vol 103, No.30, pp 11276-11281, ISSN/ISBN 0027-8424; 0027-8424.

Hughes, D., Keith, A.B., Mertin, J. & Caspary, E.A. (1980). Linoleic acid therapy in severe experimental allergic encephalomyelitis in the guinea-pig: suppression by continuous treatment. *Clinical and experimental immunology,* Vol 40, No.3, pp 523-531, ISSN/ISBN 0009-9104; 0009-9104.

James, M.J., Gibson, R.A., Neumann, M.A. & Cleland, L.G. (1993). Effect of dietary supplementation with n-9 eicosatrienoic acid on leukotriene B4 synthesis in rats: a novel approach to inhibition of eicosanoid synthesis. *The Journal of experimental medicine*, Vol 178, No.6, pp 2261-2265, ISSN/ISBN 0022-1007; 0022-1007.

Jolly, C.A., Muthukumar, A., Avula, C.P., Troyer, D. & Fernandes, G. (2001). Life span is prolonged in food-restricted autoimmune-prone (NZB x NZW)F(1) mice fed a diet enriched with (n-3) fatty acids. *The Journal of nutrition*, Vol 131, No.10, pp 2753-2760, ISSN/ISBN 0022-3166; 0022-3166.

Jolly, C.A. & Fernandes, G. (1999). Diet modulates Th-1 and Th-2 cytokine production in the peripheral blood of lupus-prone mice. *Journal of clinical immunology*, Vol 19, No.3, pp 172-178, ISSN/ISBN 0271-9142; 0271-9142.

Kagohashi, Y., Abiru, N., Kobayashi, M., Hashimoto, M., Shido, O. & Otani, H. (2010a). Maternal dietary n-6/n-3 fatty acid ratio affects type 1 diabetes development in the offspring of non-obese diabetic mice. *Congenital anomalies*, Vol 50, No.4, pp 212-220, ISSN/ISBN 1741-4520; 0914-3505.

Kagohashi, Y. & Otani, H. (2010b). Diet with a low n-6/n-3 essential fatty acid ratio when started immediately after the onset of overt diabetes prolongs survival of type 1 diabetes model NOD mice. *Congenital anomalies*, Vol 50, No.4, pp 226-231, ISSN/ISBN 1741-4520; 0914-3505.

Kaplan, G.J., Fraser, R.I. & Comstock, G.W. (1972). Tuberculosis in Alaska, 1970. The continued decline of the tuberculosis epidemic. *The American Review of Respiratory Disease*, Vol 105, No.6, pp 920-926, ISSN/ISBN 0003-0805; 0003-0805.

Kelley, D.S., Taylor, P.C., Nelson, G.J., Schmidt, P.C., Ferretti, A., Erickson, K.L., Yu, R., Chandra, R.K. & Mackey, B.E. (1999). Docosahexaenoic acid ingestion inhibits natural killer cell activity and production of inflammatory mediators in young healthy men. *Lipids*, Vol 34, No.4, pp 317-324, ISSN/ISBN 0024-4201; 0024-4201.

Kelley, V.E., Ferretti, A., Izui, S. & Strom, T.B. (1985). A fish oil diet rich in eicosapentaenoic acid reduces cyclooxygenase metabolites, and suppresses lupus in MRL-lpr mice. *Journal of immunology (Baltimore, Md.: 1950)*, Vol 134, No.3, pp 1914-1919, ISSN/ISBN 0022-1767; 0022-1767.

Kim, W., Khan, N.A., McMurray, D.N., Prior, I.A., Wang, N. & Chapkin, R.S. (2010). Regulatory activity of polyunsaturated fatty acids in T-cell signaling. *Progress in lipid research*, Vol 49, No.3, pp 250-261, ISSN/ISBN 1873-2194; 0163-7827.

Kremer, J.M., Lawrence, D.A., Jubiz, W., DiGiacomo, R., Rynes, R., Bartholomew, L.E. & Sherman, M. (1990). Dietary fish oil and olive oil supplementation in patients with rheumatoid arthritis. Clinical and immunologic effects. *Arthritis and Rheumatism*, Vol 33, No.6, pp 810-820, ISSN/ISBN 0004-3591; 0004-3591.

Kremer, J.M., Jubiz, W., Michalek, A., Rynes, R.I., Bartholomew, L.E., Bigaouette, J., Timchalk, M., Beeler, D. & Lininger, L. (1987). Fish-oil fatty acid supplementation in active rheumatoid arthritis. A double-blinded, controlled, crossover study. *Annals of Internal Medicine*, Vol 106, No.4, pp 497-503, ISSN/ISBN 0003-4819; 0003-4819.

Kremer, J.M., Bigauoette, J., Michalek, A.V., Timchalk, M.A., Lininger, L., Rynes, R.I., Huyck, C., Zieminski, J. & Bartholomew, L.E. (1985). Effects of manipulation of dietary fatty acids on clinical manifestations of rheumatoid arthritis. *Lancet,* Vol 1, No.8422, pp 184-187, ISSN/ISBN 0140-6736; 0140-6736.

Krishna Mohan, I. & Das, U.N. (2001). Prevention of chemically induced diabetes mellitus in experimental animals by polyunsaturated fatty acids. *Nutrition (Burbank, Los Angeles County, Calif.),* Vol 17, No.2, pp 126-151, ISSN/ISBN 0899-9007; 0899-9007.

Kromann, N. & Green, A. (1980). Epidemiological studies in the Upernavik district, Greenland. Incidence of some chronic diseases 1950-1974. *Acta Medica Scandinavica,* Vol 208, No.5, pp 401-406, ISSN/ISBN 0001-6101; 0001-6101.

Lefkowith, J., Schreiner, G., Cormier, J., Handler, E.S., Driscoll, H.K., Greiner, D., Mordes, J.P. & Rossini, A.A. (1990). Prevention of diabetes in the BB rat by essential fatty acid deficiency. Relationship between physiological and biochemical changes. *The Journal of experimental medicine,* Vol 171, No.3, pp 729-743, ISSN/ISBN 0022-1007; 0022-1007.

Leslie, C.A., Gonnerman, W.A., Ullman, M.D., Hayes, K.C., Franzblau, C. & Cathcart, E.S. (1985). Dietary fish oil modulates macrophage fatty acids and decreases arthritis susceptibility in mice. *The Journal of experimental medicine,* Vol 162, No.4, pp 1336-1349, ISSN/ISBN 0022-1007; 0022-1007.

Linos, A., Kaklamani, V.G., Kaklamani, E., Koumantaki, Y., Giziaki, E., Papazoglou, S. & Mantzoros, C.S. (1999). Dietary factors in relation to rheumatoid arthritis: a role for olive oil and cooked vegetables? *The American Journal of Clinical Nutrition,* Vol 70, No.6, pp 1077-1082, ISSN/ISBN 0002-9165; 0002-9165.

Linos, A., Kaklamanis, E., Kontomerkos, A., Koumantaki, Y., Gazi, S., Vaiopoulos, G., Tsokos, G.C. & Kaklamanis, P. (1991). The effect of olive oil and fish consumption on rheumatoid arthritis--a case control study. *Scandinavian journal of rheumatology,* Vol 20, No.6, pp 419-426, ISSN/ISBN 0300-9742; 0300-9742.

Loeschke, K., Ueberschaer, B., Pietsch, A., Gruber, E., Ewe, K., Wiebecke, B., Heldwein, W. & Lorenz, R. (1996). N-3 Fatty Acids Only Delay Early Relapse of Ulcerative Colitis in Remission. *Digestive diseases and sciences,* Vol 41, No.10, pp 2087-2094, ISSN/ISBN 0163-2116; 0163-2116.

Lorenz, R., Weber, P.C., Szimnau, P., Heldwein, W., Strasser, T. & Loeschke, K. (1989). Supplementation with n-3 fatty acids from fish oil in chronic inflammatory bowel disease--a randomized, placebo-controlled, double-blind cross-over trial. *Journal of internal medicine.Supplement,* Vol 731, pp 225-232, ISSN/ISBN 0955-7873; 0955-7873.

Lorenz-Meyer, H., Bauer, P., Nicolay, C., Schulz, B., Purrmann, J., Fleig, W.E., Scheurlen, C., Koop, I., Pudel, V. & Carr, L. (1996). Omega-3 fatty acids and low carbohydrate diet for maintenance of remission in Crohn's disease. A randomized controlled multicenter trial. Study Group Members (German Crohn's Disease Study Group). *Scandinavian journal of gastroenterology,* Vol 31, No.8, pp 778-785, ISSN/ISBN 0036-5521; 0036-5521.

Martinez-Dominguez, E., de la Puerta, R. & Ruiz-Gutierrez, V. (2001). Protective effects upon experimental inflammation models of a polyphenol-supplemented virgin olive oil diet. *Inflammation research : official journal of the European Histamine Research Society ...[et al.],* Vol 50, No.2, pp 102-106, ISSN/ISBN 1023-3830; 1023-3830.

Matsunaga, H., Hokari, R., Kurihara, C., Okada, Y., Takebayashi, K., Okudaira, K., Watanabe, C., Komoto, S., Nakamura, M., Tsuzuki, Y., Kawaguchi, A., Nagao, S. & Miura, S. (2009). Omega-3 polyunsaturated fatty acids ameliorate the severity of ileitis in the senescence accelerated mice (SAM)P1/Yit mice model. *Clinical and experimental immunology,* Vol 158, No.3, pp 325-333, ISSN/ISBN 1365-2249; 0009-9104.

Meade, C.J., Mertin, J., Sheena, J. & Hunt, R. (1978). Reduction by linoleic acid of the severity of experimental allergic encephalomyelitis in the guinea pig. *Journal of the neurological sciences,* Vol 35, No.2-3, pp 291-308, ISSN/ISBN 0022-510X; 0022-510X.

Meydani, S.N., Endres, S., Woods, M.M., Goldin, B.R., Soo, C., Morrill-Labrode, A., Dinarello, C.A. & Gorbach, S.L. (1991). Oral (n-3) fatty acid supplementation suppresses cytokine production and lymphocyte proliferation: comparison between young and older women. *The Journal of nutrition,* Vol 121, No.4, pp 547-555, ISSN/ISBN 0022-3166; 0022-3166.

Miles, E.A., Thies, F., Wallace, F.A., Powell, J.R., Hurst, T.L., Newsholme, E.A. & Calder, P.C. (2001). Influence of age and dietary fish oil on plasma soluble adhesion molecule concentrations. *Clinical science (London, England : 1979),* Vol 100, No.1, pp 91-100, ISSN/ISBN 0143-5221; 0143-5221.

Millar, J.H., Zilkha, K.J., Langman, M.J., Wright, H.P., Smith, A.D., Belin, J. & Thompson, R.H. (1973). Double-blind trial of linoleate supplementation of the diet in multiple sclerosis. *British medical journal,* Vol 1, No.5856, pp 765-768, ISSN/ISBN 0007-1447; 0007-1447.

Miller, M.R., Yin, X., Seifert, J., Clare-Salzler, M., Eisenbarth, G.S., Rewers, M. & Norris, J.M. (2011). Erythrocyte membrane omega-3 fatty acid levels and omega-3 fatty acid intake are not associated with conversion to type 1 diabetes in children with islet autoimmunity: The Diabetes Autoimmunity Study in the Young (DAISY). *Pediatric diabetes,* ISSN/ISBN 1399-5448; 1399-543X.

Moussa, M., Le Boucher, J., Garcia, J., Tkaczuk, J., Ragab, J., Dutot, G., Ohayon, E., Ghisolfi, J. & Thouvenot, J.P. (2000). In vivo effects of olive oil-based lipid emulsion on lymphocyte activation in rats. *Clinical nutrition (Edinburgh, Scotland),* Vol 19, No.1, pp 49-54, ISSN/ISBN 0261-5614; 0261-5614.

Nakamura, N., Kumasaka, R., Osawa, H., Yamabe, H., Shirato, K., Fujita, T., Murakami, R., Shimada, M., Nakamura, M., Okumura, K., Hamazaki, K. & Hamazaki, T. (2005). Effects of eicosapentaenoic acids on oxidative stress and plasma fatty acid composition in patients with lupus nephritis. *In vivo (Athens, Greece),* Vol 19, No.5, pp 879-882, ISSN/ISBN 0258-851X; 0258-851X.

Nieto, N., Torres, M.I., Rios, A. & Gil, A. (2002). Dietary polyunsaturated fatty acids improve histological and biochemical alterations in rats with experimental ulcerative colitis. *The Journal of nutrition,* Vol 132, No.1, pp 11-19, ISSN/ISBN 0022-3166; 0022-3166.

Norris, J.M., Yin, X., Lamb, M.M., Barriga, K., Seifert, J., Hoffman, M., Orton, H.D., Baron, A.E., Clare-Salzler, M., Chase, H.P., Szabo, N.J., Erlich, H., Eisenbarth, G.S. & Rewers, M. (2007). Omega-3 polyunsaturated fatty acid intake and islet autoimmunity in children at increased risk for type 1 diabetes. *JAMA : the journal of the American Medical Association,* Vol 298, No.12, pp 1420-1428, ISSN/ISBN 1538-3598; 0098-7484.

Owen, R.W., Mier, W., Giacosa, A., Hull, W.E., Spiegelhalder, B. & Bartsch, H. (2000). Phenolic compounds and squalene in olive oils: the concentration and antioxidant potential of total phenols, simple phenols, secoiridoids, lignansand squalene. *Food and chemical toxicology : an international journal published for the British Industrial Biological Research Association,* Vol 38, No.8, pp 647-659, ISSN/ISBN 0278-6915; 0278-6915.

Pattison, D.J., Symmons, D.P. & Young, A. (2004). Does diet have a role in the aetiology of rheumatoid arthritis? *The Proceedings of the Nutrition Society,* Vol 63, No.1, pp 137-143, ISSN/ISBN 0029-6651; 0029-6651.

Paty, D.W., Cousin, H.K., Read, S. & Adlakha, K. (1978). Linoleic acid in multiple sclerosis: failure to show any therapeutic benefit. *Acta Neurologica Scandinavica,* Vol 58, No.1, pp 53-58, ISSN/ISBN 0001-6314; 0001-6314.

Pestka, J.J. (2010). N-3 Polyunsaturated Fatty Acids and Autoimmune-Mediated Glomerulonephritis. *Prostaglandins, leukotrienes, and essential fatty acids,* Vol 82, No.4-6, pp 251-258, ISSN/ISBN 1532-2823; 0952-3278.

Prickett, J.D., Robinson, D.R. & Steinberg, A.D. (1983). Effects of dietary enrichment with eicosapentaenoic acid upon autoimmune nephritis in female NZB X NZW/F1 mice. *Arthritis and Rheumatism,* Vol 26, No.2, pp 133-139, ISSN/ISBN 0004-3591; 0004-3591.

Prickett, J.D., Robinson, D.R. & Steinberg, A.D. (1982). A diet enriched with eicosapentaenoic acid suppresses autoimmune nephritis in female (NZB x NZW) F1 mice. *Transactions of the Association of American Physicians,* Vol 95, pp 145-154, ISSN/ISBN 0066-9458; 0066-9458.

Prickett, J.D., Robinson, D.R. & Steinberg, A.D. (1981). Dietary enrichment with the polyunsaturated fatty acid eicosapentaenoic acid prevents proteinuria and prolongs survival in NZB x NZW F1 mice. *The Journal of clinical investigation,* Vol 68, No.2, pp 556-559, ISSN/ISBN 0021-9738; 0021-9738.

Puertollano, M.A., Puertollano, E. & de Pablo, M.A. (2010). Host Immune Resistance and Dietary Lipids, In: *Dietary Components and Immune Function* Watson, Zibadi & Preedy (Ed.), pp. 131-153, Humana Press Springer, NY.

Puertollano, M.A., Puertollano, E., Alvarez de Cienfuegos, G. & de Pablo, M.A. (2008). Dietary lipids, modulation of immune functions and susceptibility to infection. *Nutritional Therapy and Metabolism,* Vol 26, No.3, pp 97-108.

Puertollano, M.A., de Pablo, M.A. & Alvarez de Cienfuegos, G. (2004). Olive oil and immune system functions: potential involvement in immunonutrition. *Grasas y aceites,* No.55, pp 42-51.

Rees, D., Miles, E.A., Banerjee, T., Wells, S.J., Roynette, C.E., Wahle, K.W. & Calder, P.C. (2006). Dose-related effects of eicosapentaenoic acid on innate immune function in healthy humans: a comparison of young and older men. *The American Journal of Clinical Nutrition,* Vol 83, No.2, pp 331-342, ISSN/ISBN 0002-9165; 0002-9165.

Robinson, D.R., Prickett, J.D., Makoul, G.T., Steinberg, A.D. & Colvin, R.B. (1986). Dietary fish oil reduces progression of established renal disease in (NZB x NZW)F1 mice and delays renal disease in BXSB and MRL/1 strains. *Arthritis and Rheumatism,* Vol 29, No.4, pp 539-546, ISSN/ISBN 0004-3591; 0004-3591.

Romano, C., Cucchiara, S., Barabino, A., Annese, V. & Sferlazzas, C. (2005). Usefulness of omega-3 fatty acid supplementation in addition to mesalazine in maintaining remission in pediatric Crohn's disease: a double-blind, randomized, placebo-controlled study. *World journal of gastroenterology : WJG,* Vol 11, No.45, pp 7118-7121, ISSN/ISBN 1007-9327; 1007-9327.

Sanchez-Fidalgo, S., Villegas, I., Cardeno, A., Talero, E., Sanchez-Hidalgo, M., Motilva, V. & Alarcon de la Lastra, C. (2010). Extra-virgin olive oil-enriched diet modulates DSS-colitis-associated colon carcinogenesis in mice. *Clinical nutrition (Edinburgh, Scotland),* Vol 29, No.5, pp 663-673, ISSN/ISBN 1532-1983; 0261-5614.

Sanderson, P., Yaqoob, P. & Calder, P.C. (1995). Effects of dietary lipid manipulation upon graft vs host and host vs graft responses in the rat. *Cellular immunology,* Vol 164, No.2, pp 240-247, ISSN/ISBN 0008-8749; 0008-8749.

Sano, H., Hla, T., Maier, J.A., Crofford, L.J., Case, J.P., Maciag, T. & Wilder, R.L. (1992). In vivo cyclooxygenase expression in synovial tissues of patients with rheumatoid arthritis and osteoarthritis and rats with adjuvant and streptococcal cell wall arthritis. *The Journal of clinical investigation,* Vol 89, No.1, pp 97-108, ISSN/ISBN 0021-9738; 0021-9738.

Sharon, P. & Stenson, W.F. (1984). Enhanced synthesis of leukotriene B4 by colonic mucosa in inflammatory bowel disease. *Gastroenterology,* Vol 86, No.3, pp 453-460, ISSN/ISBN 0016-5085; 0016-5085.

Shinto, L., Marracci, G., Baldauf-Wagner, S., Strehlow, A., Yadav, V., Stuber, L. & Bourdette, D. (2009). Omega-3 fatty acid supplementation decreases matrix metalloproteinase-9 production in relapsing-remitting multiple sclerosis. *Prostaglandins, leukotrienes, and essential fatty acids,* Vol 80, No.2-3, pp 131-136, ISSN/ISBN 0952-3278; 0952-3278.

Shoda, R., Matsueda, K., Yamato, S. & Umeda, N. (1996). Epidemiologic analysis of Crohn disease in Japan: increased dietary intake of n-6 polyunsaturated fatty acids and animal protein relates to the increased incidence of Crohn disease in Japan. *The American Journal of Clinical Nutrition,* Vol 63, No.5, pp 741-745, ISSN/ISBN 0002-9165; 0002-9165.

Shoda, R., Matsueda, K., Yamato, S. & Umeda, N. (1995). Therapeutic efficacy of N-3 polyunsaturated fatty acid in experimental Crohn's disease. *Journal of gastroenterology,* Vol 30 Suppl 8, pp 98-101, ISSN/ISBN 0944-1174; 0944-1174.

Simopoulos, A.P. (2002). Omega-3 fatty acids in inflammation and autoimmune diseases. *Journal of the American College of Nutrition,* Vol 21, No.6, pp 495-505, ISSN/ISBN 0731-5724; 0731-5724.

Sperling, R.I. (1995). Eicosanoids in rheumatoid arthritis. *Rheumatic diseases clinics of North America,* Vol 21, No.3, pp 741-758, ISSN/ISBN 0889-857X; 0889-857X.

Sperling, R.I., Weinblatt, M., Robin, J.L., Ravalese, J.,3rd, Hoover, R.L., House, F., Coblyn, J.S., Fraser, P.A., Spur, B.W. & Robinson, D.R. (1987). Effects of dietary supplementation with marine fish oil on leukocyte lipid mediator generation and function in rheumatoid arthritis. *Arthritis and Rheumatism,* Vol 30, No.9, pp 988-997, ISSN/ISBN 0004-3591; 0004-3591.

Spurney, R.F., Ruiz, P., Albrightson, C.R., Pisetsky, D.S. & Coffman, T.M. (1994). Fish oil feeding modulates leukotriene production in murine lupus nephritis. *Prostaglandins,* Vol 48, No.5, pp 331-348, ISSN/ISBN 0090-6980; 0090-6980.

Stene, L.C., Joner, G. & Norwegian Childhood Diabetes Study Group. (2003). Use of cod liver oil during the first year of life is associated with lower risk of childhood-onset type 1 diabetes: a large, population-based, case-control study. *The American Journal of Clinical Nutrition,* Vol 78, No.6, pp 1128-1134, ISSN/ISBN 0002-9165; 0002-9165.

Stulnig, T.M. (2003). Immunomodulation by polyunsaturated fatty acids: mechanisms and effects. *International archives of allergy and immunology,* Vol 132, No.4, pp 310-321, ISSN/ISBN 1018-2438; 1018-2438.

Suresh, Y. & Das, U.N. (2006). Differential effect of saturated, monounsaturated, and polyunsaturated fatty acids on alloxan-induced diabetes mellitus. *Prostaglandins, leukotrienes, and essential fatty acids,* Vol 74, No.3, pp 199-213, ISSN/ISBN 0952-3278; 0952-3278.

Swank, R.L. (1950). Multiple sclerosis; a correlation of its incidence with dietary fat. *The American Journal of the Medical Sciences,* Vol 220, No.4, pp 421-430, ISSN/ISBN 0002-9629; 0002-9629.

Trebble, T.M., Stroud, M.A., Wootton, S.A., Calder, P.C., Fine, D.R., Mullee, M.A., Moniz, C. & Arden, N.K. (2005). High-dose fish oil and antioxidants in Crohn's disease and the response of bone turnover: a randomised controlled trial. *The British journal of nutrition,* Vol 94, No.2, pp 253-261, ISSN/ISBN 0007-1145; 0007-1145.

Trebble, T.M., Wootton, S.A., Miles, E.A., Mullee, M., Arden, N.K., Ballinger, A.B., Stroud, M.A., Burdge, G.C. & Calder, P.C. (2003). Prostaglandin E2 production and T cell function after fish-oil supplementation: response to antioxidant cosupplementation. *The American Journal of Clinical Nutrition,* Vol 78, No.3, pp 376-382, ISSN/ISBN 0002-9165; 0002-9165.

Tulleken, J.E., Limburg, P.C., Muskiet, F.A. & van Rijswijk, M.H. (1990). Vitamin E status during dietary fish oil supplementation in rheumatoid arthritis. *Arthritis and Rheumatism,* Vol 33, No.9, pp 1416-1419, ISSN/ISBN 0004-3591; 0004-3591.

van der Tempel, H., Tulleken, J.E., Limburg, P.C., Muskiet, F.A. & van Rijswijk, M.H. (1990). Effects of fish oil supplementation in rheumatoid arthritis. *Annals of the Rheumatic Diseases,* Vol 49, No.2, pp 76-80, ISSN/ISBN 0003-4967; 0003-4967.

Venkatraman, J.T. & Chu, W.C. (1999). Effects of dietary omega-3 and omega-6 lipids and vitamin E on serum cytokines, lipid mediators and anti-DNA antibodies in a mouse model for rheumatoid arthritis. *Journal of the American College of Nutrition,* Vol 18, No.6, pp 602-613, ISSN/ISBN 0731-5724; 0731-5724.

Vilaseca, J., Salas, A., Guarner, F., Rodriguez, R., Martinez, M. & Malagelada, J.R. (1990). Dietary fish oil reduces progression of chronic inflammatory lesions in a rat model of granulomatous colitis. *Gut,* Vol 31, No.5, pp 539-544, ISSN/ISBN 0017-5749; 0017-5749.

Volker, D.H., FitzGerald, P.E. & Garg, M.L. (2000). The eicosapentaenoic to docosahexaenoic acid ratio of diets affects the pathogenesis of arthritis in Lew/SSN rats. *The Journal of nutrition,* Vol 130, No.3, pp 559-565, ISSN/ISBN 0022-3166; 0022-3166.

Wallace, F.A., Miles, E.A., Evans, C., Stock, T.E., Yaqoob, P. & Calder, P.C. (2001). Dietary fatty acids influence the production of Th1- but not Th2-type cytokines. *Journal of leukocyte biology,* Vol 69, No.3, pp 449-457, ISSN/ISBN 0741-5400; 0741-5400.

Walton, A.J., Snaith, M.L., Locniskar, M., Cumberland, A.G., Morrow, W.J. & Isenberg, D.A. (1991). Dietary fish oil and the severity of symptoms in patients with systemic lupus erythematosus. *Annals of the Rheumatic Diseases,* Vol 50, No.7, pp 463-466, ISSN/ISBN 0003-4967; 0003-4967.

Weinstock-Guttman, B., Baier, M., Park, Y., Feichter, J., Lee-Kwen, P., Gallagher, E., Venkatraman, J., Meksawan, K., Deinehert, S., Pendergast, D., Awad, A.B., Ramanathan, M., Munschauer, F. & Rudick, R. (2005). Low fat dietary intervention with omega-3 fatty acid supplementation in multiple sclerosis patients. *Prostaglandins, leukotrienes, and essential fatty acids,* Vol 73, No.5, pp 397-404, ISSN/ISBN 0952-3278; 0952-3278.

Westberg, G. & Tarkowski, A. (1990). Effect of MaxEPA in patients with SLE. A double-blind, crossover study. *Scandinavian journal of rheumatology,* Vol 19, No.2, pp 137-143, ISSN/ISBN 0300-9742; 0300-9742.

Whiting, C.V., Bland, P.W. & Tarlton, J.F. (2005). Dietary n-3 polyunsaturated fatty acids reduce disease and colonic proinflammatory cytokines in a mouse model of colitis. *Inflammatory bowel diseases,* Vol 11, No.4, pp 340-349, ISSN/ISBN 1078-0998; 1078-0998.

Wright, J.R.,Jr, Fraser, R.B., Kapoor, S. & Cook, H.W. (1995). Essential fatty acid deficiency prevents multiple low-dose streptozotocin-induced diabetes in naive and cyclosporin-treated low-responder murine strains. *Acta Diabetologica,* Vol 32, No.2, pp 125-130, ISSN/ISBN 0940-5429; 0940-5429.

Wright, S.A., O'Prey, F.M., McHenry, M.T., Leahey, W.J., Devine, A.B., Duffy, E.M., Johnston, D.G., Finch, M.B., Bell, A.L. & McVeigh, G.E. (2008). A randomised interventional trial of omega-3-polyunsaturated fatty acids on endothelial function and disease activity in systemic lupus erythematosus. *Annals of the Rheumatic Diseases,* Vol 67, No.6, pp 841-848, ISSN/ISBN 1468-2060; 0003-4967.

Yaqoob, P. (2002). Monounsaturated fatty acids and immune function. *European journal of clinical nutrition,* Vol 56 Suppl 3, pp S9-S13, ISSN/ISBN 0954-3007; 0954-3007.

Yaqoob, P., Newsholme, E.A. & Calder, P.C. (1994). Inhibition of natural killer cell activity by dietary lipids. *Immunology letters,* Vol 41, No.2-3, pp 241-247, ISSN/ISBN 0165-2478; 0165-2478.

Yuceyar, H., Ozutemiz, O., Huseyinov, A., Saruc, M., Alkanat, M., Bor, S., Coker, I. & Batur, Y. (1999). Is administration of n-3 fatty acids by mucosal enema protective against trinitrobenzene-induced colitis in rats? *Prostaglandins, leukotrienes, and essential fatty acids,* Vol 61, No.6, pp 339-345, ISSN/ISBN 0952-3278; 0952-3278.

10

The Ectopic Germinal Centre Response in Autoimmune Disease and Cancer

David I. Stott and Donna McIntyre
Institute of Infection, Immunity & Inflammation, University of Glasgow, Glasgow, Scotland, U.K.

1. Introduction

1.1 The B-cell response in autoimmune disease

The pathological effects of autoimmune diseases on the target tissues can be mediated by autoantibodies, cell-mediated immune responses, or both. It is increasingly evident that some autoimmune diseases previously thought to be essentially T-cell-mediated also have a B-cell component, which may involve direct effects of autoantibody secreted by plasma cells, pro- or anti-inflammatory cytokines secreted by activated effector or regulatory B-cells, or through the highly efficient antigen presentation function of B-cells enabling them to activate $CD4^+$ T-cells and *vice versa.* The number of autoimmune diseases known to be mediated partly or largely through autoantibodies has increased markedly in recent times. Systemic lupus erythematosus (SLE)[1], in which the pathology is mediated via Type II & III hypersensitivity reactions involving anti-DNA autoantibodies, has long been known to fall into this category. Many other autoantibodies are produced by these patients, principally against nuclear antigens, but most are not thought to be involved in pathology. Hashimoto's thyroiditis and Graves' disease patients produce pathogenic autoantibodies against thyroid antigens, the latter being a rare example of an activating autoantibody inducing signalling via the thyroid stimulating hormone receptor. Myasthenia gravis patients produce autoantibodies against the acetylcholine receptor (AChR), present on the motor muscle endplates, thereby inhibiting muscle contraction. Anti-SS-A and anti-SS-B (anti-Ro & anti-La) autoantibodies are implicated in congenital heart block in children born to mothers with Sjögren's Syndrome due to transplacental uptake of IgG autoantibodies; autoantibodies against α-fodrin are also believed to be pathogenic in these patients. Rheumatoid arthritis (RA), one member of the group of systemic rheumatic autoimmune diseases that also includes SLE, psoriatic arthritis and the various forms of myositis, has now gone full cycle in views on its pathological mechanisms.

---

[1] Abbreviations: AChR, Acetylcholine Receptor; AID, Activation Induced Cytidine Deaminase; AMC, Arthrogryposis Multiplex Congenita; ARS, Anti-amino acyl-tRNA Synthetase; Bmem, Memory B-cell; CDR, Complementarity Determining Region; DM, Dermatomyositis; EOMG, Early Onset Myasthenia Gravis; FDC, Follicular Dendritic Cell; G.C., Germinal Centre; IBM, Inclusion Body Myositis; IM, Inflammatory Myopathies; LOMG, Late Onset Myasthenia Gravis; MAA, Myositis-Associated Autoantibodies; MAb, Monoclonal Antibody; MIR, Main Immunogenic Region; MSA, Myositis Specific Autoantibodies; PM, Polymyositis; RA, Rheumatoid Arthritis; SLE, Systemic Lupus Erythematosus; TAA, Tumour-Associated Antigen; TIL, Tumour-Infiltrating Lymphocytes; Tfh, Follicular T helper cell; UNG, Uracil Nucleotidyl Glycosylase.

Initially thought to be caused by the anti-IgG Fc antibody (rheumatoid factor), although approximately 25% of RA patients are rheumatoid factor negative, the evidence then swung in favour of a cell mediated autoimmune response involving effector T-cells and cytokines, principally TNFα. Although these are clearly involved in joint pathology, autoantibodies against cyclic citrullinated proteins are a much better diagnostic marker for RA than rheumatoid factor and there is some limited evidence that they may be pathogenic. It is also now recognised that B-cells play an important role in the pathogenic autoimmune response, as clearly demonstrated by the marked clinical improvement in patients treated with Rituximab®, an anti-CD20 chimaeric (human/mouse) monoclonal antibody that suppresses B-cell responses. Other autoimmune diseases with B-cell involvement include autoimmune haemolytic anaemia, idiopathic thrombocytopaenia, Type I diabetes, and some subtypes of myositis, although the situation is often confused by the presence of non-pathogenic autoantibodies.

1.2 The germinal centre response to foreign antigens

Germinal centres (g.c.) are the main sites of generation of high affinity, antibody-secreting plasma cells and Ig class-switched memory B-cells during T-cell-dependent immune responses, extensively reviewed by others (Allen, Okada, & Cyster, 2007; Brink, 2007; Hauser, Shlomchik, & Haberman, 2007; Klein & Dalla-Favera, 2008; Leavy, 2010; Minton, 2011). Here we shall summarise briefly the principal features of the g.c. response. The response is initiated by B-cells binding to their cognate antigen on the surface of antigen presenting cells, such as dendritic cells, in a secondary lymphoid organ (lymph node, spleen, Peyer's patches or human tonsil). The antigen becomes internalised, degraded into peptides which are expressed on the cell surface bound to MHC Class II and presented to a helper T (T_h) cell that provides costimulatory activation signals, including binding of the B-cell surface molecule CD40 to its ligand, CD154, on the T-cell membrane.

This interaction takes place at or near the interface between the B-cell follicle and the T-cell area and some activated B-cells proliferate outside the follicle and differentiate into short-lived plasma cells secreting IgM antibodies. Others migrate into the B-cell follicle where they proliferate and differentiate into centroblasts expressing low levels of surface Ig. This region develops into a germinal centre with a dark zone of densely packed, proliferating centroblasts, and a light zone of more loosely packed B-cells (centrocytes) interspersed with the processes of follicular dendritic cells (FDC, Figure 1A). These have distinct stromal origins, unlike the bone marrow derived, extra-follicular dendritic cells; almost uniquely, their C′ and Fc receptors trap immune complexes and retain antigens in their native state for months.

The pre-existing IgM^+,IgD^+ follicle B-cells are pushed out to form a mantle zone around the developing germinal centre, the whole structure being termed a secondary follicle. Proliferation of the dark zone centroblasts is extremely rapid, with cell cycle times estimated at between 6 and 12 hours. These proliferating clones of B-cells switch on the molecular machinery required for somatic hypermutation of their rearranged, expressed, Ig V-genes, including expression of activation-induced cytidine deaminase (AID). This induces mutations specifically targeted to the Ig V-genes at a frequency of 1 per 1000 base pairs per cell division, although much lower levels of mutation can also occur in some other, non-Ig genes such as Bcl-2 & Bcl-6. AID deaminates cytidine to uracil at C/G base pairs, introducing mismatches in the DNA that can be replaced by T/A base pairs. Uracil nucleotidyl glycosylase (UNG) can remove the uracil leading to insertion of any of the four bases at the abasic site; mismatch repair enzymes also recognise the mismatch and induce single strand breaks which are repaired by error prone DNA polymerases (Di Noia & Neuberger, 2007). The mutations are targeted mainly to the complementarity determining regions (CDRs) which are intimately involved in binding to the epitope and therefore determine specificity and affinity of the antibody. Combined with the rapid proliferation, this results in clones of B-cells expressing receptors with a variety of affinities for the antigen, some high, some low; some will have lost the ability to bind to the antigen altogether and rare B-cells may cross-react with a self-antigen.

Several clones of proliferating, mutating B-cells are usually present within each germinal centre. These cells differentiate into centrocytes expressing mutated antigen receptors and migrate into the light zone. The centrocytes move through the light zone, acquire antigen for a second time from immune complexes on the follicular dendritic cells, which they internalise, process and present to follicular helper T-cells (T_{fh}-cells) (Patakas *et al.*, 2011), thereby receiving survival signals, probably via costimulatory molecule interactions including CD40/CD154 and CD80/CD28 binding. These signals, together with T_{fh}-cell cytokines (IL-4 and IFNγ) and AID deamination of cytidines, promote induction of class switch recombination (Patakas *et al.*, 2011). Some of these centrocytes differentiate directly into plasmablasts and antibody-secreting plasma cells; others differentiate into Ig class switched memory B-cells, both of which migrate out of the follicle. Competition for limiting availability of antigen results in selection of B-cells expressing high affinity antigen receptors; recent evidence has shown that a broad range of mutations is involved in selection, not only for high affinity receptors but also for stability and expression of the B-cell receptor (Weiser *et al.*, 2011). Cells expressing antigen receptors with low affinity are unable to compete for survival signals and the default response is that they die by apoptosis and are engulfed by macrophages, in which their degenerating nuclei are visible as tingible bodies. Most of this information is derived from studies in mice, in which the germinal centres reach maximum size about two weeks after immunisation and then gradually decline in the absence of further immunisation, disappearing after several weeks. Although the cell composition and structure of secondary follicles appear similar in Man, the kinetics and some of the detailed cellular interactions may differ.

Detailed studies of the kinetics and cellular interactions within germinal centres using multiphoton microscopy of living tissue in combination with B & T-lymphocytes expressing defined antigen receptors from transgenic animals have revealed much more dynamic activity than was previously suspected. It is now recognised that there is less distinction between the dark and light zones than suggested by static immunohistological examination, and there is continual recycling of B-cells both between and within the two zones, although there is net migration from the dark zone to the light zone (Beltman *et al.*, 2011)(Figure 1B). Centrocytes move rapidly through the network of follicular dendritic cell processes, apparently sampling the immune complexes attached to their membranes and some of these cells return to the dark zone for further rounds of proliferation and somatic hypermutation. Migration of B-cells between the zones is controlled by chemokines, possibly secreted by stromal cells within the germinal centre. T_{fh}-cells are present mainly in the light zone and recent data suggest that affinity selection of B-cells may involve competition for signals from cognate T_{fh}-cells via peptide/MHC Class II binding as well as, or instead of, competition for antigen on the surface of follicular dendritic cells (Victora *et al.*, 2010). Anti-self B-cells that have escaped negative selection in the bone marrow, or have arisen in the germinal centre due to somatic hypermutation, are either eliminated at this stage, suppressed by regulatory T-cells, or alter their antigen specificity by receptor revision, a process similar to V-gene rearrangement in developing B-cells. This involves re-expression of RAG1 and RAG2 and rearrangement of an upstream light chain V-gene to an unused J exon (Nemazee, 2006). Despite the absence of D exons in the rearranged heavy chain locus, we have shown that an upstream heavy chain V-gene can also replace all or part of a rearranged V_H-gene, thereby altering the specificity of the receptor away from self antigen (Darlow & Stott, 2005). The architecture, cellular components and processes occurring in a typical germinal centre are summarised in Figure 1.

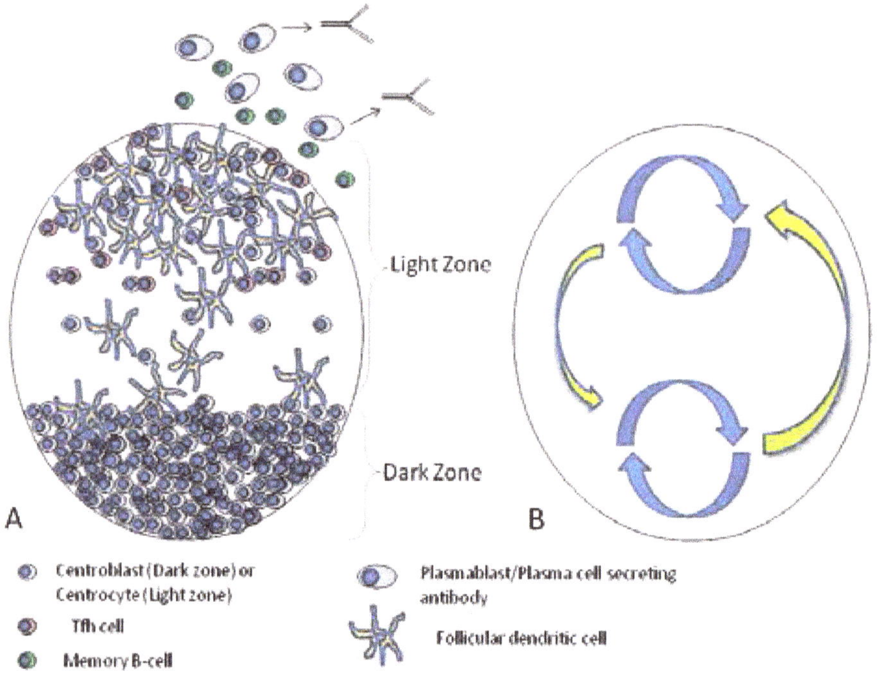

Fig. 1. Diagrammatic representation of a germinal centre in a lymph node.

A: Showing a dark zone containing proliferating clones of mutating centroblasts and a light zone containing centrocytes in contact with follicular dendritic cells and follicular helper T-cells (Tfh cells). Long-lived memory B-cells, plasmablasts and plasma cells secreting antibody molecules migrate out of the g.c. and leave the lymph node via the efferent lymphatic vessel. Apoptotic B-cells, macrophages containing tingible bodies and the mantle zone are not shown.

B: The same germinal centre showing recirculation of B-cells within and between the dark and light zones.

1.3 The ectopic germinal centre response in autoimmune disease

It has been known for many years that the target tissues of autoimmune diseases contain infiltrating lymphocytes and other immune cells, including T-cells, B-cells, plasma cells, macrophages, dendritic and follicular dendritic cells. In many cases the infiltrating cells organise themselves into structures resembling germinal centres. Some of these have a mantle zone, suggesting that they were formed from a primary follicle whereas, even when absent, it is often possible to distinguish a dark zone, containing few or no $CD4^+$ T-cells or follicular dendritic cells, and a light zone containing both. Autoantigens have been identified on the finger-like processes of follicular dendritic cells (Shiono *et al.*, 2003) and, in some cases, autoantibodies have been identified in g.c. B-cells. Separate T-cell areas containing dendritic cells and, sometimes, high endothelial venules, can also be seen. The stage of lymphoid neogenesis appears to be directly related to the extent of infiltration of lymphoid and other immune cells (Aloisi & Pujol-Borrell, 2006). Examples of autoimmune diseases in which germinal centre-like structures have been identified in the target, or disease-related tissues are shown in Table 1. It is now apparent that ectopic germinal centres, also known as tertiary lymphoid organs, can also develop in other chronic inflammatory diseases, such as the gut in Crohn's disease and ulcerative colitis patients, in chronic infections (Aloisi & Pujol-Borrell, 2006) and some types of cancer (Table 1). The questions these observations raise are: 1. How do they develop?; 2. How closely do they resemble germinal centres in secondary lymphoid organs?; 3. Are the B-cells within them undergoing a germinal centre response, as described in section 1.2 above?; 4. Are they generating plasma cells secreting pathogenic autoantibodies?; 5. What role do they play in the pathogenesis of autoimmune disease?

Autoimmune Diseases	**Organ containing Germinal Centres**	**Antigen(s) Recognised by GC B-cells**	**Reference**
Hashimoto's thyroiditis	Thyroid	Thyroglobulin, Thyroperoxidase	(Knecht, Saremaslani, & Hedinger, 1981) (Armengol *et al.*, 2001)
Graves' disease	Thyroid	Thyroglobulin, Thyroperoxidase	(Armengol *et al.*, 2001)
Myasthenia gravis	Thymus	Acetylcholine receptor	(Yoshitake *et al.*, 1994) (SHIONO *et al.*, 2003)
Sjögren's syndrome	Salivary glands	SS-A (Ro), SS-B (La)	(Stott *et al.*, 1998)
Rheumatoid arthritis	Synovial membranes of joints	IgG Fc, Cyclic citrullinated protein/peptide	(Manzo & Pitzalis, 2007) (Humby *et al.*, 2009)
Psoriatic arthritis	Synovial membranes of joints	?	(Canete *et al.*, 2007) (Gerhard *et al.*, 2002)
Cryptogenic fibrosing alveolitis	Lungs	?	(Wallace *et al.*, 1996)
Uveoretinits	Choroid of the eye	?	(Liversidge *et al.*, 1993)
Autoimmune hepatitis	Liver	?	(Mosnier *et al.*, 1993)
Multiple sclerosis	Meninges (?)	?	(Prineas, 1979) (Serafini *et al.*, 2004)
Chronic Inflammatory Diseases			
Crohn's disease	Gastrointestinal tract	?	(Kaiserling, 2001)
Ulcerative colitis	Descending colon	?	(Kaiserling, 2001)
Infectious Diseases			
Chronic hepatitis C infection	Liver	?	(Mosnier *et al.*, 1993)
Helicobacter pylori or *Campylobacter* gastritis	Stomach	Bacterial antigens	(Genta, Hamner, & Graham, 1993) (Stolte & Eidt, 1989)
Chronic Lyme disease	Synovial membranes of joints	?	(Ghosh *et al.*, 2005)
Oncocerciasis	Skin	?	(Brattig *et al.*, 2010)
Cancers			
Lymphoma of MALT associated with Sjögren's Syndrome	Lymphoma	?	(Bombardieri *et al.*, 2007a)
Ductal breast carcinoma	Breast tumour	Epidermal growth factor receptor family	(Coronella *et al.*, 2002) (Nzula, Going, & Stott, 2003a) (Simsa *et al.*, 2005) and section 5.
Medullary breast carcinoma	Breast tumour	Ganglioside	(Coronella *et al.*, 2001) (Kotlan *et al.*, 2005)

Table 1. Diseases in which ectopic germinal centres have been observed.

It has now been shown by combined immunohistochemistry, identification of antigen specificity of B-cells and plasma cells in and around ectopic germinal centres, and sequence analysis of expressed, rearranged Ig V-genes and their somatic mutations, that germinal centre B-cells in the target tissues of several autoimmune diseases are undergoing clonal expansion, somatic hypermutation and affinity selection, in a similar manner to that seen in the germinal centres of secondary lymphoid organs (Table 1 and section 1.2). This has been demonstrated in Sjögren's syndrome, rheumatoid arthritis, psoriatic arthritis, myasthenia gravis, multiple sclerosis and also in breast cancer. In some of these cases, expression of RAG1 and 2 have been observed (Armengol *et al.*, 2001), indicating that receptor revision also takes place in ectopic germinal centres and therefore the generation and attempted elimination of self-reactive B-cells. The signals involved in tertiary lymphoid organ neogenesis appear to be similar to those in development of secondary lymphoid organs, although the temporal and causal relationship between appearance of these structures in the target tissue and autoimmune pathology-related tissue damage is unclear. One scenario is that an initial event in the tissue, which could, in some cases, include microbial infection, leads to the release of molecules seen by the immune system as "danger signals" (Matzinger, 2007) thereby inducing infiltration of inflammatory cells and subsequent lymphoid neogenesis, causing further tissue damage with concomitant release of self-antigens, more danger signals and a vicious cycle, perpetuating a chronic autoimmune reaction. Alternatively, initial tissue damage may be caused by an autoimmune response commencing in the secondary lymphoid organs, with subsequent events following a similar course to that described above. Lymphotoxins α, β, $\alpha_1\beta_2$ and TNFα have been shown to be required for development of ectopic germinal centres. Growth-factor receptor-bound protein-2 (Grb2) has recently been shown to control orthotopic lymphoid follicle organisation and the germinal centre response by inducing production of lymphotoxin-α via CXCR5 signalling (Jang *et al.*, 2011). These molecules are secreted by infiltrating B and T_h1-cells and activated NK cells; on binding to their receptor on stromal cells they induce expression of adhesion molecules and secretion of chemokines which induce further lymphocyte infiltration and segregation into B-cell follicles, formation of a follicular dendritic cell network and T-cell areas. It has also recently been proposed that overexpression of costimulatory molecules on T_{fh}-cells may contribute to overcoming B-cell tolerance (Patakas *et al.*, 2011). This may be a contributory factor in ectopic as well as orthotopic germinal centres. Primary B-cell follicles are rarely seen in autoimmune disease target tissues but this may be because chronic antigen stimulation has been in progress for a considerable time before biopsies are taken. For example, in type I diabetes mellitus there is evidence that the autoimmune response develops long before overt disease is diagnosed. Whether ectopic germinal centres are initiated by naïve or memory B-cells is unclear but recent evidence shows that at least some B-cell clones arise *de novo* from naïve B-cells (Sims *et al.*, 2001; Nzula, Going, & Stott, 2003b; Nzula, Going, & Stott, 2003a).

The frequency of ectopic germinal centres varies markedly between autoimmune diseases; as one might expect, the highest incidence is in diseases where pathogenic autoantibodies are most strongly implicated. Thus, they have been identified in thyroid tissues of 100% of Hashimoto's thyroiditis patients and 54 - 63% of Graves' disease cases; in rheumatoid arthritis the figure is 25 - 50% but in Sjögren's syndrome it is only 17%, although variations may to some extent reflect differences in the difficulty of finding the germinal centres. In Sjögren's syndrome, the source is usually biopsies of the small labial salivary glands of which there is a large number; as g.c.s are only present in some of the many small labial salivary glands, they may easily be overlooked. Tissues containing different types of cells respond in a variety of ways to inflammatory signals and this may also determine whether, and to what extent, lymphoid organ neogenesis occurs. The origin of follicular dendritic cells is unclear but it has been proposed that they develop from precursor cells already present in the tissue, either fibroblasts or fibroblast precursor cells (Park & Choi, 2005). Alternatively, the precursor cells may be induced to migrate into the tissue by the same or similar chemokines as those attracting the B and T-lymphocytes. In several autoimmune diseases (Table 1) and animal models of autoimmune diseases (Astorri *et al.*, 2010; Nacionales *et al.*, 2009), it has been demonstrated that ectopic germinal centres are generating plasma cells secreting pathogenic autoantibodies and, almost certainly, memory B-cells bearing anti-self antigen receptors, implying that they aid the diversification of the autoantibody repertoire and contribute to the maintenance of immune pathology. In addition to autoantibody production, self-reactive B-cells generated in ectopic germinal centres may also contribute to autoimmune pathology by secretion of pro-inflammatory cytokines and activation of pathogenic T-cells by presentation of processed self-antigens. B-cells may contribute in this way to immune pathology in autoimmune diseases generally considered to be principally T-cell mediated, and may be one explanation for the efficacy of Rituximab therapy for rheumatoid arthritis.

2. Methods

2.1 Identification and cellular composition of ectopic germinal centres

The methods we used to identify ectopic germinal centres, characterise their cellular composition, analyse the rearranged Ig V-gene sequences expressed by germinal centre B-cells and identify their antibody specificity have been described in detail in previously published papers (Nzula, Going, & Stott, 2003a; Sims *et al.*, 2001). Briefly, sections were cut from snap frozen tissue biopsies and every tenth section stained for B-cells with anti-CD20. Sections containing germinal centre-like structures or B-cell aggregates were further characterised by staining for T-cells (anti-CD3, CD4, CD8), regulatory T-cells (anti-FoxP3), follicular dendritic cells (anti-FDC (DAKO) or anti-CD35), plasma cells (DAKO), macrophages (anti-CD68) and proliferating cells (anti-Ki67). Double immunofluorescent staining with the above cell subset-specific antibodies and Ki67 was used to identify dividing cells. Acetylcholine receptor-specific B-cells in germinal centres from the thymus of myasthenia gravis patients were identified by ^{125}I-α-bungarotoxin-labelled acetylcholine receptor and autoradiography (Shiono *et al.*, 2003; Hill *et al.*, 2008); other autoantibody-producing cells were identified by immunofluorescence staining with the relevant antigen.

2.2 Cloning and sequence analysis of rearranged Ig V-genes

Ectopic germinal centres and B-cell aggregates were excised by microdissection, digested with proteinase K and the released DNA used as a template for amplification of the rearranged Ig V-genes by nested PCR. Details of the method and the primers are described in Sims *et al.* (2001) and Nzula *et al.* (2003). Amplified DNA was purified by agarose gel electrophoresis, ligated into plasmid DNA and cloned in *E. coli*. Cloned plasmid DNA was purified and the Ig V-genes sequenced in both directions using primers complementary to sequences flanking the cloning site. The best matching germline V, D & J sequences were identified initially by comparison with the VBASE directory of human Ig V-genes and later, after VBASE ceased to be updated, using the Immunogenetics (IMGT) Database of Human

Immunoglobulin Sequences (http://www.imgt.org/). Sequences were analysed using JOINSOLVER (http://joinsolver.niaid.nih.gov/) and IMGTV-QUEST. Silent and replacement somatic mutations were identified by comparison with the germline gene sequence; in early experiments the ratio of replacement to silent mutations was considered to be evidence of affinity selection if significantly higher than 3:1. To correct for the inherent bias towards replacement mutations in CDRs, we have more recently applied the method of Hershberg to determine whether affinity selection has occurred in B-cell clones from ectopic germinal centres (Hershberg *et al.*, 2008). This method employs an algorithm that allows for the effects of microsequences in the complementarity determining regions (CDRs) and the bias towards transition mutations. Clonally related sets of rearranged V-genes were identified by their use of the same germline V, (D) and J exons and shared junctional sequences. Genealogical trees were constructed by analysis of shared and unshared mutations using the parsimony method of phylogenetic analysis (PAUP, (Swofford, 1993)), enabling the assignment of sequences from parent and daughter cells that have been produced during clonal proliferation, thus providing clear evidence of the presence of clonally proliferating, somatically mutating B-cells within the germinal centre.

2.3 Cloning antigen-specific autoantibodies from germinal centre B-cells by 'phage display

In order to confirm the antigen specificity of B-cells generated in ectopic germinal centres, and to analyse in detail the relationship between their mutations and antigen specificity, we reconstituted the rearranged Ig V-genes as single chain Fv (scFv) or Fab antibodies by 'phage display. Single chain Fv antibodies comprise the heavy and light chain variable region domains linked by a short peptide. Although linked together by a short additional peptide sequence, the V_H and V_L domains are able to fold into their natural 3-dimensional conformation and pair correctly, as the antibody produced by a B-cell or plasma cell. They contain the antigen binding site, and therefore mimic the antigen specificity of the original antibodies from which they were derived. A caveat that must be born in mind is that the original H and L chain pairings are unknown, except when both genes are cloned from a single cell. The detailed methodology has been described elsewhere (Stott & Sims, 2000; Matthews *et al.*, 2002). Rearranged V_H and V_L-genes amplified either from microdissected germinal centres or pooled V-genes from the same B-cell clone, were used to construct scFvs using a $(Gly_4Ser)_3$ linker DNA. The resulting scFv library, comprising a pool of randomly linked V_H-V_L genes, was then inserted into the phagemids pCANTAB6 or pHEN2 continuously with the gene encoding the bacteriophage coat protein P3, and grown in *E. coli* in the presence of helper phage. The resulting scFv-P3 fusion protein was expressed on the surface of bacteriophage or as soluble scFv by transfection into a non-permissive, or permissive, strain of *E. coli* respectively. Alternatively, Fab libraries were constructed using whole light chain cDNA and DNA encoding the V_H region and the first constant region domain of the heavy chain by similar techniques (Matthews et al., 2002). An advantage of amplifying directly from genomic DNA is that the distribution of cloned V-genes reflects the usage of those genes by B-cells and plasma cells more accurately than amplification from cDNA, which is biased towards plasma cells. The library of scFvs or Fabs attached to bacteriophage by the P3 'phage coat protein was then panned on plastic plates coated with either a whole extract of the target tissue, or purified recombinant antigen, to identify self-reactive antibodies. Bound 'phage were washed, eluted, re-grown in *E. coli* and panning repeated until the eluate had become enriched with a small number of 'phage clones. These were recloned and their H & L chains sequenced and used to investigate the specificity and properties of their antigen-binding sites.

2.4 Statistical analysis

The method of Hershberg *et al.* (2008), described in section 2.2 above, was used to determine the significance of replacement mutations in rearranged Ig V-genes cloned from germinal centre B-cells, as evidence for affinity maturation of the antibodies expressed by them. The distribution of V_H gene families and individual V, D and J exons was assessed using two-tailed χ^2 analysis, corrected for multiple comparisons.

3. The ectopic germinal centre response in myasthenia gravis

3.1 Pathology of myasthenia gravis

Myasthenia gravis is an organ-specific autoimmune disease characterised by weakness of striated muscles and thymic hyperplasia (Vincent, 2002). Patients are generally divided into subgroups with early-onset (EOMG, pre-40 years) or late onset (LOMG, post-40 years) forms of the disease, or with thymoma in about 10% of patients. It is a classic autoantibody-mediated autoimmune disease, caused by autoantibodies directed against the postsynaptic nicotinic acetylcholine receptor (AChR) at the neuromuscular junction. Many thymoma patients and some late onset patients also have serum antibodies against striated muscle antigens, interferon-α and IL-12. Loss of functional AChRs leads to muscle weakness, usually first evident in weakness of eye movement. This can progress to other striated muscles of the body, causing problems with breathing due to effects on the diaphragm, swallowing difficulties and paralysis. These effects can be life-threatening if untreated. Evidence that the effects are mediated by autoantibodies against the AChR include induction of similar symptoms by: their transfer from mother to baby *in utero*; passive transfer from patients to mice; immunisation of animals with AChR; and marked improvement of symptoms in patients after removal of circulating IgG antibodies by plasmapheresis. Several pathogenic mechanisms are involved (Vincent, 2002; Drachman, 1994): (i) Cross-linking of the receptor by autoantibodies causes loss of AChR by antigenic modulation, leading to internalisation and degradation of the receptors; (ii) The majority of anti-AChR antibodies are of the IgG1 and IgG3 subclasses, which are particularly efficient at complement activation, resulting in lysis and damage to the muscle membrane; (iii) Less commonly, some antibodies cause direct inhibition of the ion channel function of the AChR; (iv) Antibody-dependent cell-mediated cytotoxicity has also been implicated, although there is little direct evidence for this mechanism. The IgG autoantibodies can cross the placenta of pregnant mothers with myasthenia gravis by an active transport mechanism involving the neonatal Fc receptor, FcRn, resulting in transient symptoms of myasthenia gravis in the newborn infant. The symptoms gradually ameliorate as the maternal antibodies are catabolised and replaced by the infant's own antibodies. More rarely, the autoantibodies produced by multiparous mothers can induce severe, often fatal, developmental abnormalities, termed arthrogryposis multiplex congenita, due to paralysis of fetal muscles *in utero* (see section 3.4.5).

3.2 Structure and epitopes of the acetylcholine receptor

The AChR is a pentameric transmembrane glycoprotein found almost exclusively at the muscle endplate, comprising two α polypeptide subunits, one β, one δ and, in the adult, one ε subunit; in the fetus there is also one γ subunit, which is gradually replaced by an ε from the third trimester onwards (Fig. 2) (Vincent, 2002). The five subunits are combined into a cylindrical structure with a central cation channel that is closed in the inactive conformation. There are two binding sites for acetylcholine, formed at the interfaces between one α and δ subunit and the second α and ε or γ subunits. Electrical impulses passing down the motor nerve trigger release of acetylcholine molecules at the nerve termini. When these bind to the two receptor binding sites, they cause the central cation channel to open and sodium ions to flood into the muscle resulting in local membrane depolarisation. When this reaches threshold the resulting action potential spreads across the muscle triggering it to contract. Loss of at least 50% of receptors is required to produce overt muscle weakness.

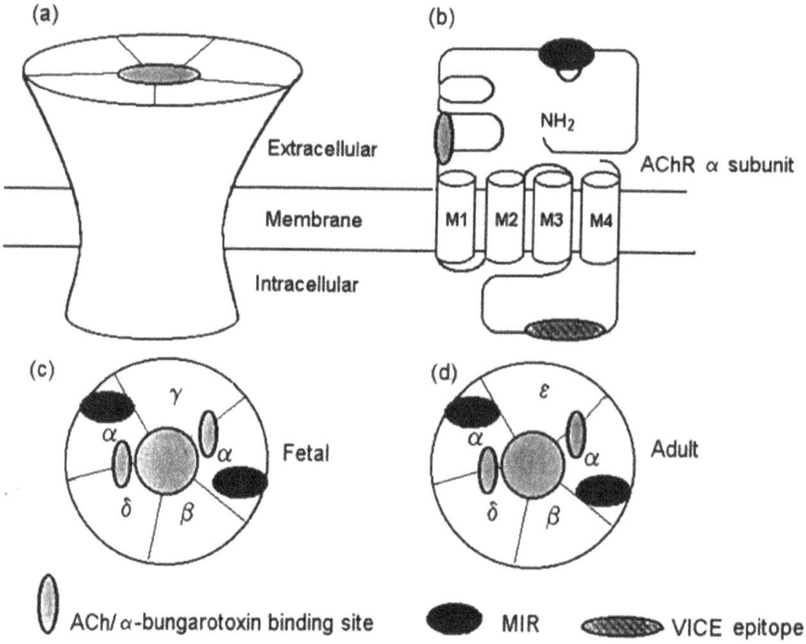

Fig. 2. Diagrammatic representation of the structure of the acetylcholine receptor:

(a) the complete pentameric molecule in the cell membrane; (b) the topology of the subunits, illustrated for the α subunit that contributes to the acetylcholine/α-bungarotoxin binding site, the main immunogenic region (MIR) and the very immunogenic cytoplasmic epitope (VICE); It is doubtful whether the latter plays any significant role in pathogenesis; (c and d) the fetal and adult subtypes of AChR. Reproduced with permission from (Vincent et al., 1997), Plenum Press.

Since the patients' autoantibodies are almost exclusively specific for the complex native conformation of the extracellular AChR subunit domains, and not short peptides or even whole subunit polypeptides, mapping of the autoantibody epitopes has proved to be difficult. The antibodies are mainly IgG1 or IgG3, of high avidity and heterogeneous in their sequences and fine specificity. Disease severity correlates poorly with autoantibody titre, suggesting that pathogenicity may depend upon precise epitope specificity. Many of the antibodies bind to a region of the extracellular domain of the α chain, the main immunogenic region or MIR. Its conformation is affected by the ε ↔ γ interchange, as demonstrated by the observation that some antibodies bind better to the MIR of the fetal AChR than the adult form, even though the γ and ε subunits do not contribute directly to the MIR (Fostieri, Beeson, & Tzartos, 2000). Titres of MIR antibodies vary considerably between patients and other antibodies may play an equally important role in some individuals. Some patients also produce autoantibodies against the acetylcholine binding sites (that also bind α-bungarotoxin); these are the blocking antibodies described above.

3.3 Role of the thymus

Early onset myasthenia gravis is associated with thymic hyperplasia characterized by secondary lymphoid organ-like structures in the medulla of >90% of patients. These include T-cell areas containing AChR-specific helper T-cells and large numbers of germinal centres with clearly defined mantle, dark and light zones. Plasmablasts and plasma cells secreting autoantibodies against AChR are also detectable within and around the germinal centres (Hill *et al.*, 2008; SHIONO *et al.*, 2003). Approximately 20% of germinal centres contain plasmablasts positive for antibodies against AChR and AChR is trapped on follicular dendritic cells in c.50% of thymic germinal centres (SHIONO *et al.*, 2003). Anti-AChR-secreting hybridomas and AChR-specific Fabs have been cloned from thymic B-cells and thymectomy results in a reduction in the serum anti-AChR titre and reduced clinical symptoms in some patients, although the benefits of thymectomy have never been rigorously proved (Cardona *et al.*, 1994; Farrar *et al.*, 1997; Graus *et al.*, 1997). The relative contribution of the thymus to production of anti-AChR autoantibodies compared with the secondary lymphoid organs is unknown, but it appears to play a significant role. Therefore, using the methods described in section 2, we tested the hypothesis that thymic germinal centres are sites of ongoing autoimmune responses driven by autoantigen, i.e. sites of activated B-cells, clonally proliferating, somatically mutating their expressed Ig V-genes and undergoing affinity maturation, driven by the acetylcholine receptor.

3.4 The thymic germinal centre response in myasthenia gravis

3.4.1 Germinal centres in the thymus

Thymi from 5 EOMG patients were examined by immunohistology. All 5 contained large numbers of germinal centres with typical mantle zones within the thymic medulla, histologically indistinguishable from germinal centres in human tonsil controls. The mantle zones contained densely packed $CD20^+$ B-cells surrounding the germinal centre B-cells (Fig. 3A). These were interspersed with a network of follicular dendritic cells extending throughout the dark and light zones (Fig. 3C) and a crescent of T-cells can be seen at the apex of the light zone (Fig. 3B). Proliferating B-cells were distributed throughout the germinal centre but in larger numbers within the dark zone (Fig. 3D). Autoradiography with ^{125}I-α-bungarotoxin alone, which binds to AChR, diffusely labelled c.50% of germinal centres and appeared to be associated with the follicular dendritic cell processes. No labelling was seen in human tonsils or thymi from two seronegative myasthenia patients and bungarotoxin binding was blocked by the cholinergic drug, carbamyl choline, which is structurally similar to AChR, indicating that the follicular dendritic network contained membrane-bound antigen or immune complexes.

In contrast, ^{125}I-α-bungarotoxin-labelled AChR bound to individual cells in 20% of germinal centres, including large numbers of moderately labelled centrocytes in the light zone, smaller numbers in the dark zone, and heavily labelled plasmablasts/plasma cells in and around the germinal centres (Fig. 3E & F).

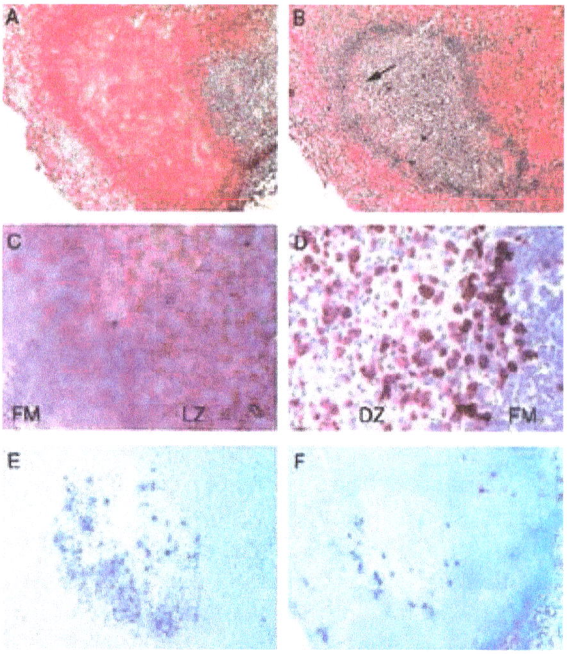

Fig. 3. Immunohistochemically stained serial sections through thymic germinal centres.

A & B: Germinal centres stained (red) with anti-CD20 and anti-CD3 for B and T-cells respectively. The arrow (B) shows a crescent of T-cells in the light zone. C: A network of follicular dendritic cell processes is spread throughout the germinal centre, including both the light and dark zones. D: Germinal centre cells stained with an antibody against proliferating cell nuclear antigen, revealing dividing B-cells in both areas but more concentrated in the dark zone. E & F: ^{125}I-α-bungarotoxin-labelled AChR reveals individual AChR-specific plasmablasts/plasma cells in and around germinal centres (detected by autoradiography). Diffuse labelling in the light zone probably indicates binding of free ^{125}I-α-bungarotoxin to AChR trapped on follicular dendritic cells (see text). Reproduced from Sims *et al* (2001).

3.4.2 Ig V-gene expression by thymic germinal centre B-cells

In order to determine whether thymic germinal centre B-cells are subjected to antigen-driven clonal proliferation, somatic hypermutation and affinity selection, as seen in the orthotopic germinal centres of secondary lymphoid organs, we cloned and sequenced rearranged Ig heavy chain V-genes from multiple sections through four thymic germinal centres (A - D) and the follicular mantle surrounding one of them (A). 216 rearranged V_H-genes, derived from 61 independently rearranged, functional sequences, were obtained from the four germinal centres and 46 V_H-genes from the follicular mantle were derived from 24 functional V_H-genes. Since the PCR error rate in control experiments was estimated to be less than one base per four V_H-genes, only sequences using the same V, D & J exons, the same junctional sequences and a minimum of one base difference per gene, were accepted as mutated members of a clonally related set of B-cells. This conservative assessment almost certainly discards some B-cell clones with low frequencies of somatic mutation and therefore underestimates the true B-cell diversity. When calculating the number of V_H-genes used, members of the same B-cell clone were counted only once. However, this reflects the number of individual B-cell clones and non-dividing B-cells rather than the total number of B-cells using a particular gene.

The distribution of V_H-gene families was similar in the follicular mantle and all four germinal centres, with predominant use of members of the V_H3 gene family compared with the number of germline V_H-genes in this family (Fig. 4A). However, since this gene family is also predominantly used by the peripheral blood B-cells of healthy individuals, it was not considered to be significant. No V_H6, V_H7 or J_H2 genes were isolated and J_H1 was under-used, but the rarely used V_H5-51 gene and the J_H4 exon (Fig. 4B) were over-represented, both being used by rearranged V-genes from three different germinal centres in combination with different D exons (D_H2-2, D_H5-12 and D_H-6-19). In many cases the D exon could not be identified due to junctional diversity and removal of bases during recombination. Of those that could be identified, D_H3 and D_H6 were the most commonly used. These data strongly imply selection for B-cells expressing antigen receptors using particular combinations of V, D and J segments, despite the heterogeneity of the germinal centre B-cells. This would be even more apparent if individual members of the same B-cell clone were counted separately.

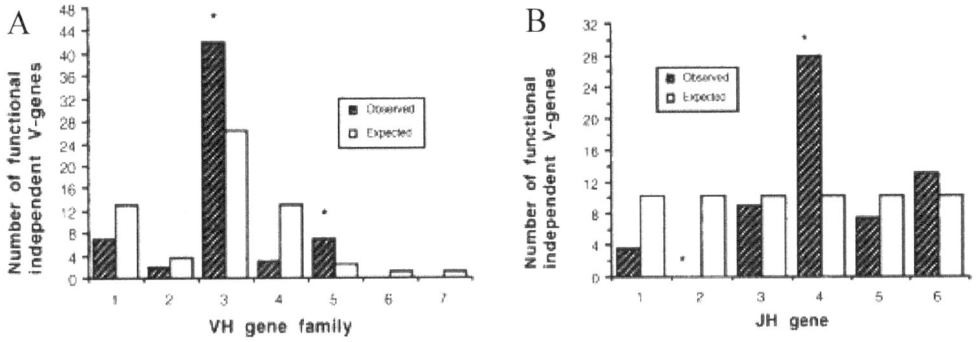

Fig. 4. Frequency of usage of V_H and J_H germline genes by thymic germinal centre B-cells.

A: The frequency of VH gene family usage in all germinal centres analysed differs significantly from predictions from the number of members of each family in the germline. Members of clonally related sets were only counted once. B: The frequency of individual JH exon usage in all germinal centres analysed differs significantly from the number of JH exons in the germline (*$p<0.01$). Reproduced from Sims *et al* (2001).

3.4.3 Somatic hypermutation and clonal proliferation of B-cells in thymic germinal centres

All the germinal centres and the follicular mantle contained B-cells expressing both mutated and unmutated Ig V-genes, the latter presumably coming from naïve B-cells. The majority of V-genes from the germinal centres and the follicular mantle were mutated, with considerable variation in the number of mutations, ranging from 0 - 52. Some of the rearranged V-genes in clonally related sets had high ratios of replacement to silent mutations from 4.7:1 to 7.0:1 in the CDRs, which form the antigen-binding site, suggesting affinity selection of mutated antigen receptors is taking place in the germinal centre. Some other sequences had low numbers of replacement mutations, suggesting selection against replacement mutations, as also found by (Zuckerman *et al.*, 2010). 18 different sets of functionally rearranged V_H-genes included two or more related sequences sharing the same V, D and J segments and junctional sequences but with significantly more than one mutation per V-gene and, in three cases, they were cloned in separate amplifications from different sections through the same germinal centre and therefore could only be from different B-cells.

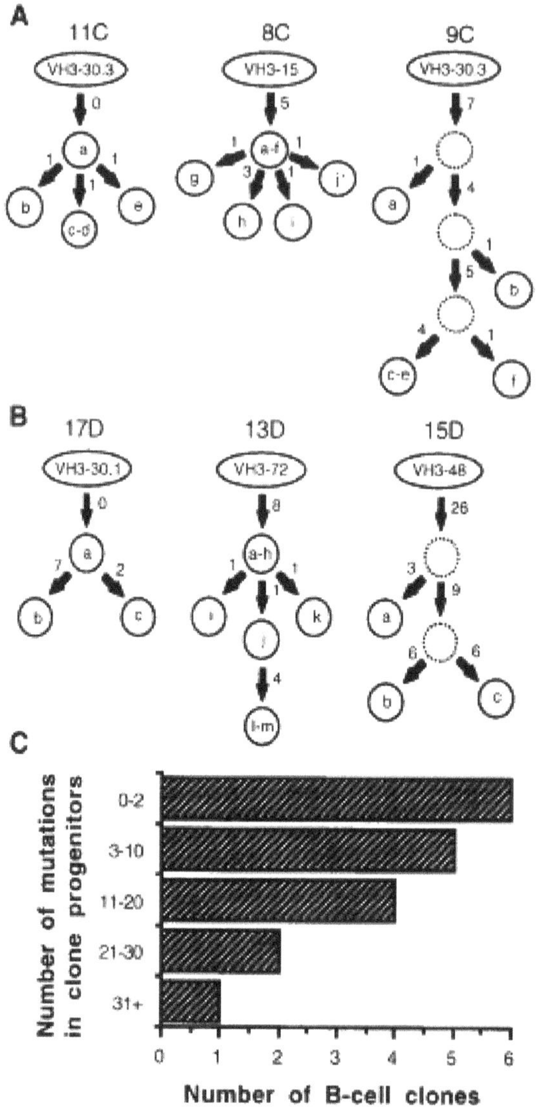

Fig. 5. Examples of clonally related sets of rearranged V_H genes isolated from thymic germinal centres C and D.

The genealogical trees were constructed using the most parsimonious parent-daughter cell relationships of clonally related sets of sequences (section 2.2). The best matching germline gene is depicted as an ellipse. Letters in the circles refer to individual sequences from the same clonally related set. Deduced intermediates are shown as dotted circles. Numbers at the side of the arrows indicate the minimum number of mutations required to generate a daughter cell from the immediate parental cell. The results show that the B-cells from which they were derived are undergoing antigen-driven clonal proliferation and somatic hypermutation from both naïve and memory B-cell precursors. A: B-cell clones from germinal centre C; B: B-cell clones from germinal centre D; C: Frequency of mutations in the V_H genes expressed by the most probable progenitor cells of all 18 B-cell clones analysed. Reproduced from Sims *et al.* (2001).

These related sets of V-genes were therefore derived from members of the same proliferating B-cell clone, showing that antigen-driven B-cell proliferation and somatic hypermutation are taking place within the thymic germinal centres. All of the isolated B-cell clones were small, containing a maximum of five members.

We do not know the total number of clones proliferating within a single germinal centre. We examined every tenth section but may have missed small B-cell clones, so there are likely to be more than we detected. Genealogical trees of related sets of V-genes were constructed by the most parsimonious relationship on the basis of shared and unshared mutations (section 2.5). Six of the 18 clones isolated from two germinal centres containing AChR-specific B-cells were derived from unmutated precursors, i.e. naïve B-cells, whereas the V_H-genes of the earliest founder cells isolated from the other 12 clones contained from 5 to >30 mutations. Examples of six of these clones are shown in Fig. 5. Although we cannot rule out the possibility that some of these clones were also derived from unidentified naïve B-cells, it is most probable that the majority were generated from founder memory B-cells. Thus, both memory and naïve B-cells have been stimulated by antigen and are proliferating and mutating their antigen receptors within thymic germinal centres of myasthenia patients.

3.4.4 Evidence for selection of AChR-specific B-cell clones in thymic germinal centres

Three B-cell clones from 3 different AChR positive germinal centres expressed the rarely used V_H5-51 genes. Furthermore, these three independent sets of V-genes exhibited the same amino acid replacements at three positions. Comparison of our V-gene sequences with those of heavy chains from known AChR-specific hybridomas and Fabs revealed some common features. Germline genes used by four of our B-cell clones also encode anti-AChR antibodies cloned from other EOMG patients, and several of the amino acid substitutions in CDR1 and CDR2 from two B-cell clones were also present in an anti-AChR Fab (Sims *et al.*, 2001; Matthews *et al.*, 2002). It is therefore unlikely that these mutations occurred by chance, suggesting that a common selection process for mutants with high affinity for the AChR is in operation.

3.4.5 Evidence for immunisation by the fetal form of acetylcholine receptor

Babies born to mothers with myasthenia gravis can develop transient symptoms due to transplacental transfer of the maternal autoantibodies and, in rare cases, they have severe developmental abnormalities, arthrogryposis multiplex congenita (AMC), caused by maternal anti-AChR antibodies that inhibit the ion channel function of the fetal AChR, causing paralysis during fetal development *in utero*, whereas the adult form of the mother's AChR is relatively unaffected. Fetal AChR-specific antibodies are particularly prevalent in women who have had babies, suggesting that they may be induced by the fetus.

In order to determine the specificity and clonal origins of fetal AChR-specific autoantibodies, combinatorial Fab libraries were constructed from cDNA prepared from thymic cells of two mothers (M2 and M6) of AMC babies. 25 Fab clones were isolated and two clonally related sets were examined in greater detail. All Fabs bound specifically to the γ subunit of fetal AChR, except one that recognised the β subunit also present in the adult receptor. Sequencing of the fetal-specific Fabs revealed clearly restricted usage of V_H, J_H, $V\kappa$ & J_κ gene segments and convergent coding mutations. All the Fabs from AMC mother M2 used the V_H3-07 gene recombined with J_H6b and an unidentified D exon in combination with various V_κ genes, suggesting that the heavy chain is the major contributor to AChR binding, at least in this case. The V_H3-07 segments were mutated and clonally related. Most of the Fabs from AMC mother M6 used the same combination of mutated V_H3-21 and J_H5b, with an unidentified D exon, plus a Vκ02-12/J_κ4 light chain, which was also used in two of the Fabs from M2. In this case, both the V_H3-21 and V_κ02-12 sets of sequences were clonally related, suggesting that they may both be derived from the same B-cell clone. The clonally related sequences from both sets of Fabs from M2 and M6 contained many shared and unshared coding mutations. The apparent founder member of each set of sequences had a large number of base differences from the best matching germline V-gene, suggesting that the clones were derived from mutated memory B-cells (Fig. 6).

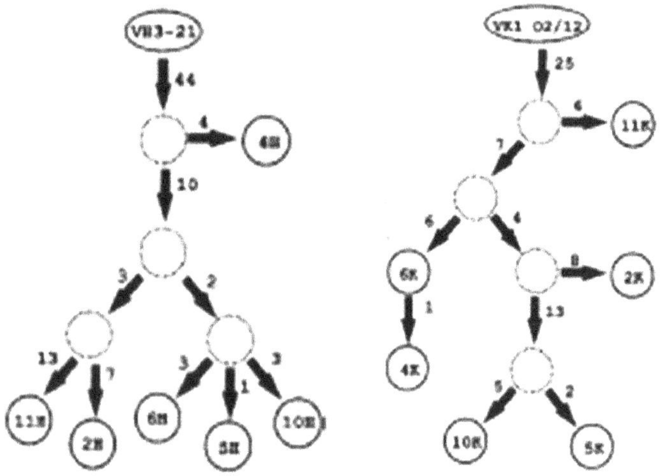

Fig. 6. Clonally related sets of rearranged V_H & V_κ genes encoding AChR-binding Fabs cloned from thymic cells from AMC mother M6.

The heavy and light chains were from the same set of Fabs. Genealogical trees were constructed and mutations numbered as described in the legend to figure 5. Fab names are shown in the circles, H referring to the heavy chain and K referring to the κ light chain. Dotted circles represent hypothetical intermediates. Numbers at the side of arrows show the minimum number of mutations required to generate a daughter cell from its immediate parent. Reproduced from Matthews *et al.* (2002).

Several sequences from both clonally related sets of Fabs had many more replacement mutations than expected by chance, indicating affinity selection. There was also clear evidence of convergent mutations. Many independently rearranged sequences from both patients shared consensus mutations. All the Fabs using V_H3 genes contained the same 31S→T mutation and most of the Vκ02-12 genes contained a 22SRASET28 motif in CDR1. A search of the GenBank database of all human Ig sequences found only two other κ chains containing this motif, suggesting that it is important in determining the specificity of the anti-AChR autoantibodies.

3.5 Conclusions

Since the EOMG thymus contains many typical germinal centres surrounded by mantle zones, including clones of proliferating, AChR-specific B-cells, it is clearly a site of autoantibody diversification. The B-cells are undergoing somatic hypermutation and affinity selection by cognate binding to AChR bound to the membrane processes of follicular dendritic cells, which form a network surrounding B and T-cells in the germinal centres. B-cells expressing high affinity, AChR-specific antigen receptors receive rescue signals from follicular dendritic and helper T-cells inducing them to differentiate into antibody-secreting plasmablasts and plasma cells that migrate out of the follicles and leave the thymus to enter the circulation, in a classical germinal centre type response. The numerous mutations seen in some V-gene sequences suggests that Ig class-switched memory B-cells are also generated and either leave the thymus, or some may recirculate within the germinal centre, undergoing further rounds of somatic hypermutation and affinity selection, consistent with the observations of others that recirculation of centrocytes between the light and dark zones occurs in orthotopic germinal centres. Several of the B-cell clones we identified were derived from highly mutated precursors, which supports this hypothesis. The autoantibodies produced by mothers of AMC babies included antibodies specific for the fetal form of the AChR, directed against the γ subunit.

The reason why large numbers of germinal centres producing AChR-specific B-cells and plasma cells develop in the thymi of myasthenia gravis patients is unclear, but it is possible that the rare thymic myoid cells may be involved. The induction of fetal AChR-specific antibodies in parous women suggests, at least in some cases, that expression of the fetal AChR on thymic epithelial and myoid cells may initiate an immune response, for which the patient's immune system has not been tolerised. Furthermore, generation of thymic germinal centres may be induced by a pre-existing proinflammatory cytokine environment, including IFNγ and TNFα. These molecules have been shown to upregulate expression of AChR subunits in thymic epithelial cells and on the membranes of myoid cells (Poea-Guyon *et al.*, 2005). The chemokines CXCL13 AND CCL21 are produced by endothelial cells of the afferent lymphatic vessels in the thymus, attracting activated T and B-cells, including naïve B-cells, suggesting that this is the mechanism of induction of thymic germinal centres (Berrih-Aknin *et al.*, 2009; Le Panse *et al.*, 2006; Meraouna *et al.*, 2006; Le Panse *et al.*, 2010).

We therefore propose a two step process for initiation of the autoimmune response in myasthenia gravis (SHIONO *et al.*, 2003). In step 1, there is hyperplasia of thymic epithelial cells expressing linear AChR epitopes, including the α and ε subunits, in the context of the MHC Class II antigen HLA-DR52a, a susceptibility factor for EOMG patients. Whereas these peptides would normally induce tolerance, an imbalance in regulatory factors and expression of costimulatory molecules results in activation of thymic T_h-cells against AChR epitopes. In step 2, the T_h-cells induce an early B-cell response against the linear peptides and some of the resulting antibodies cross-react with conformational epitopes of the native AChR expressed on the thymic myoid cells, leading to myoid cell damage, release of AChR/antibody immune complexes, danger signals, and recruitment of professional antigen presenting cells. These stimulate an enhanced B-cell response accompanied by formation of germinal centres with production of high affinity, class switched, pathogenic autoantibodies. Although some aspects of this hypothesis are conjectural, they are also testable.

4. Tissue-infiltrating B-cells in inflammatory myopathies

4.1 Introduction

The inflammatory myopathies (IM), collectively called myositis, are classified into three principal subsets, Dermatomyositis (DM), Polymyositis (PM) and Inclusion Body Myositis (IBM) (Bohan & Peter, 1975a; Bohan & Peter, 1975b; Dalakas & Hohlfeld, 2003). Each of these disorders is characterised by moderate to severe muscle weakness and muscle fatigue with inflammatory mononuclear cell infiltration within the muscle, but each disorder has distinct clinical and pathological features. IM can be associated with various autoimmune and connective tissue disorders as well as malignancies, the latter being associated with up to 45% of adult DM patients.

DM, the most common of the inflammatory myopathies, is a multi-organ disease not only affecting skeletal muscle but, often, the skin as well as other tissues and is more commonly found in women than men; it also accounts for up to c.85% of all juvenile IM (Rider, 2007). DM is characterised by a heliotrope rash on the upper eyelid, face or upper trunk accompanying, or more commonly preceding, proximal muscle weakness. Muscle inflammation is predominantly perivascular and/or perimysial or in the interfascicular septae and around, rather than within, the muscle fascicles. Perivascular atrophy is a characteristic feature of DM patients, often in groups at the periphery of the fascicle. In DM, muscle lymphocytic infiltrates consist largely of B-cells and $CD4^{+}$ T-cells (Arahata & Engel, 1984; Engel & Arahata, 1984) suggesting that DM may be a humorally mediated immune response.

PM and IBM, though separate disorders, are both characterised by scattered necrotic and regenerating muscle fibres and endomysial inflammation with invasion and destruction of non-necrotic muscle fibres. PM generally becomes evident in adulthood and is best defined as a subacute myopathy that evolves over weeks to months and presents with symmetrical weakness of the proximal muscles. Its clinical onset is hard to define with no early recognition signs such as the rash observed in DM. PM is uncommon as a stand-alone disorder and more commonly associates with other autoimmune and connective tissue disorders.

Onset of IBM is usually after the age of 50 and occurs more frequently in men. Muscle weakness can be both proximal and distal and is often asymmetrical. Despite similarities with PM, distinctive features of IBM include: rimmed vacuoles; groups of atrophic fibres; increased lymphocytic invasion of non-necrotic fibres; less frequent myofibre necrosis; and a more slowly progressing clinical course with patients being unresponsive to treatment. In both disorders, inflammatory infiltrates typically consist of $CD8^{+}$ T-cells and macrophages (Arahata & Engel, 1984; Engel & Arahata, 1984) which invade MHC Class 1 antigen-expressing muscle fibres, a feature absent in normal muscle tissue, leading to fibre necrosis. The muscle fibre invading $CD8^{+}$ T-cells can be clonally expanded in both PM and IBM (Dalakas, 2004; Fyhr *et al.*, 1997; Hofbauer *et al.*, 2003; Mantegazza *et al.*, 1993; Seitz *et al.*, 2006), which persists over time (Amemiya, Granger, & Dalakas, 2000).

4.1.1 Autoantibodies associated with myositis

As with most autoimmune disorders, different autoantibody specificities have been described in DM and PM; autoantibodies are generally absent from IBM although they have been detected in a small number of cases (Dalakas *et al.*, 1997). They can either be myositis-specific (MSAs) or myositis-associated autoantibodies (MAAs), which can also be associated with other autoimmune diseases. Most bind to protein or ribonucleoprotein complexes involved in protein synthesis, translocation or elongation; MAA target antigens are primarily located in the nucleoplasm or nucleolus. The most prevalent MSAs are directed against amino-acyl-tRNA-synthetases (ARS), and are associated with a distinctive clinical phenotype, anti-synthetase syndrome, characterised by myositis, Raynaud's phenomenon and interstitial lung disease, with a higher mortality. Anti-Jo-1 (anti-histidyl-tRNA synthetase) antibodies are the most prevalent in myositis patients (20-30% of patients), while the other anti-ARS antibodies are only present in 1-3% of IM patients, and are a diagnostic and prognostic marker for disease severity (Mielnik *et al.*, 2006; Zampieri *et al.*, 2005).

4.1.2 Muscle-infiltrating B-cells in myositis

As described above B-cells have been found to be prominent within the muscle infiltrating cell populations of DM patients and are rarely found, or absent, in the inflamed muscle of PM and IBM patients. CD138$^+$ plasma cells have been identified within the infiltrating populations, predominantly in the endomysial areas of muscle tissue of PM and IBM patients (Greenberg *et al.*, 2002; Greenberg *et al.*, 2005). This was confirmed by sequence analysis of immunoglobulin V-genes expressed by laser dissected cells as well as microarray studies which showed an abundance of immunoglobulin transcripts.

The role for B-cells and plasma cells in IM is still currently unresolved, with continuing studies providing further insight into the immune mechanisms. The identification of muscle infiltrating B-cells, plasma cells and autoantibodies suggests that these diseases may be at least partly driven by a loss of B-cell tolerance and, in the case of PM and IBM patients, not solely by the oligoclonal expansion of T-cells. We therefore investigated whether there is clonal expansion of infiltrating, autoantibody producing B-cells *in situ* in IM.

4.2 The muscle infiltrating B-cell response in myositis

4.2.1 The cellular composition of infiltrating lymphoid cells in myositis

To determine whether specific, antigen-driven, B-cell adaptive immune responses were occurring *in situ*, we used the methods described in section 2 to study the cellular composition of muscle infiltrating cells in twelve different muscle samples (2 DM, 9 PM, 1 IBM); we also examined their Ig V-gene repertoire and the processes of somatic hypermutation and clonal diversification of the rearranged V-genes. In contrast with other autoimmune diseases (see above), no classical ectopic germinal centre structures were observed within the inflamed muscle; instead, muscle-infiltrating cells were present in cellular aggregations which varied from loose to dense in the appropriate perivascular/perimysial or endomysial locations, as in previous studies. B-cells were a significant component of the inflammatory infiltrate in all samples examined for all three myositis subsets, either as CD20$^+$ B-cells or differentiated plasma cells (Figure 7A-D), although the most significant infiltration of CD20$^+$ B-cells was observed within the muscles of the two DM patients. FDCs were rare, and were seen only in one IBM and three PM samples, and not at all in DM. In addition to these cell phenotypes, CD3$^+$, CD4$^+$, CD8$^+$, CD68$^+$ and FoxP3$^+$ cells were also present. Double immunofluorescence staining of cell phenotypes with the proliferating cell marker Ki67 identified proliferating cells within the infiltrating population. In addition to CD20$^+$ B-cells (Figure 7E & F), proliferating CD3$^+$, CD4$^+$, CD8$^+$ and CD68$^+$ cells were observed, as well as FoxP3$^+$ cells in one DM patient.

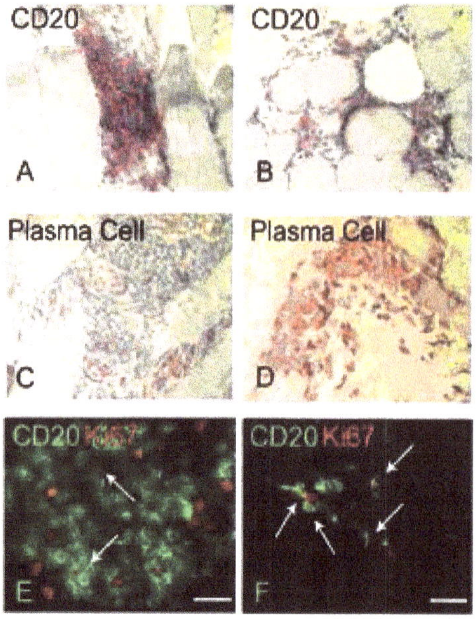

Fig. 7. Immunohistochemical staining of antigen-specific muscle-infiltrating B-cells and plasma cells.

A - D: Infiltrating B-cells and plasma cells (red) within inflamed muscle; E & F: Proliferating B-cells ($CD20^+$ B-cells - Fluorescein-Avidin D (green), $Ki67^+$ - Texas Red-Avidin D (red)). Slides A, B, C & E are from 2 DM patients; D & F are from a PM patient. Original magnification for images A - D: 400x; E & F: 630x. Scale Bar (E & F) represents 15 μm. Arrows indicate double positive staining.

4.2.2 The Ig V-gene repertoire and clonally proliferating, muscle-infiltrating B-cells

Analysis of the repertoire of rearranged Ig V-genes expressed by infiltrating B-cells and plasma cells revealed significant biases for and against individual gene segments and families relative to the normal peripheral blood B-cell and the germline gene repertoires. V-gene usage varied between patients and myositis subsets and, in a few instances, differed significantly between the DM and PM subsets. Interestingly, naïve or unmutated B-cells (0-2 mutations per V_H gene) constituted almost 50% of the B-cells in DM, but <10% in PM, where a large proportion of sequences was highly mutated (c.30% >20 mutations). As expected, mutations were prevalent within CDRs 1 & 2. A total of nine clonally related sequences was found in five of the IM patients studied; 2 DM and 3 PM patients, each with up to four different clones comprising between two and ten clonal variants (Figure 8). These clonally related sequences provide evidence for specific, antigen-driven B-cell immune responses within the inflamed muscle. However, using the method of Hershberg *et al.* (2008), we found no evidence of positive selection in the CDRs of clonally related sequences, nor in any sequences isolated from the DM patients, and only in a small percentage from the PM patients. Finally, using biotinylated recombinant antigens, we identified antigen-specific B and plasma cells in infiltrates from the five out of twelve patients whose autoantibody specificities were known, including Jo-1 (Figure 9).

Parallel studies (Bradshaw *et al.*, 2007) also demonstrated B-cell responses in muscle of 3 DM, 2 PM and 7 IBM patients but very few $CD19^+$ or $CD20^+$ cells were observed, the majority of B-lineage cells being CD138+ plasma cells that had class switched to either IgG or IgA. Clonally related sequences were isolated from whole muscle sections from ten of the twelve myositis patients, with up to four different clonal sets isolated from each muscle sample. Further studies also support the absence of classical ectopic germinal centre structures and the clonal expansion and maturation of B-cells within inflamed muscle (Salajegheh *et al.*, 2010). Collectively this and our work strongly suggest the participation of antigen-specific B-cell immune responses within the muscle.

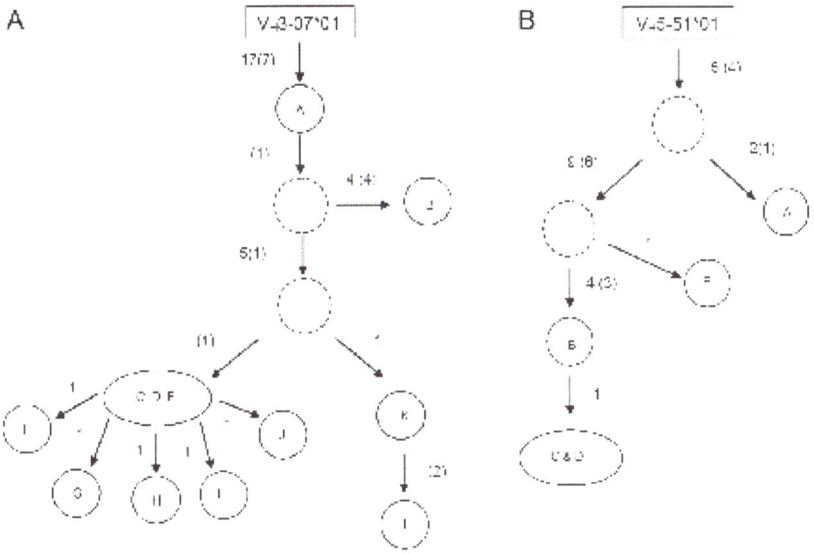

Fig. 8. Oligoclonal expansion of B-cells and plasma cells in inflammatory myopathies

Representative examples of clonal genealogical trees constructed from sequences isolated from muscle-infiltrating B-cells and plasma cells in individual patients, representing the minimum number of cell divisions required to generate each daughter cell. Clone A from a DM patient; clone B from a PM patient. The letters in the circles refer to individual sequences isolated from each B-cell clone. Genealogical trees were constructed and mutations numbered as described in the legend to Figure 5. Bracketed figures representing additional silent mutations. Dashed circles represent hypothetical intermediates whose sequences were not isolated from the muscle-infiltrating population.

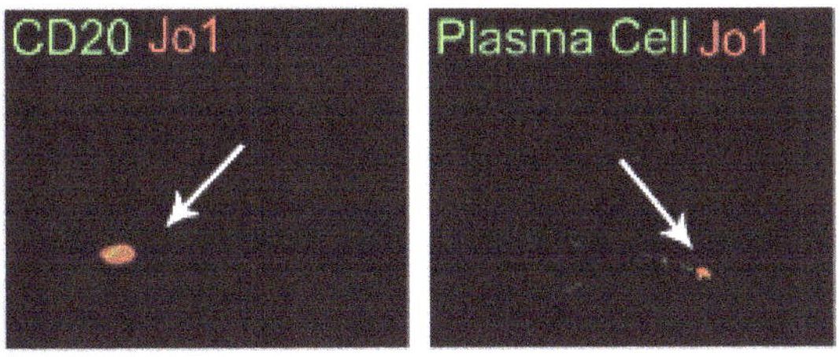

Fig. 9. Infiltrating antigen-specific B-cells and plasma cells in inflammatory myopathies

CD20+ B-cells and antigen-specific cells were visualised by Fluorescein-Avidin D (green) and Texas Red-Avidin D (red) respectively. Original magnification was 630X. Arrows identify antigen-specific cells within the muscle-infiltrating population of polymyositis patients.

4.3 Conclusions

As previously described in other autoimmune diseases, a role for B-cells in IM is implied by the clinical improvement in patients administered Rituximab® therapy, including improvements in muscle strength. Some patients relapsed as their B-cell pools repopulated and depletion of autoantibody titres was variable (Chung, Genovese, & Fiorentino, 2007; Cooper et al., 2007; Levine, 2005). The potential of B-cells as therapeutic targets is further supported by the elevations in serum levels and gene expression of B-cell activating factor (BAFF) in IM patients, a cytokine crucial for B-cell maturation and survival, which is also thought to play a role in autoantibody production (Krystufkova *et al.*, 2008; Salajegheh *et al.*, 2010).

Despite all the evidence described here implicating B-cells and loss of B-cell tolerance in the IM, numerous questions still remain to be resolved, including identification of the stimulating antigens and epitopes, sequence characteristics and pathogenicity of high-affinity, antigen-specific antibodies produced *in situ*, and the factors regulating and controlling these autoimmune reactions. The resolution of these questions will enhance our understanding of the immune pathology of IM and facilitate the diagnosis, treatment and management of these diseases.

5. The ectopic germinal centre response in breast cancer

In autoimmune diseases there is a failure of immunological tolerance resulting in an immune response to self-antigens, causing pathological damage to the target organ and tissues, the nature of the target tissue depending on the specificity of the response. In malignancy the immune response, if it occurs, is similar in that it is essentially directed against self, i.e. tumour-associated, antigens. These antigens may be mutated, altered by metabolic processes, or merely aberrantly or over-expressed on the tumour. The problem, however, is converse to autoimmune disease in that, whereas in autoimmune disease the aim is to suppress the immune response, preferably specifically against the target organ, in cancer the hope is that it will be possible to boost the immune response which is often too weak to overcome the rapidly growing tumour.

Several autoimmune disorders sometimes associate with certain tumours, most often small cell lung cancer, breast or ovarian carcinomas, ovarian teratomas, neuroblastomas and lymphomas (with Sjögren's syndrome), reviewed by Lang & Vincent and Rosenfeld *et al.* (Lang & Vincent, 2009; Rosenfeld & Dalmau, 2010). In the examples studied, the target autoantigen(s) are expressed on the tumour which seems to autoimmunise against them. Indeed, if the tumour is removed, autoantibody levels often decline (Chalk *et al.*, 1990). In many syndromes, the autoimmune disorder serves as a valuable early warning of the associated tumour, and may even slow its growth (Maddison & Lang, 2008).

5.1 Pathology of breast cancer

Breast cancer is the second most common malignancy in women, accounting for 31% of all types of cancer, with a lifetime incidence in the U.K. of 1/8 in women and c.1/1000 in men. Despite advances in screening, diagnosis and therapy, 12,000 women die of breast cancer each year in the U.K. and the global incidence in females is 23%, but there are marked variations between different regions, it being the highest in Western Europe, Australia, New Zealand and North America. The incidence is relatively low in Asian and African countries (figures from Cancer Research UK). There are several different histopathological types of breast cancer, of which the major types are the ductal and lobular carcinomas, either of which can be *in situ* or invasive, the *in situ* type being considered a possible precursor of invasive carcinoma. Ductal and lobular carcinomas *in situ* are confined to the mammary ducts and lobules and have a very high cure rate, approaching 100%. Invasive carcinomas account for the majority of breast cancers and have a much poorer prognosis. Malignant cell growth appears to start in the ducts and lobules and then invades the surrounding tissues and ultimately metastasises to other tissues and organs. A less common type is medullary carcinoma, comprising only c.1 - 5% of breast cancers; this typically has heavy infiltrates of B-lymphocytes and a significantly better prognosis than the invasive ductal and lobular types. Length of disease free survival in breast cancer is unpredictable, with relapse occurring up to ten years post treatment and even beyond; it has been postulated that this may be due to host factors, including the nature and extent of the immune response.

5.2 The immune response to breast cancer

Most breast cancers contain infiltrates of lymphoid cells with large numbers of T-cells, including $CD4^+$ and $CD8^+$ T-cells, and variable numbers of B-cells, natural killer cells and macrophages. The degree of infiltration varies between different types of breast cancer with extensive lymphoid cell infiltrates in ductal carcinoma *in situ* and some invasive ductal and lobular carcinomas (Ben Hur *et al.*, 2002). Most studies have focused on the role of cytotoxic T-cells in tumour immunity, with variable success in attempting to suppress tumour growth by boosting the T-cell response to tumour-associated antigens. Relatively few studies have addressed the role of B-cells and humoral immunity in response to cancers, including breast cancer, despite the observation that c.40% of ductal breast carcinomas have significant B-cell infiltration.

There is increasing evidence that B-cells play important dual opposing roles in the immune response to tumours; on the one hand as antigen presenting cells and producers of cytotoxic antibodies effective at killing tumour cells by antibody-dependent cell-mediated cytotoxicity (ADCC) and complement-dependent cell lysis, and as tumour antigen-presenting cells capable of very efficient T-cell activation; on the other hand as promoters of inflammation aiding tumour progression (de Visser, Korets, & Coussens, 2005; de Visser, Eichten, & Coussens, 2006). These seemingly contradictory effects may be due to the difference between a specific, high affinity immune response to antigen versus a low affinity, polyclonal response, or even suppression of the cytotoxic immune response via regulatory B-cells (Mauri, 2010). The importance of antibodies in eliminating tumours is clearly demonstrated by the results of treatment of breast cancer patients with humanised monoclonal antibodies (MAbs) specific for the epidermal growth factor receptor HER-2 (trastuzumab/herceptin and pertuzumab). Not only is herceptin effective in slowing down the progression of established metastatic disease, it has also recently been demonstrated to prevent the emergence of metastases when given as an adjuvant treatment (Hortobagyi, 2005). Pertuzumab has also yielded promising results in clinical trials (Bianco, 2004). Synergistic effects between herceptin and pertuzumab suggest promising new approaches to therapy using cocktails of antibodies (Nahta, Hung, & Esteva, 2004) and elucidation of the molecular structure of the herceptin Fab/HER-2 complex (Cho *et al.*, 2003) allows rational design of therapeutic anti-HER-2 antibodies. MAbs specific for other tumour-associated antigens (TAAs) are needed to work synergistically with trastuzumab and to treat patients who do not overexpress HER-2.

Several molecules have been identified that are either over-expressed, mutated, or structurally modified on tumour cells and are therefore potential targets for immunotherapy, including HER-1, HER-2, MUC-1 and p53 (Taylor-Papadimitriou *et al.*, 2002). Some TAAs appear to overcome tolerance and induce a natural immune response as a result of mutation or altered expression; humoral immune responses to these antigens in breast cancer patients are associated with better early disease stage-specific survival (Angelopoulou *et al.*, 2000;Visco *et al.*, 2000; von Mensdorff-Pouilly *et al.*, 2000) and anti-MUC-1 antibodies are cytotoxic to tumour cells (Snijdewint *et al.*, 2001). TAA-specific tumour infiltrating (TIL) B-lymphocytes and recombinant antibodies have been isolated from both tumour (Kotlan *et al.*, 2000; Kotlan *et al.*, 2005) and lymph nodes (Petrarca *et al.*, 1999; Rothe *et al.*, 2004) of medullary and ductal carcinoma patients, showing that they are responding specifically to the tumour. Evasion of the immune response by the tumour can be overcome by passive immunotherapy or active immunisation regimes. B-cells actively responding in the draining lymph node and tumour are therefore ideal sources to study the immune response to the tumour and provide the most relevant source of potentially therapeutic antibodies.

5.3 Ductal carcinoma infiltrating lymphocytes are clustered into germinal centres

We and others found infiltrating lymphocytes in ductal carcinomas were aggregated into clusters containing T-cells, B-cells and follicular dendritic cells with plasmablasts/plasma cells in and around the aggregates (Coronella *et al.*, 2002; Nzula, Going, & Stott, 2003a). These cell clusters appeared to be similar to those seen in the target tissues of autoimmune diseases except that there was no mantle zone (also absent in the salivary glands of patients with Sjögren's syndrome (Stott *et al.*, 1998)), so we examined whether they were responding as germinal centres.

5.4 The Ig V-gene repertoire and clonal proliferation of B-cells in ductal carcinoma

We cloned and sequenced 401 rearranged Ig V_H-genes from microdissected tumour-infiltrating B-cell foci of 7 patients with invasive ductal carcinoma and 271 V_H-genes from paired sentinel lymph nodes of 3 of the patients. 15 sets of V_H-genes from clonally related B-cells within individual foci were identified by their shared V_H, D, J_H and CDR3 sequences, showing that proliferating, mutating B-cell clones were present in lymphoid foci and that these foci were undergoing a germinal centre response within the tumour, similar to the ectopic germinal centres we have observed in the target tissues of autoimmune diseases (Fig. 10). There was preferential usage of certain V_H, D & J_H exons, indicating selection of B-cells expressing antigen receptors encoded by these gene combinations. V_H & V_L-genes from proliferating B-cell clones contained numerous mutations, demonstrating that the somatic hypermutation machinery was switched on within the cell cluster, again characteristic of a germinal centre response. Analysis of the pattern of mutations showed that the B-cell clones are undergoing an antigen-driven response accompanied by selection of specific mutations and affinity maturation *in situ*. Clone founder cells were of both naïve and memory B-cell type, showing that a secondary response involving memory B-cells was taking place, but also new B-cells that had not previously encountered antigen moved into cell clusters and were stimulated by antigen. We also cloned rearranged V_H-genes from microdissected germinal centres in the paired sentinel lymph node and identified proliferating, hypermutating B-cell clones there too. These also revealed selection for particular V_H & J_H-genes showing selection by antigen for B-cells expressing these genes during the immune response but we did not find evidence that members of the same B-cell clones had migrated from the sentinel node to the tumour; this could have been due to insufficient sample sizes (Nzula, Going & Stott, 2003a; Simsa *et al.*, 2005).

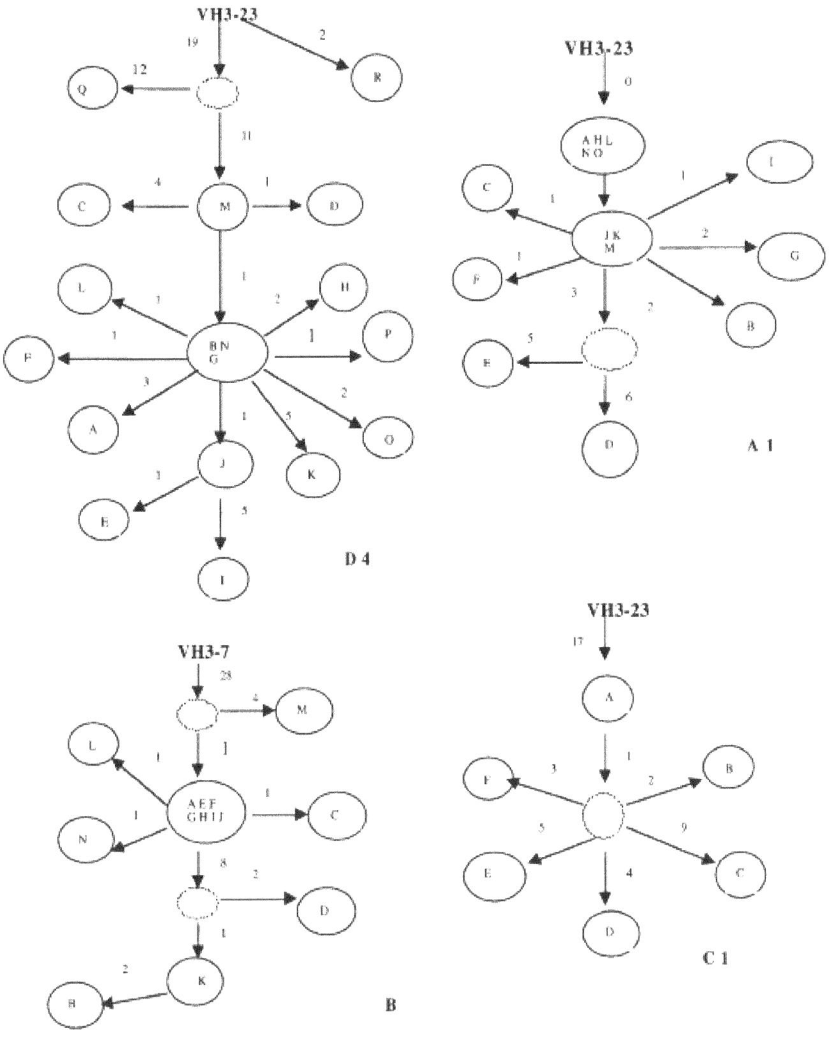

Fig. 10. Examples of proliferating, hypermutating B-cell clones from the breast tumours of four ductal carcinoma patients.

The best matching germline V_H-gene is shown at the origin of each tree. The founder rearranged V_H-genes of three of these B-cell clones already appear to be mutated, implying that they originated from memory B-cells, whereas clone A1 appears to have been founded by a naïve B-cell. Genealogical trees were constructed and mutations numbered as described in the legend to Figure 5. Reproduced from Nzula *et al.* (2003).

5.5 Cloning and characterisation of scFv antibodies

In order to identify the antigens driving the immune response within the tumour, we reconstructed the antigen receptors expressed by germinal centre B-cells as scFv antibodies by cloning V_H and V_L-genes into phagemid (pHEN2), as described in section 2.3, to generate scFv-phage libraries expressing randomly assorted combinations of V_H and V_L-genes. These "mini-libraries" were made from the B-cells in individual germinal centres within the tumour and are therefore much smaller and more restricted than the very large libraries normally made by random combination of large pools of V_H and V_L-genes. Two scFv-phage mini-libraries were constructed from a germinal centre incorporating all the V_H-genes pooled from the largest proliferating B-cell clone (D4 in Fig. 10) linked randomly to either the rearranged V_κ-genes or the rearranged V_λ-genes amplified from the same germinal centre.

Tumour-binding scFv were selected from the mini-libraries by three or four cycles of panning and elution on a heterologous tumour homogenate pooled from breast tumours of 5 patients. During the panning cycles we observed exponential enrichment of the V_λ mini-library, but not the V_κ mini-library, indicating that scFv within the V_λ mini-library bind specifically to tumour-associated antigens (Fig. 11A). This is consistent with the scFv-libraries being derived from the same B-cell clone, since a single B-cell clone uses either a κ or λ light chain, not both. 13 scFv-phages binding to the tumour extract were cloned and their specificity for tumour tissue confirmed by ELISA. 7 scFv-phage clones that bound to the tumour extract were identified for further characterisation. All 7 used the same combination of V_H3-23 with exons D1-26 & J_H2, expressed by B-cell clone D4, and the light chain gene V_λ1c with J_λ3b.

We also constructed two scFv-phage libraries from DNA extracted from a whole sample of tumour tissue, as described for the mini-libraries. The 2 libraries were panned on the same heterologous tumour homogenate as used with the mini-libraries. After 4 cycles of panning we observed an enrichment of several logs for both libraries, indicating the presence of tumour-specific antibodies (Fig. 11B). The enrichment of both global libraries shows that tumour-specific B-cells derived from independent B-cell clones were present in the tumour, as expected. 19 scFv-phages were cloned from the 2 global libraries and their specificity for tumour tissue confirmed by ELISA using the same tumour homogenate as source of antigen.

5.6 Identification of the specificity of proliferating B-cells

Since the scFvs from the V_H/V_λ mini-library were derived from proliferating B-cell clone D4, their sequences and antigen specificities reveal the nature of the genes and antigen receptor specificities of the original germinal centre B-cells. We therefore sequenced the scFv clones that showed the strongest binding to the tumour extract and performed a Blast search of the Genbank gene database. The V_HDJ_H heavy chain gene used by all members of B-cell clone D4 exhibited 89% homology with a human anti-HER3 MAb (AF048774) and the $V_\lambda J_\lambda$ light chain gene, also used by the same B-cells, matched a human anti-EGFR antibody (DQ666353.1) with 96% homology. These, and scFvs from the global libraries, were tested for binding to recombinant antigens from the epidermal growth factor receptor family: HER-2, HER-3 and HER-4, kindly provided by Genentech (San Francisco, USA) and Pharmexa A/S (Hørsholm, Denmark) by ELISA. Six scFvs from B-cell clone D4 and one from the global tumour library bound to recombinant HER-2, HER-3 & HER-4, indicating that they recognised a shared epitope expressed by all three members of this EGFR family of receptors (Fig. 12). Specificity for HER-2, HER-3 & HER-4 was confirmed using soluble scFv produced in the non-suppressor strain of *E.coli*.

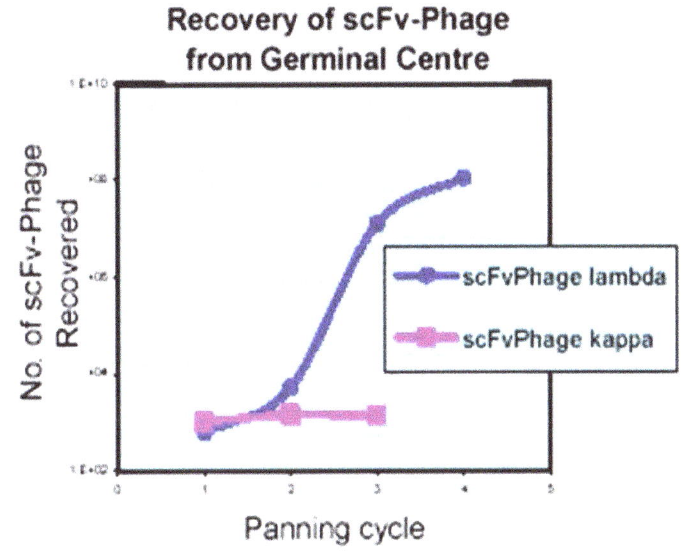

A

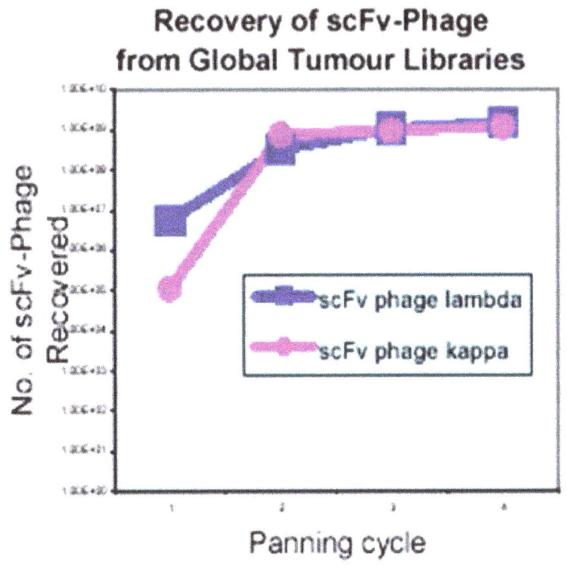

B

Fig. 11. Exponential enrichment of scFv-phage after panning and elution on a breast tumour extract

A. $V_H/V\kappa$ and $V_H/V\lambda$ scFv mini-libraries, using V_H-genes from B-cell clone D4, panned on pooled heterologous tumour extract The eluate from each panning was then subjected to further cycles of panning and elution; B. Global $V_H/V\kappa$ and $V_H/V\lambda$ scFv-phage libraries from a human breast tumour, panned on the same heterologous tumour extract as in A.

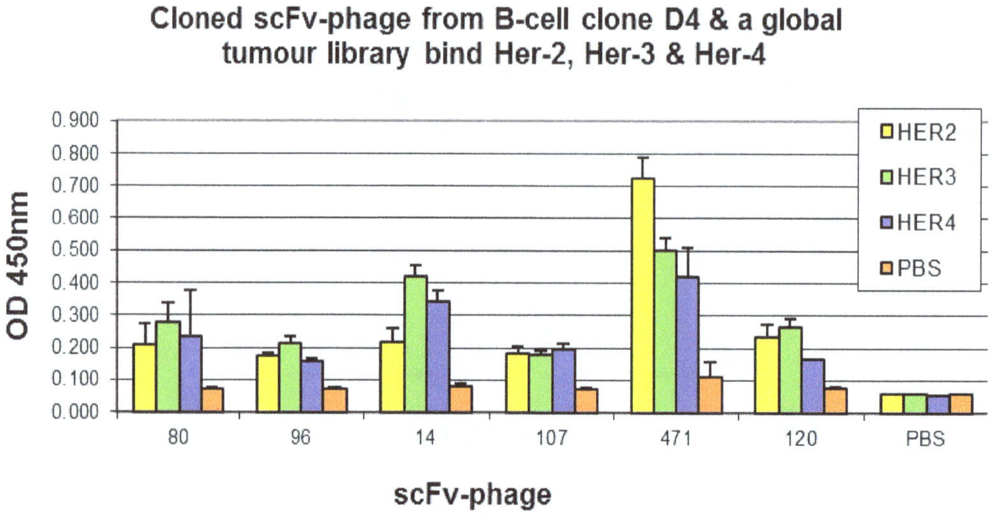

Fig. 12. EGFR family specificity of scFv antibodies cloned from a mammary carcinoma germinal centre.

Individual scFv-phage (80, 96, 14 & 107 & 120) from B-cell clone D4, proliferating and mutating in a breast tumour, and scFv-phage (471), cloned from whole breast tumour tissue, bind to members of the epidermal growth factor receptor family Her-2, Her-3 & Her-4.

5.7 Conclusions

Clusters of B-cells, T-cells and follicular dendritic cells form within human ductal breast carcinomas, resembling the ectopic germinal centres observed in the target tissues of patients with autoimmune diseases. These clusters of lymphoid cells contain clones of proliferating B-cells that are undergoing somatic hypermutation of their rearranged, Ig V-(D)-J-genes and affinity selection of their B-cell receptors driven, in the case described here, by members of the epidermal growth factor receptor family, viz. HER2, HER3 and HER4. The antibodies produced during this response recognise an epitope shared by these 3 cell surface receptors, which are known to be overexpressed on breast carcinoma cells and several other types of carcinoma, including ovarian cancer. It is very probable that other tumour associated antigens are also able to stimulate a local B-cell response within the tumour, e.g. antibodies specific for a ganglioside were cloned from medullary carcinoma B-cells, although it is not clear whether these are involved in attacking the tumour (Kotlan *et al.*, 2005).

Single chain Fv antibodies cloned from tumour germinal centre B-cells can readily be converted to complete antibodies by splicing their V-genes on to Ig constant regions of any desired isotype. These fully human antibodies can be produced in large quantities in a protein expression system and are therefore potential candidates for diagnosis, monitoring and therapy of breast and other types of cancer.

6. General conclusions

It has become increasingly clear that infiltrating B- and T-lymphocytes organise themselves into ectopic lymphoid follicles and germinal centres within tissues undergoing inflammatory processes. This has been observed in several autoimmune diseases (Table 1), usually within the target organ or tissue, myasthenia gravis being the exception to the rule for reasons discussed in section 3.5. However, ectopic g.c.s are not restricted to autoimmune diseases but can also develop in other chronic inflammatory diseases, such as Crohn's disease and ulcerative colitis; at sites of infection such as the liver during chronic hepatitis C virus infection and the skin of oncocerciasis patients (Brattig *et al.*, 2010); and in neoplasias, including lymphoma of the mucosal-associated lymphoid tissue associated with Sjögren's syndrome (Bombardieri *et al.*, 2007a) and, as shown here, in breast cancer (Table 1).

How these ectopic g.c.s develop, their role in the pathology of autoimmune diseases, and in combating infections and malignancies is still unclear but evidence is beginning to emerge. Cytokines, chemokines and signalling molecules involved in lymphoid neogenesis in the secondary lymphoid organs also appear to be required for ectopic g.c. formation, including lymphotoxins-α, β and $\alpha_1\beta_2$, TNFα, Grb2, the chemokine receptor CXCR5, its ligand CXCL15, and the B-cell attracting chemokines CXCL13 and CCL21, in this case due to release of these molecules within the inflammatory environment, suggesting that g.c. formation may be secondary to inflammation (Aloisi & Pujol-Borrell, 2006).

When reports first emerged of germinal centre-like structures within the target tissues of autoimmune diseases, there was some scepticism regarding whether these structures were involved in true germinal centre reactions. These doubts have now been dispelled. Identification of dark and light zones and a follicular dendritic cell network in intimate contact with B-cells was highly suggestive of a germinal centre reaction, especially when it was shown that autoantigen was trapped on the follicular dendritic cell processes, e.g. (SHIONO *et al.*, 2003). Studies by us and other researchers have shown that the B-cells within ectopic germinal centres are activated to antigen-driven clonal proliferation, somatic hypermutation and class switching, similar to the response in orthotopic g.c.s responding to foreign antigens. That they switch on the somatic hypermutation machinery has been shown in several autoimmune diseases by sequencing studies of the expressed, rearranged Ig V-genes cloned from microdissected g.c.s. This has been confirmed in the salivary gland g.c.s of Sjögren's patients and the synovial g.c.s of rheumatoid arthritis patients by identification of activation induced cytidine deaminase (AID), a key enzyme in somatic hypermutation and class switch recombination (Bombardieri *et al.*, 2007b; Humby *et al.*, 2009). Interestingly, expression of AID has recently been observed in hyperplastic fibroblasts of rheumatoid arthritis patients (Igarashi et al., 2010). Expression correlated with mutations in the *p53* gene and was induced by TNFα *in vitro*. AID is known to induce mutations in non-Ig genes at a lower frequency and it was suggested that the mutations of this tumour suppressor gene may be the cause of the fibroblast hyperplasia. Affinity maturation of B-cell receptors during somatic hypermutation has been demonstrated by analysis of replacement mutations, although early analyses failed to take into account the bias towards replacement mutations in the CDRs resulting from targeting of AID to sequence motifs such as RGYW. Final confirmation requires direct affinity measurements of autoantibodies cloned from germinal centre B-cells and/or by 3-D molecular modelling of the antigen-binding site bound to its epitope, as we have shown for anti-hen egg lysozyme antibodies produced in an orthotopic germinal centre reaction (Adams *et al.*, 2003).

In several cases it has been shown that the autoantibodies generated in ectopic g.c.s have similar specificities to the autoantibodies found in the blood, notably in Hashimoto's thyroiditis, Sjögren's syndrome and rheumatoid arthritis, suggesting that the g.c.s contribute to pathological mechanisms, although whether they are critical in the early stages of development of the disease, or only contribute to its maintenance once the initial tissue damage has commenced, has yet to be established. Production of cytokines and chemokines at sites of damage that attract lymphocytes and contribute to lymphoid neogenesis suggests that the latter may be the more likely scenario. Nevertheless, a detailed understanding of the mechanisms involved in generation of ectopic g.c. structures and maintenance of production of plasma cells and memory B-cells producing potentially pathogenic antibodies is essential for a full understanding of the pathology of autoimmune disease and holds promise for developing new methods of therapy, based on controlling this response or inducing immunological tolerance to the autoantigens.

Even more work needs to be done to determine the role of ectopic g.c.s in other diseases, including sterile and infectious chronic inflammatory diseases and cancer. What other types of cancer, in addition to breast cancer and lymphoma, induce germinal centre reactions within the tumour and the nature of their response in elimination of cancer cells have yet to be determined. The identification of intra-tumour g.c.s producing antibodies and memory B-cells with specificity for members of the epidermal growth factor receptor family holds out hope that therapeutic vaccines can be developed to boost this response for therapy of breast cancer and, potentially other neoplasias, such as ovarian cancer, in which these molecules are overexpressed. Experimental approaches using mouse models of breast cancer support this optimism (Renard *et al.*, 2003; Renard & Leach, 2007; Mukhopadhyay, MS in preparation). Cloning of antibodies against tumour-associated antigens from intra-tumour g.c.s is also a novel way of producing fully human antibodies for passive immunotherapy.

7. Acknowledgements

We wish to thank Professors Nick Willcox and Angela Vincent, F.R.S. (Institute for Molecular Medicine, University of Oxford, U.K.), Paul Garside and Iain McInnes (Institute of Infection, Immunity & Inflammation, University of Glasgow, U.K.) for critically reading the manuscript and their helpful suggestions. We also wish to thank all the people who have worked in D.I. Stott's research group and those of his collaborators whose work contributed to the results described here, especially Gary Sims, Michael Matthews, Sazini Nzula and Anne-Sophie Rouziere, whose data on myasthenia gravis and ductal carcinoma are presented in this chapter. Any errors and oversights are entirely our own.

The original research described in this chapter was funded by The Wellcome Trust, the Scottish Executive Health Dept. Chief Scientist Office, Cancer Research UK, the Dr. Robert Mairs Trust and the Medical Research Council.

8. References

Adams, C. L., MacLeod, M. K. L., Milner-White, E. J., Aitken, R., Garside, P., & Stott, D. I. 2003, "Complete analysis of the B-cell response to a protein antigen, from *in vivo* germinal centre formation to 3-D modelling of affinity maturation", *Immunology*, vol. 108, pp. 274-287.

Allen, C. D. C., Okada, T., & Cyster, J. G. 2007, "Germinal-Center Organization and Cellular Dynamics", *Immunity*, vol. 27, pp. 190-202.

Aloisi, F. & Pujol-Borrell, R. 2006, "Lymphoid neogenesis in chronic inflammatory diseases", *Nature Reviews Immunology*, vol. 6, pp. 205-217.

Amemiya, K., Granger, R. P., & Dalakas, M. C. 2000, "Clonal restriction of T-cell receptor expression by infiltrating lymphocytes in inclusion body myositis persists over time. Studies in repeated muscle biopsies", *Brain*, vol. 123 (Pt 10), pp. 2030-2039.

Angelopoulou, K., Yu, H., Bharaj, B., Giai, M., & Diamandis, E. P. 2000, "p53 gene mutation, tumor p53 protein overexpression, and serum p53 autoantibody generation in patients with breast cancer.", *Clin.Biochem.*, vol. 33, pp. 53-62.

Arahata, K. & Engel, A. G. 1984, "Monoclonal antibody analysis of mononuclear cells in myopathies. I: Quantitation of subsets according to diagnosis and sites of accumulation and demonstration and counts of muscle fibers invaded by T cells", *Ann.Neurol.*, vol. 16, no. 2, pp. 193-208.

Armengol, M. P., Juan, M., Lucas-Martin, A., Fernandez-Figueras, M. T., Jaraquemada, D., Gallart, T., & Pujol-Borrell, R. 2001, "Thyroid autoimmune disease: demonstration of thyroid antigen-specific B cells and recombination-activating gene expression in chemokine-containing active intrathyroidal germinal centers", *American Journal of Pathology*, vol. 159, pp. 861-873.

Astorri, E., Bombardieri, M., Gabba, S., Peakman, M., Pozzilli, P., & Pitzalis, C. 2010, "Evolution of Ectopic Lymphoid Neogenesis and In Situ Autoantibody Production in Autoimmune Nonobese Diabetic Mice: Cellular and Molecular Characterization of Tertiary Lymphoid Structures in Pancreatic Islets", *The Journal of Immunology*, vol. 185, pp. 3359-3368.

Beltman, J. B., Allen, C. D. C., Cyster, J. G., & de Boer, R. J. 2011, "B cells within germinal centers migrate preferentially from dark to light zone", *Proceedings of the National Academy of Sciences*, vol. 108, pp. 8755-8760.

Ben Hur, H., Cohen, O., Schneider, D., Gurevich, P., Halperin, R., Bala, U., Mozes, M., & Zusman, I. 2002, "The role of lymphocytes and macrophages in human breast tumorigenesis: an immunohistochemical and morphometric study", *Anticancer Res*, vol. 22, pp. 1231-1238.

Berrih-Aknin, S., Ruhlmann, N., Bismuth, J., Cizeron-Clairac, G., Zelman, E., Shachar, I., Dartevelle, P., De Rosbo, N. K., & Le Panse, R. 2009, "CCL21 overexpressed on lymphatic vessels drives thymic hyperplasia in myasthenia", *Ann.Neurol.*, vol. 66, pp. 521-531.

Bianco, A. R. 2004, "Targeting c-erbB2 and other receptors of the c-erbB family: rationale and clinical applications", *J Chemother.*, vol. 16 Suppl 4, pp. 52-54.

Bohan, A. & Peter, J. B. 1975a, "Polymyositis and dermatomyositis (first of two parts)", *N.Engl.J.Med.*, vol. 292, no. 7, pp. 344-347.

Bohan, A. & Peter, J. B. 1975b, "Polymyositis and dermatomyositis (second of two parts)", *N.Engl.J.Med.*, vol. 292, no. 8, pp. 403-407.

Bombardieri, M., Barone, F., Humby, F., Kelly, S., McGurk, M., Morgan, P., Challacombe, S., De Vita, S., Valesini, G., Spencer, J., & Pitzalis, C. 2007a, "Activation-induced cytidine deaminase expression in follicular dendritic cell networks and interfollicular large B cells supports functionality of ectopic lymphoid neogenesis in autoimmune sialoadenitis and MALT lymphoma in Sjogren's syndrome", *The Journal of Immunology*, vol. 179, pp. 4929-4938.

Bombardieri, M., Barone, F., Humby, F., Kelly, S., McGurk, M., Morgan, P., Challacombe, S., De Vita, S., Valesini, G., Spencer, J., & Pitzalis, C. 2007b, "Activation-Induced Cytidine Deaminase Expression in Follicular Dendritic Cell Networks and Interfollicular Large B Cells Supports Functionality of Ectopic Lymphoid Neogenesis in Autoimmune Sialoadenitis and MALT Lymphoma in Sjogren's Syndrome", *The Journal of Immunology*, vol. 179, pp. 4929-4938.

Bradshaw, E. M., Orihuela, A., McArdel, S. L., Salajegheh, M., Amato, A. A., Hafler, D. A., Greenberg, S. A., & O'Connor, K. C. 2007, "A local antigen-driven humoral response is present in the inflammatory myopathies", *The Journal of Immunology*, vol. 178, no. 1, pp. 547-556.

Brattig, N. W., Tenner-Racz, K., Korten, S., Hoerauf, A., & Buttner, D. W. 2010, "Immunohistology of ectopic secondary lymph follicles in subcutaneous nodules from patients with hyperreactive onchocerciasis (sowda)", *Parasitol.Res*, vol. 107, pp. 657-666.

Brink, R. 2007, "Germinal-Center B Cells in the Zone", *Immunity*, vol. 26, pp. 552-554.

Canete, J. D., Santiago, B., Cantaert, T., Sanmarti, R., Palacin, A., Celis, R., Graell, E., Gil-Torregrosa, B., Baeten, D., & Pablos, J. L. 2007, "Ectopic lymphoid neogenesis in psoriatic arthritis", *Annals Rheumatic Disease*, vol. 66, pp. 720-726.

Cardona, A., Garchon, B., Vernet der Garabedian, E., Morel, P., Gajdos, P., & Bach, J.-F. 1994, "Human IgG monoclonal autoantibodies against muscle acetylcholine receptor: direct evidence for clonal heterogeneity of the anti-self humoral response in myasthenia gravis", *J.Neuroimmunol.*, vol. 53, p. 9.

Chalk, C. H., Murray, N. M., Newsom-Davis, J., O'Neill, J. H., & Spiro, S. G. 1990, "Response of the Lambert-Eaton myasthenic syndrome to treatment of associated small-cell lung carcinoma", *Neurology*, vol. 40, pp. 1552-1556.

Cho, H. S., Mason, K., Ramyar, K. X., Stanley, A. M., Gabelli, S. B., Denney, D. W., Jr., & Leahy, D. J. 2003, "Structure of the extracellular region of HER2 alone and in complex with the Herceptin Fab", *Nature*, vol. 421, pp. 756-760.

Chung, L., Genovese, M. C., & Fiorentino, D. F. 2007, "A pilot trial of rituximab in the treatment of patients with dermatomyositis", *Arch.Dermatol.*, vol. 143, no. 6, pp. 763-767.

Cooper, M. A., Willingham, D. L., Brown, D. E., French, A. R., Shih, F. F., & White, A. J. 2007, "Rituximab for the treatment of juvenile dermatomyositis: a report of four pediatric patients", *Arthritis Rheum.*, vol. 56, no. 9, pp. 3107-3111.

Coronella, J. A., Spier, C., Welch, M., Trevor, K. T., Stopeck, A. T., Villar, H., & Hersh, E. M. 2002, "Antigen-Driven Oligoclonal Expansion of Tumor-Infiltrating B Cells in Infiltrating Ductal Carcinoma of the Breast", *The Journal of Immunology*, vol. 169, pp. 1829-1836.

Coronella, J. A., Telleman, P., Kingsbury, G. A., Truong, T. D., Hays, S., & Junghans, R. P. 2001, "Evidence for an antigen-driven humoral immune response in medullary ductal breast cancer", *Cancer Research*, vol. 61, pp. 7889-7899.

Dalakas, M. C. 2004, "The molecular pathophysiology in inflammatory myopathies", *La Revue de Medecine Interne*, vol. 25, no. Supplement 1, p. S14-S16.

Dalakas, M. C. & Hohlfeld, R. 2003, "Polymyositis and dermatomyositis.", *Lancet.362(9388):971-82.*

Dalakas, M. C., Illa, I., Gallardo, E., & Juarez, C. 1997, "Inclusion body myositis and paraproteinemia: incidence and immunopathologic correlations", *Ann.Neurol.*, vol. 41, no. 1, pp. 100-104.

Darlow, J. M. & Stott, D. I. 2005, "VH replacement in immunoglobulin genes", *Immunology*, vol. 114, pp. 155-165.

de Visser, K. E., Korets, L. V., & Coussens, L. M. 2005, "De novo carcinogenesis promoted by chronic inflammation is B lymphocyte dependent", *Cancer Cell*, vol. 7, pp. 411-423.

de Visser, K. E., Eichten, A., & Coussens, L. M. 2006, "Paradoxical roles of the immune system during cancer development", *Nature Reviews Cancer*, vol. 6, pp. 24-37.

Di Noia, J. M. & Neuberger, M. S. 2007, "Molecular Mechanisms of Antibody Somatic Hypermutation", *Annual Review of Biochemistry*, vol. 76, pp. 1-22.

Drachman, D. B. 1994, "Myasthenia gravis", *New England J.Med.*, vol. 330, pp. 1797-1810.

Engel, A. G. & Arahata, K. 1984, "Monoclonal antibody analysis of mononuclear cells in myopathies. II: Phenotypes of autoinvasive cells in polymyositis and inclusion body myositis", *Ann.Neurol.*, vol. 16, no. 2, pp. 209-215.

Farrar, J., Portolano, S., Willcox, N., Vincent, A., Jacobson, L., Newsom-Davis, J., Rapoport, B., & McLachlan, S. M. 1997, "Diverse Fab specific for acetylcholine receptor epitopes from a myasthenia gravis thymus combinatorial library.", *International Immunology*, vol. 9, pp. 1311-1318.

Fostieri, E., Beeson, D., & Tzartos, S. J. 2000, "The conformation of the main immunogenic region on the alpha-subunit of muscle acetylcholine receptor is affected by neighboring receptor subunits", *FEBS Lett.*, vol. 481, pp. 127-130.

Fyhr, I. M., Moslemi, A. R., Mosavi, A. A., Lindberg, C., Tarkowski, A., & Oldfors, A. 1997, "Oligoclonal expansion of muscle infiltrating T cells in inclusion body myositis", *J.Neuroimmunol.*, vol. 79, no. 2, pp. 185-189.

Genta, R. M., Hamner, H. W., & Graham, D. Y. 1993, "Gastric lymphoid follicles in Helicobacter pylori infection: frequency, distribution, and response to triple therapy", *Hum.Pathol.*, vol. 24, pp. 577-583.

Gerhard, N., Krenn, V., Magalhaes, R., Morawietz, L., Brandlein, S., & Konig, A. 2002, "IgVH-genes analysis from psoriatic arthritis shows involvement of antigen-activated synovial B-lymphocytes", *Z.Rheumatol.*, vol. 61, pp. 718-727.

Ghosh, S., Steere, A. C., Stollar, B. D., & Huber, B. T. 2005, "In situ diversification of the antibody repertoire in chronic Lyme arthritis synovium", *J.Immunol.*, vol. 174, pp. 2860-2869.

Graus, Y. F., de Baets, M. H., Parren, P. W. H. I., Berrih-Aknin, S., Wokke, J., van Breda Vriesman, P. J., & Burton, D. R. 1997, "Human anti-nicotinic acetylcholine receptor recombinant Fab fragments isolated from thymus-derived phage display libraries from myasthenia gravis patients reflect predominant specificities in serum and block the action of pathogenic serum antibodies", *J.Immunol.*, vol. 158, pp. 1919-1929.

Greenberg, S. A., Bradshaw, E. M., Pinkus, J. L., Pinkus, G. S., Burleson, T., Due, B., Bregoli, L., O'Connor, K. C., & Amato, A. A. 2005, "Plasma cells in muscle in inclusion body myositis and polymyositis", *Neurology*, vol. 65, no. 11, pp. 1782-1787.

Greenberg, S. A., Sanoudou, D., Haslett, J. N., Kohane, I. S., Kunkel, L. M., Beggs, A. H., & Amato, A. A. 2002, "Molecular profiles of inflammatory myopathies", *Neurology*, vol. 59, no. 8, pp. 1170-1182.

Hauser, A. E., Shlomchik, M. J., & Haberman, A. M. 2007, "In vivo imaging studies shed light on germinal-centre development", *Nature Reviews Immunology*, vol. 7, pp. 499-504.

Hershberg, U., Uduman, M., Shlomchik, M. J., & Kleinstein, S. H. 2008, "Improved methods for detecting selection by mutation analysis of Ig V region sequences", *International Immunology*, vol. 20, pp. 683-694.

Hill, M. E., SHIONO, H., Newsom-Davis, J., & Willcox, N. 2008, "The myasthenia gravis thymus: a rare source of human autoantibody-secreting plasma cells for testing potential therapeutics", *J.Neuroimmunol.*, vol. 201-202, pp. 50-56.

Hofbauer, M., Wiesener, S., Babbe, H., Roers, A., Wekerle, H., Dornmair, K., Hohlfeld, R., & Goebels, N. 2003, "Clonal tracking of autoaggressive T cells in polymyositis by combining laser microdissection, single-cell PCR, and CDR3-spectratype analysis", *Proc.Natl.Acad.Sci.U.S.A*, vol. 100, no. 7, pp. 4090-4095.

Hortobagyi, G. N. 2005, "Trastuzumab in the Treatment of Breast Cancer", *The New England Journal of Medicine*, vol. 353, pp. 1734-1736.

Humby, F., Bombardieri, M., Manzo, A., Kelly, S., Blades, M. C., Kirkham, B., Spencer, J., & Pitzalis, C. 2009, "Ectopic Lymphoid Structures Support Ongoing Production of Class-Switched Autoantibodies in Rheumatoid Synovium", *PLoS Medicine*, vol. 6, pp. 0001-0017.

Igarashi, H., Hashimoto, J., Tomita, T., YOSHIKAWA, H., & Ishihara, K. 2010, "TP53 mutations coincide with the ectopic expression of activation-induced cytidine deaminase in the fibroblast-like synoviocytes derived from a fraction of patients with rheumatoid arthritis", *Clinical & Experimental Immunology*, vol. 161, pp. 71-80.

Jang, I. K., Cronshaw, D. G., Xie, L. k., Fang, G., Zhang, J., Oh, H., Fu, Y. X., Gu, H., & Zou, Y. 2011, "Growth-factor receptor-bound protein-2 (Grb2) signaling in B cells controls lymphoid follicle organization and germinal center reaction", *Proceedings of the National Academy of Sciences*, vol. 108, pp. 7926-7931.

Kaiserling, E. 2001, "Newly-formed lymph nodes in the submucosa in chronic inflammatory bowel disease", *Lymphology*, vol. 34, pp. 22-29.

Klein, U. & Dalla-Favera, R. 2008, "Germinal centres: role in B-cell physiology and malignancy", *Nature Reviews Immunology*, vol. 8, pp. 22-33.

Knecht, H., Saremaslani, P., & Hedinger, C. 1981, "Immunohistological findings in Hashimoto's thyroiditis, focal lymphocytic thyroiditis and thyroiditis de Quervain. Comparative study", *Virchows Archiv - Abteilung A Pathologische Anatomie*, vol. 393, pp. 215-231.

Kotlan, B., Simsa, P., Gruel, N., Foldi, J., Fridman, W. H., Petranyi, G., & Teillaud, J. L. 2000, "A scFv phage display mini library generated from the immunoglobulin repertoire of breast medullary carcinoma infiltrating B lymphocytes", *Dis.Markers*, vol. 16, pp. 25-27.

Kotlan, B., Simsa, P., Teillaud, J. L., Fridman, W. H., Toth, J., McKnight, M., & Glassy, M. C. 2005, "Novel Ganglioside Antigen Identified by B Cells in Human Medullary Breast Carcinomas: The Proof of Principle Concerning the Tumor-Infiltrating B Lymphocytes", *The Journal of Immunology*, vol. 175, pp. 2278-2285.

Krystufkova, O., Vallerskog, T., Barbasso, H. S., Mann, H., Putova, I., Belacek, J., Malmstrom, V., Trollmo, C., Vencovsky, J., & Lundberg, I. E. 2008, "Increased serum levels of B-cell activating factor (BAFF) in subsets of patients with idiopathic inflammatory myopathies", *Annals of the Rheumatic Diseases.*

Lang, B. & Vincent, A. 2009, "Autoimmune disorders of the neuromuscular junction", *Curr.Opin.Pharmacol.*, vol. 9, pp. 336-340.

Le Panse, R., Bismuth, J., Cizeron-Clairac, G., Weiss, J. M., Cufi, P., Dartevelle, P., De Rosbo, N. K., & Berrih-Aknin, S. 2010, "Thymic remodeling associated with hyperplasia in myasthenia gravis", *Autoimmunity*, vol. 43, pp. 401-412.

Le Panse, R., Cizeron-Clairac, G., Bismuth, J., & Berrih-Aknin, S. 2006, "Microarrays reveal distinct gene signatures in the thymus of seropositive and seronegative myasthenia gravis patients and the role of CC chemokine ligand 21 in thymic hyperplasia", *The Journal of Immunology*, vol. 177, pp. 7868-7879.

Leavy, O. 2010, "B cells: Illuminating the dark zone", *Nature Reviews Immunology*, vol. 11, p. 8.

Levine, T. D. M. 2005, "Rituximab in the Treatment of Dermatomyositis: An Open-Label Pilot Study.", *Arthritis & Rheumatism*, vol. 52, no. 2, pp. 601-607.

Liversidge, J., Dick, A., Cheng, Y.-F., Scott, G. B., & Forrester, J. V. 1993, "Retinal antigen specific lymphocytes, TCR-gamma delta T cells and CD5+ B cells cultured from the vitreous in acute sympathetic ophthalmitis", *Autoimmunity*, vol. 15, pp. 257-266.

Maddison, P. & Lang, B. 2008, "Paraneoplastic neurological autoimmunity and survival in small-cell lung cancer", *J.Neuroimmunol.*, vol. 201-202, pp. 159-162.

Mantegazza, R., Andreetta, F., Bernasconi, P., Baggi, F., Oksenberg, J. R., Simoncini, O., Mora, M., Cornelio, F., & Steinman, L. 1993, "Analysis of T cell receptor repertoire of muscle-infiltrating T lymphocytes in polymyositis. Restricted V alpha/beta rearrangements may indicate antigen-driven selection", *J.Clin.Invest*, vol. 91, no. 6, pp. 2880-2886.

Manzo, A. & Pitzalis, C. 2007, "Lymphoid tissue reactions in rheumatoid arthritis", *Autoimmunity Reviews*, vol. 7, pp. 30-34.

Matthews, I., Sims, G. P., Ledwidge, S., Stott, D. I., Beeson, D., Willcox, N., & Vincent, A. 2002, "Antibodies to Acetylcholine Receptor in Parous Women with Myasthenia: Evidence for Immunization by Fetal Antigen", *Laboratory Investigation*, vol. 82, pp. 1407-1417.

Matzinger, P. 2007, "Friendly and dangerous signals: is the tissue in control?", *Nat Immunol*, vol. 8, pp. 11-13.

Mauri, C. 2010, "Regulation of immunity and autoimmunity by B cells", *Current Opinion in Immunology*, vol. 22, pp. 761-767.

Meraouna, A., Cizeron-Clairac, G., Panse, R. L., Bismuth, J., Truffault, F., Tallaksen, C., & Berrih-Aknin, S. 2006, "The chemokine CXCL13 is a key molecule in autoimmune myasthenia gravis", *Blood*, vol. 108, pp. 432-440.

Mielnik, P., Wiesik-Szewczyk, E., Olesinska, M., Chwalinska-Sadowska, H., & Zabek, J. 2006, "Clinical features and prognosis of patients with idiopathic inflammatory myopathies and anti-Jo-1 antibodies", *Autoimmunity*, vol. 39, no. 3, pp. 243-247.

Minton, K. 2011, "B cells: Short- and long-term memory", *Nature Reviews Immunology*, vol. 11, pp. 160-161.

Mosnier, J.-F., Degott, C., Marcellin, P., Henin, D., Erlinger, S., & Benhamou, J.-P. 1993, "The intraportal lymphoid nodule and its environment in chronic active hepatitis C: An Immunohistochemical study", *Hepatology*, vol. 17, pp. 366-371.

Nacionales, D. C., Weinstein, J. S., Yan, X. J., Albesiano, E., Lee, P. Y., Kelly-Scumpia, K. M., Lyons, R., Satoh, M., Chiorazzi, N., & Reeves, W. H. 2009, "B Cell Proliferation, Somatic Hypermutation, Class Switch Recombination, and Autoantibody Production in Ectopic Lymphoid Tissue in Murine Lupus", *The Journal of Immunology*, vol. 182, pp. 4226-4236.

Nahta, R., Hung, M. C., & Esteva, F. J. 2004, "The HER-2-Targeting Antibodies Trastuzumab and Pertuzumab Synergistically Inhibit the Survival of Breast Cancer Cells", *Cancer Research*, vol. 64, pp. 2343-2346.

Nemazee, D. 2006, "Receptor editing in lymphocyte development and central tolerance", *Nature Reviews Immunology*, vol. 6, pp. 728-740.

Nzula, S., Going, J. J., & Stott, D. I. 2003a, "Antigen-driven clonal proliferation, somatic hypermutation and selection of B-lymphocytes infiltrating human ductal breast carcinoma", *Cancer Res.*, vol. 63, pp. 3275-3280.

Nzula, S., Going, J. J., & Stott, D. I. 2003b, "The role of B lymphocytes in breast cancer: a review and current status", *Cancer Therapy*, vol. 1, pp. 353-362.

Park, C. S. & Choi, Y. S. 2005, "How do follicular dendritic cells interact intimately with B cells in the germinal centre?", *Immunology*, vol. 114, pp. 2-10.

Patakas, A., Platt, A. M., Butcher, J. P., Maffia, P., McInnes, I. B., Brewer, J. M., Garside, P., & Benson, R. A. 2011, "Putative existence of reciprocal dialogue between Tfh and B cells and its impact on infectious and autoimmune disease", *Immunol Lett.*, vol. In press.

Petrarca, C., Casalino, B., Mensdorff-Pouilly, S., Rughetti, A., Rahimi, H., Scambia, G., Hilgers, J., Frati, L., & Nuti, M. 1999, "Isolation of MUC1-primed B lymphocytes from tumour-draining lymph nodes by immunomagnetic beads", *Cancer Immunology, Immunotherapy*, vol. 47, pp. 272-277.

Poea-Guyon, S., Christadoss, P., Le Panse, R., Guyon, T., De Baets, M., Wakkach, A., Bidault, J., Tzartos, S., & Berrih-Aknin, S. 2005, "Effects of cytokines on acetylcholine receptor expression: implications for myasthenia gravis", *The Journal of Immunology*, vol. 174, pp. 5941-5949.

Prineas, J. W. 1979, "Multiple sclerosis: presence of lymphatic capillaries and lymphoid tissue in the brain and spinal cord", *Science*, vol. 203, pp. 1123-1125.

Renard, V. & Leach, D. R. 2007, "Perspectives on the development of a therapeutic HER-2 cancer vaccine", *Vaccine*, vol. 25 Suppl 2, p. B17-B23.

Renard, V., Sonderbye, L., Ebbehoj, K., Rasmussen, P. B., Gregorius, K., Gottschalk, T., Mouritsen, S., Gautam, A., & Leach, D. R. 2003, "HER-2 DNA and Protein Vaccines Containing Potent Th Cell Epitopes Induce Distinct Protective and Therapeutic Antitumor Responses in HER-2 Transgenic Mice", *The Journal of Immunology*, vol. 171, pp. 1588-1595.

Rider, L. G. 2007, "The heterogeneity of juvenile myositis", *Autoimmun.Rev.*, vol. 6, no. 4, pp. 241-247.

Rosenfeld, M. R. & Dalmau, J. 2010, "Update on paraneoplastic and autoimmune disorders of the central nervous system", *Semin.Neurol.*, vol. 30, pp. 320-331.

Rothe, A., Klimka, A., Tur, M. K., Pfitzner, T., Huhn, M., Sasse, S., Mallmann, P., Engert, A., & Barth, S. 2004, "Construction of phage display libraries from reactive lymph nodes of breast carcinoma patients and selection for specifically binding human single chain Fv on cell lines", *Int.J Mol.Med*, vol. 14, pp. 729-735.

Salajegheh, M., Pinkus, J. L., Amato, A. A., Morehouse, C., Jallal, B., Yao, Y., & Greenberg, S. A. 2010, "Permissive environment for B-cell maturation in myositis muscle in the absence of B-cell follicles", *Muscle & Nerve*, vol. 42, no. 4, pp. 576-583.

Seitz, S., Schneider, C. K., Malotka, J., Nong, X., Engel, A. G., Wekerle, H., Hohlfeld, R., & Dornmair, K. 2006, "Reconstitution of paired T cell receptor alpha- and beta-chains from microdissected single cells of human inflammatory tissues", *Proc.Natl.Acad.Sci.U.S.A*, vol. 103, no. 32, pp. 12057-12062.

Serafini, B., Rosicarelli, B., Magliozzi, R., Stigliano, E., & Aloisi, F. 2004, "Detection of ectopic B-cell follicles with germinal centers in the meninges of patients with secondary progressive multiple sclerosis", *Brain Pathol.*, vol. 14, pp. 164-174.

Shiono, H., Roxanis, I., Zhang, W., Sims, G. P., Meager, A., Jacobson, L. W., Liu, J. L., Matthews, I., Wong, Y. L., Bonifati, M., Micklem, K., Stott, D. I., Todd, J. A., Beeson, D., Vincent, A., & Willcox, N. 2003, "Scenarios for autoimmunization of T and B cells in myasthenia gravis", *Ann.N.Y.Acad.Sci.*, vol. 998, pp. 237-256.

Sims, G. P., Hiroyuki, S., Willcox, N., & Stott, D. I. 2001, "Somatic Hypermutation and Selection of B Cells in Thymic Germinal Centers Responding to Acetyl Choline Receptor in Myasthenia Gravis", *J.Immunol.*, vol. 167, pp. 1935-1944.

Simsa, P., Teillaud, J. L., Stott, D. I., Toth, J., & Kotlan, B. 2005, "Tumor-infiltrating B cell immunoglobulin variable region gene usage in invasive ductal breast carcinoma", *Pathol Oncol.Res*, vol. 11, pp. 92-97.

Snijdewint, F. G., Mensdorff-Pouilly, S., Karuntu-Wanamarta, A. H., Verstraeten, A. A., Livingston, P. O., Hilgers, J., & Kenemans, P. 2001, "Antibody-dependent cell-mediated cytotoxicity can be induced by MUC1 peptide vaccination of breast cancer patients", *Int.J Cancer*, vol. 93, pp. 97-106.

Stolte, M. & Eidt, S. 1989, "Lymphoid follicles in antral mucosa: immune response to Campylobacter pylori?", *J Clin.Pathol.*, vol. 42, pp. 1269-1271.

Stott, D. I., Hiepe, F., Hummel, M., Steinhauser, G., & Berek, C. 1998, "Antigen-driven clonal proliferation of B cells within the target tissue of an autoimmune disease . The salivary glands of patients with Sjögren's syndrome.", *J.Clin.Invest.*, vol. 102, pp. 938-946.

Stott, D. I. & Sims, G. P. 2000, "Application of scFv-phage display to analysis of B-cell clones proliferating in the salivary glands of a patient with Sjögren's syndrome", *Disease Markers*, vol. 16, pp. 21-23.

Swofford, D. L. 1993, "PAUP: Phylogenetic analysis using parsimony, version 3.1,".

Taylor-Papadimitriou, J., Burchell, J. M., Plunkett, T., Graham, R., Correa, I., Miles, D., & Smith, M. 2002, "MUC1 and the immunobiology of cancer", *J Mammary.Gland.Biol.Neoplasia.*, vol. 7, pp. 209-221.

Victora, G. D., Schwickert, T. A., Fooksman, D. R., Kamphorst, A. O., Meyer-Hermann, M., Dustin, M. L., & Nussenzweig, M. C. (12-11-2010)Germinal Center Dynamics Revealed by Multiphoton Microscopy withàa Photoactivatable Fluorescent Reporter. Cell 143[4], 592-605.

Vincent, A. 2002, "Unravelling the pathogenesis of myasthenia gravis", *Nature Revs.Immunol.*, vol. 2, pp. 797-804.

Vincent, A. & et al. 1997, "Thymoma and autoimmune neurological disorders," in *Epithelial Tumours of the Thymus*, A. Marx & H. K. Muller-Hermelink, eds., Plenum Press, New York, pp. 195-204.

Visco, V., Bei, R., Moriconi, E., Gianni, W., Kraus, M. H., & Muraro, R. 2000, "ErbB2 immune response in breast cancer patients with soluble receptor ectodomain.", *Am.J.Pathol.*, vol. 156, pp. 1417-1424.

von Mensdorff-Pouilly, S., Verstraeten, A. A., Kenemans, P., Snijdewint, F. G. M., Kok, A., Van Kamp, G. J., Paul, M. A., Van Diest, P. J., Meijer, S., & Hilgers, J. 2000, "Survival in Early Breast Cancer Patients Is Favorably Influenced by a Natural Humoral Immune Response to Polymorphic Epithelial Mucin", *Journal of Clinical Oncology*, vol. 18, p. 574.

Wallace, W. A. H., Howie, S. E. M., Krajewski, A. S., & Lamb, D. 1996, "The immunological architecture of B-lymphocyte aggregates in cryptogenic fibrosing alveolitis", *J.Pathol.*, vol. 178, pp. 323-329.

Weiser, A. A., Wittenbrink, N., Zhang, L., Schmelzer, A. I., Valai, A., & Or-Guil, M. 2011, "Affinity maturation of B cells involves not only a few but a whole spectrum of relevant mutations", *International Immunology*, vol. 23, pp. 345-356.

Yoshitake, T., Masunaga, A., Sugawara, I., Nakamura, H., Itoyama, S., & Oka, T. 1994, "A comparative histological and immunohistochemical study of thymomas with and without myasthenia gravis", *Surgery Today*, vol. 24, pp. 1044-1049.

Zampieri, S., Ghirardello, A., Iaccarino, L., Tarricone, E., Gambari, P. F., & Doria, A. 2005, "Anti-Jo-1 antibodies", *Autoimmunity*, vol. 38, no. 1, pp. 73-78.

Zuckerman, N. S., Howard, W. A., Bismuth, J., Gibson, K., Edelman, H., Berrih-Aknin, S., Dunn-Walters, D., & Mehr, R. 2010, "Ectopic GC in the thymus of myasthenia gravis patients show characteristics of normal GC", *Eur.J Immunol*, vol. 40, pp. 1150-1161.

11

Autoimmune Disorder and Autism

Xiaohong Li and Hua Zou
New York State Institute for Basic Research in Developmental Disabilities
USA

1. Introduction

1.1 Diagnosis of ASD

Autism (also known as classic autism or autism disorder) is a common neurodevelopmental disorder. Typically diagnosed before three years old, autistic children usually present with significant language delays, social and communication impairments, as well as abnormal repetitive and restrictive behaviors. Autism spectrum disorders (ASD) however, refers to a boarder definition of autism. Based on the severity of the clinical conditions, ASD is further divided into three subgroups namely autism (the most severe type of ASD), Asperger syndrome and pervasive developmental disorder - not otherwise specified (PDD-NOS; also called atypical autism) [1-3].

Of note, current diagnosis criteria of these disorders are based on behavior tests, no single biomarker has been clinically accepted, which mainly due to the difficulties for studying cellular and molecular etiology of ASD. First, subjects among different researches lack of comparability because of the diagnostic heterogeneity [4]. Second, the prevalence of ASD is relatively low therefore sample sizes are usually too small for statistical analysis. Third, comparing with other diseases, the young ages of the autistic subjects make biological study difficult. Forth, valid control groups require age-, gender-, IQ- and socioeconomic status-matched developmentally normal subjects, which most studies failed to satisfy with [5].

1.2 Epidemiology

ASD is reported to occur in all racial, ethnic and socioeconomic groups, and are about four times more likely to occur in boys than in girls probably due to the extremes of typical male neuroanatomy of autism [6, 7]. Studies in Asia, Europe and North America have identified individuals with ASD with an approximate prevalence of 6/1,000 to over 10/1,000 [8]. Chronologically, the prevalence of ASD increased from 0.8/1,000 in 1983 to 4.6/1,000 in 1999 in Western Australia, while this ratio increased from 6.6/1,000 in 2000 to 9/1,000 in 2006 in United States [9-11]. This increase is probably because of changes and broadening of the diagnostic criteria and due to heightened awareness, but may also reflect, in part, a true increase due to environmental factors acting upon a genetically vulnerable background [12, 13].

2. Immune disorders and autism

The relationship between immune disorders and ASD has been proposed for decades. Based on the epidemiological data, higher rate of autoimmune conditions, such as rheumatoid arthritis, autoimmune thyroid disease, asthma, ulcerative colitis, exits in parents of autistic children [14-17]. Another line of evidence supporting immune dysfunction at least partly responsible for ASD comes from large population studies, which suggest maternal immune dysfunctions may be related to a later diagnosis of ASD in the offspring [18]. Furthermore, cumulative evidences support the theory that ASD is caused by a loss of self-tolerance to one or more neural antigens during early childhood. Using western blot for the presence of IgG antibodies against protein extracts from human brain or sera, multiple brain-specific autoantibodies are detected [19, 20]. Other groups measured the plasma concentration of immunoglobulins and/or cytokines, autistic subjects exclusively exhibited abnormal immunoglobin and/or cytokine profiles [21-24]. It's not known yet whether immune activation plays an initiating or ongoing role in the pathology of ASD. But investigations of dynamic adaptive cellular immune function suggested dysfunctional immune activation, which may be linked to disturbances in behavior and developmental functioning [25].

2.1 Autoimmune diseases

Autoimmune diseases are the most common type of immune disorders. And its relationship with autism has been widely studied. Very early study reported an increased number of autoimmune disorders in some families with autism, suggesting immune dysfunction plays a role in autism pathogenesis [26]. Consistent with this result, Sweeten et al investigated the frequency of autoimmune disorders in families that have probands with pervasive developmental disorders and autism, compared with control groups. Autoimmunity was increased significantly in families with pervasive developmental disorders compared with those of healthy and autoimmune control subjects [27]. More persuasive evidence comes from a multicenter study of 308 children with Autism Spectrum Disorder. Regression was significantly associated with a family history of autoimmune disorders. But the only specific autoimmune disorder found to be associated with regression was autoimmune thyroid disease [28].

2.2 Cytokines and chemokines

Cytokines and chemokines are thought to mediate the pathogenesis of autism, although the exact mechanism remains unclear. Jyonouchi group determined innate and adaptive immune responses in children with developmental regression and autism spectrum disorders, developmentally normal siblings, and controls. Their results indicated excessive innate immune responses in a number of ASD children that may be most evident in TNF-alpha production [29]. Similarly, Molloy et al reported children with ASD had increased activation of both Th2 and Th1 arms of the adaptive immune response, with a Th2 predominance, and without the compensatory increase in the regulatory cytokine IL-10 [30]. But Li et al showed that proinflammatory cytokines (TNF-alpha, IL-6 and GM-CSF), Th1 cytokine (IFN-gamma) and chemokine (IL-8) were significantly increased in the brains of ASD patients compared with the controls, but not the Th2 cytokines (IL-4, IL-5 and IL-10). The Th1/Th2 ratio was also significantly increased in ASD patients. Based on these results, the author concluded that ASD patients displayed an increased innate and adaptive immune response through the Th1 pathway, suggesting that localized brain inflammation and autoimmune disorder may be involved in the pathogenesis of ASD [31]. Most recently, Ashwood group used larger number of participants than previous studies and found that significant increases in plasma levels of a number of cytokines, including IL-1beta, IL-6, IL-8 and IL-12p40 in the ASD group compared with typically developing controls [32]. All these findings suggest that inflammatory responses may be related to disturbances in behavior. And the characterization of immunological parameters in ASD has important implications for diagnosis, therefore should be considered when designing therapeutic strategies to treat ASD.

2.3 Immunoglobulin

Using human fetal and adult brains as antigenic substrates, maternal serum antibodies transferred through placenta are detected by four independent research groups, suggesting an association between the transfer of IgG autoantibodies during early neurodevelopment and the risk of developing of autism in some children [33-37].

Singh et al provided more confirmative evidence by studying regional distribution of antibodies to rat caudate nucleus, cerebral cortex, cerebellum, brain stem and hippocampus of 30 normal and 68 autistic children. Autistic children, but not normal children, had antibodies to caudate nucleus (49% positive sera), cerebral cortex (18% positive sera) and cerebellum (9% positive sera). Brain stem and hippocampus were negative. Since a significant number of autistic children had antibodies to caudate nucleus, the author proposed that an autoimmune reaction to this brain region may cause neurological impairments in autistic children [38]. Agreed with this result, Trajkovski et al measured plasma concentration of IgA, IgM, IgG classes, and IgG1, IgG2, IgG3, and IgG4 subclasses in children with autism. Plasma concentrations of IgM and IgG in autistic children were significantly higher in comparison with their healthy brothers or sisters. Children with autism had significantly higher plasma concentrations of IgG4 compared to their siblings. Increased plasma concentration of IgG1 was found in autistic males as compared with their healthy brothers. Plasma concentrations of IgG and IgG1 in autistic females were increased in comparison with IgG and IgG1 in their healthy sisters [39]. More recently, Enstrom et al report significantly increased levels of the IgG4 subclass in children with autism compared with typically developing control children and compared with developmental delayed controls [40].

However, No consensus has been reached regarding the immunoglobin levels in autistic subjects. Morris and colleagues failed to find any useful biomarker in a small group of subjects, posing question to the current theory [41]. Stern et al found in their study most of the autistic children had normal immune function, suggesting that routine immunologic investigation is unlikely to be of benefit in most autistic children [42].

2.4 Gastrointestinal disorders

The report regarding the relationship between autism and gastrointestinal disorders was seen as early as 1971, when Goodwin et al described 6 of 15 randomly selected autistic children with symptoms of malabsorption [43]. Later Horvath et al investigated 412 autistic children, of which 84.1% had at least one of the eight abnormal gastrointestinal symptoms, comparing with 31.2% of the healthy siblings [44]. However, disagreements exit. Kuddo group and Molloy group failed to find any association between chronic gastrointestinal symptoms and autism based on the literature search or their own sample [45, 46]. Fernell et al tested two independent biomarkers of inflammatory reactions (faecal calprotectin and rectal nitric oxide) in 24 autistic children, but didn't find clear link between active intestinal inflammation and autism [47].

Morphological and histological studies provided consistent results with the clinical manifestations. Ileocolonoscopic examinations in 60 children with autism and other developmental disorders revealed that 8% (4/51) affected children but none in controls presented with active ileitis. Chronic colitis was identified in 88% (53/60) affected children compared with 4.5% (1/22) controls [48]. Similarly, another group conducted upper gastrointestinal endoscopy in 36 autistic subjects. 69.4% (25/36) of whom presented with grade I or II reflux esophagitis, 41.7% (15/36) with chronic gastritis, and 66.7% with chronic duodenitis [49].

In addition, biochemical researches reported evidences of abnormal intestinal cytokine profiles. Ashwood et al found enhanced pro-inflammatory cytokine production present in 21 ASD children compared with 65 controls [50]. Furthermore, they investigated the peripheral blood and mucosal CD3+ lymphocyte cytokine profiles in 18 autistic children with gastrointestinal symptoms. In both peripheral blood and mucosa, CD3+ TNFalpha+ and CD3+ IFNgamma+ were increased, while CD3+ IL-10+ were markedly lower in ASD children. And mucosal CD3+ IL-4+ cells were increased in ASD compared with NIC [51]. Similarly, Jyonouchi et al provided evidence that intrinsic defects of innate immune responses in ASD children with gastrointestinal symptoms, suggesting a possible link between GI and behavioral symptoms mediated by innate immune abnormalities [52]. However, DeFelice et al assessed levels of proinflammatory cytokines, interleukin (IL)-6, IL-8, and IL-1beta, produced by intestinal biopsies of children with pervasive developmental disorders but failed to find significant difference between autistic and control groups [53].

How do the gastrointestinal disorders affect brain functions? Currently available pathophysiological studies provided partial explanations. D'Eufemia et al investigated the occurrence of gut mucosal damage using the intestinal permeability test in 21 autistic children without known intestinal disorders. They found increased intestinal permeability in 43% (9/21) autistic patients, but in none of the 40 controls, which suggested an altered intestinal permeability could represent a possible mechanism for the increased passage through the gut mucosa of peptides derived from foods with subsequent behavioral abnormalities [54].

3. Genetics of autism

Similar to several other complex diseases, autism was not widely considered to have a strong genetic component until the 1980s. But increasing numbers of epidemiological and genetic studies are deepening our understanding of the genetic contribution autism. First, it is estimated that about 10% of children with ASD have an identifiable co-occuring genetic, neurologic or metabolic disorder, such as the fragile X syndrome and tuberous sclerosis [55]. Second, the relative risk of a newborn child to have autism, if he or she has an affected sibling, increases at least 25 folds comparing with general population [56]. Third, independent twin studies have suggested identical twins have a 60-90% chance to be concordantly diagnosed with autism, and this risk decreases sharply to the sibling risk of 0-24% in non-identical twins [57, 58]. However, based on a large scale study of 503 ASD twins in California, Liu *et al* suggest the heritability has been largely overestimated [59]. They found the concordance rate for monozygotic male twins was 57% and for females 67%, while for same sex dizygotic twins the rate was 33%. Fourth, cumulative reports have confirmed mutations or structural variations of a number of specific genes significantly increase the risk of ASD [56].

3.1 Genetic methodology

However, unlike monogenic Mendelian disorders, the genetic and clinical heterogeneity of ASD poses a difficult challenge to precisely define the underlying genetics. This complexity has been blamed for the lack of replicability of the many reported chromosomal susceptibility regions. Therefore, multiple parallel approaches are needed for the exploration of the potential loci underlying the etiology of ASD. In general, there are a number of methods available for genetic studies of ASD, with each having different advantages as well as limitations. The most widely used methods include cytogenetic analysis, linkage and association studies, copy number variation and DNA micro-array analysis.

A cytogenetic study is the most "classic" of genetic methods. Based on the assumption that ASD is a result of unique rare mutations that present sporadically or "de novo" in the population and are not usually inherited, cytogenetics helps to determine the contribution of chromosomal abnormalities in childhood diseases. Cytogenetics has transitioned from light microscopy to molecular cytogenetics to DNA-based microarray detections of structural variations [60]. Copy number variation (CNV) analysis is a newer molecular cytogenetic approach, aiming to detect the insertion or deletion of DNA fragments typically larger than 50 kb [61]. However, extreme caution must be paid when interpreting CNV analysis since it is very dependent on the specific methods employed, which may partly account for the low replicability among studies [62].

Differing from cytogenetics, linkage studies trace genetic loci that are transmitted with autism in the families of affected individuals. Parametric and non-parametric linkage studies are two typical designs. While parametric analysis requires a model for the disease (i.e. frequency of disease alleles and penetrance for each genotype), and therefore is typically employed for single gene disorders and Mendelian forms of complex disorders, "model-free" non-parametric linkage analysis evaluates whether segregation at specific locations is "not-random". Given the uncertainty of the mode of inheritance in ASD, non-parametric linkage is more widely used, providing suggestive evidence of linkage on almost all of the chromosomes [63]. However, linkage studies are unable to identify mutations in critical genes in highly heterogeneous disorders involving many different genes and chromosomal loci [64].

Genetic association studies, including case-control and family-based studies, examine differences in allele or genotype frequencies between two groups [63]. Typically, several microsatellite markers or SNPs are chosen based on linkage studies or biological evidence. The seemingly countless potential candidates make it hard to determine the causative relations between genes and ASD [61]. In addition, although association studies are suitable to identify common susceptibility alleles present in large numbers of patients compared to controls, they usually fail to identify rare, causal mutations [63, 64].

Rapid advances in micro-array technologies have substantially improved our ability to detect submicroscopic chromosomal abnormalities. These tools have allowed for high-output and high-resolution detection of rare and de novo changes in a genome-wide manner. Moreover, newly developed, commercially available whole-exome arrays are increasingly being employed to detect de novo mutations in complex disorders. Based on the fact that the protein coding regions of genes (i.e. exons) habor 85% of the mutations of disease-related traits, whole-exome sequencing offers the possibility to identify disease-causing sequence variations in small kindreds for phenotypically complicated, genetically heterogeneous diseases when traditional linkage studies are impossible [65-69]. As such, studies in this realm have been increasing in the past several years and there will surely benefit the etiological diagnosis and genetic counseling of ASD in the near future [70].

3.2 Potential loci in autism

3.2.1 Genome wide linkage analysis

Although there is accumulating evidence supporting a genetic component to ASD, the specific genes involved have yet to be totally clarified. Genome-wide screening of autistic subjects and their first-degree relatives offers an attractive means to search for susceptibility genes. However there has been a disappointing lack of replication of many of the reported susceptibility regions. The reason for this could be due to the epistasis of many interacting genes. But it may also be due to the genetic and clinical heterogeneity present in ASD [71]. The noted effects of heterogeneity of the samples on the corresponding results, have led to attempts to decrease sample heterogeneity by various ways which include narrowing inclusion criteria and studies of specific, autism-related endophenotypes.

A substantial body of evidence has resulted from genome-wide screening for the susceptibility genes of ASD (table 1). Significant replicability has been found for several chromosomal loci including 2q, 5, 7q, 15q and 16p. Two studies provided suggestive evidence for linkage to chromosome 2q using a two-stage genome screen [71, 72], while association tests for specific candidate genes in the chromosome 2q31-q33 region led to negative results [73]. Additional support for the presence of susceptibility loci on chromosome 2q is given by overlapping positive linkage findings in four other independent genomic scans [74-77].

There are three reports about gene variants on chromosome 5. Philippi found strong association with autism for allelic variants of "paired-like homeodomain transcription factor 1" (*PITX1*), a key regulator of hormones within the pituitary-hypothalamic axis [78]. Two other groups used genome-wide linkage and association mapping studies to analyze chromosome 5 gene variations finding that SNPs located at 5p14.1 and 5q15 respectively were significantly associated with autism [79, 80].

Chromosome 16 linkage results have been fairly consistent in showing a peak at 16p11-13, which strongly suggested a gene in this region may contribute to the risk of ASD [81, 82]. 15q11-q13 is another frequently identified locus by linkage studies. Several genes located in this region have been intensively studied and some have provided very promising results [83-86]. But in all of these linkage reports there is a certain lack of reproducibility, and therefore they require further validation based on using a combination of several methods.

Besides these "hot spots", there are other reports regarding associations of other loci with ASD [80, 87-90], including some evidence of linkage to the X chromosome [91]. However, there is little overlap of these potential loci involving potential candidate genes, suggesting that the genetic background of ASD is full of complexity.

3.2.2 Copy number variation (CNV)

Rapid advances in genomic DNA microarray technologies have substantially improved our ability to detect submicroscopic chromosomal abnormalities. Novel rare variants have been detected in association with ASD and these can be either *de novo* or inherited. *De novo* or noninherited CNVs are found in 7%-10% of ASD samples from simplex families (having only one child affected, the majority), in 2%-3% from multiplex families, and in ~1% in non-ASD controls. Further, about 10% of ASD subjects with *de novo* CNVs carry two or more CNVs [100-102]. Inherited CNVs reportedly are found in up to 50% of ASD subjects for whom one of the presumably normal parents also has the duplication/deletion. These familial CNVs may include candidate genes relevant to ASD where they are rare in the normal population.

Chromosome	Loci	Candidate genes	Ref.
1	1p34.2	Regulating Synaptic Membrane Exocytosis 3(*RIMS3*)	[90]
2	2q		[71, 72]
	2q31-2q33	*GAD1,STK17B,ABI2,CTLA4,CD28,NEUROD1, PDE1A,HOXD1, DLX2*	[73]
	2q31	*SLC25A12*	[92]
	2q24-2q33	*SLC25A12, CMYA3*	[75]
	2q24-2q33	*SLC25A12, STK39, ITGA4*	[77]
	2q34	Neuropilin-2 (*NRP2*)	[74]
3	3q25-3q27	HTR3C	[48]
5	5q31	Paired-like homeodomain transcription factor 1(*PITX1*)	[78]
	5p14.1		[79]
	5p15	*SEMA5A*	[80]
6	6q	Abelson's Helper Integration 1 (*AHI1*)	[88]
	6q27		[80]
7	7q22.1-7q31		[93]
	7q31	Laminin Beta-1 (*LAMB1*), Neuronal cell adhesion molecule (*NRCAM*)	[94, 95][96]
	7q32	NADH-ubiquinone oxidoreductase 1 alpha subcomplex 5 *(NDUFA5)*	[48]
	7q31-7q33	wingless-type MMTV integration site family member 2 (*WNT2*)	[97]
11	11p12-p13		[76]
12	12q14		[87]
15	15q11-q13	Angelman syndrome gene (*UBE3A*)	[85]
	15q11-q13		[83]
	15q13	Amyloid precursor protein-binding protein A2 (*APBA2*)	[84]
16	16p11-13	4-Aminobutyrate Aminotransferase (*ABAT),* CREB-binding protein *(CREBBP),* Glutamate receptor, ionotropic, NMDA 2A *(GRIN2A)*	[98]
	16p11.2		[81, 82, 90]
17	17q11.2		[99]
19	19p13		[99]
20	20q13		[80]
22	22q13	*SHANK3*	[89]
X	Xp22.11	*PTCHD1*	[91]

Table 1. Loci identified by genome wide linkage analysis

Array comparative genomic hybridization (aCGH) is the most widely used method for detection of CNVs. A seminal early report used aCGH, with a mean resolution of one probe every 35 kb, to study a sample of 264 ASD families. After validation by higher-resolution microarray scans, G-banded karyotype, FISH, and microsatellite genotyping, 17 *de novo*

CNVs were confirmed [102]. A Korean group recently reported deletion CNVs at 8p23.1 and 17p11.2 using whole-genome aCGH [103]. Using aCGH with a mean 19 kb resolution, 51 autism-specific CNV were identified in 397 unrelated ASD subjects [100]. Similarly, Qiao and colleagues performed aCGH on 100 autistic subjects and identified 9 CNVs, three of which were unique to their cohort [104]. A Spanish group recently reported the identification of 13 CNVs containing 24 different genes in their sample of 96 ASD subjects [105].

Single-nucleotide polymorphism (SNP) array analysis, primarily developed to determine linkage, now is also employed to determine genomic CNVs [106]. Marshall performed a genome-wide assessment via SNP array analysis. They genotyped proximately 500,000 SNPs for each sample and detected 13 loci with recurrent or overlapping CNVs in a sample of 427 ASD cases [101]. Using SNP markers, another group identified 6 CNVs within a 2.2-megabase (Mb) intergenic Chr 2 region between cadherin 10 (CDH10) and cadherin 9 (CDH9) in a combined sample set of 1,984 ASD probands of European ancestry [107]. In addition, SNP array analysis offers some special advantages in the exploration of potentially relevant gene networks. Two recent reports have provided strong evidence for the involvement of certain genes in important gene networks including neuronal cell-adhesion, ubiquitin degradation and GTPase/Ras signaling [108, 109].

Currently available aCGH methods for identifying CNV typically assay the genome in the 40-kb to several Mb range. Methodological improvements that employ oligonucleotides are providing a high potential resolution down to approximately the 5-kb resolution level for aCGH with genome-wide detection of CNVs [106]. Thus, SNP or oligonucleotide aCGH analysis can detect a CNV as small as a few kilobases. Therefore, it is clear that the higher-density oligonucleotide or SNP arrays offer the higher resolution for analysis of CNVs in the future.

3.3 Selected candidate genes

As it is becoming apparent, a genetic predisposition to ASD may involve one or more interconnected genetic networks involving neurogenesis, neuronal migration, synaptogenesis, axon pathfinding and neuronal or glial structure regionalization [110]. Function-targeted studies, mainly by association that focus exclusively on the candidate genes, including some of the most widely studied will be reviewed in the following section (table 2).

Reelin is an extracellular matrix glycoprotein responsible for guiding the migration of several neural cell types and the establishment of neural connection. In the 1980s, it was discovered that reelin plays important roles in the positioning of neuronal cells in the inferior olivery complex, cerebral cortex and cerebellum early in embryonic development [203-205]. Further research has confirmed and further extended our knowledge about the widespread functions reelin plays in laminated regions of the brain, both embryonically and postnatally [206-208].

Given the critical functions of reelin in brain development, and knowing there are neuroanatomical abnormities in autism [209], the reelin gene (*RELN*) was a plausible candidate to investigate in ASDs. Significantly reduced levels of reelin in the human cortex, cerebellum and peripheral blood were confirmed in ASD at both the protein and mRNA levels [210-212]. Genome-wide scans also identified 7q22 as an autism critical region, where *RELN* is located [213].

Genes	Loci	Positive results	Negative/Unconfirmed results
RELN	7q22	[111-120]	
SLC6A4	17q11.1-17q12	[121-127]	[128-140]
GABR	15q11-15q13	[141-154]	[155-157]
NLGN	3q26(*NLGN1*), 17p13 (*NLGN2*), Xq13 (*NLGN3*), Xp22.3 (*NLGN4*), Yq11.2 (*NLGN4Y*)	[158-163]	[164-169]
OXTR	3p24-3p25	[170-174]	
MET	7q31.2	[175-179]	
SLC25A12	2q31	[180-183]	[184-186]
GluR6	6q21	[187-189]	[190]
CNTNAP2	7q35	[191-196]	
GLO1	6p21.3-6p21.2	[197, 198]	[199, 200]
TPH2	12q21.1	[201]	[197, 202]

Table 2. Selected candidate genes

i. Reelin gene (RELN)

Additionally, case-control and family-based studies provided further evidence supporting the association of *RELN* and ASD. Persico identified a *RELN*-related polymorphic GGC repeat located immediately 5′ of the ATG initiator codon in Italian and American subjects [120]. Using the similar methods and 126 multiplex ASD families, Zhang *et al* examined the polymorphic CGG-repeat of *RELN* [118]. Family-based association tests showed that larger *RELN* alleles (≥11 repeats) were transmitted more often than expected to autistic children. Independant studies regarding the CGG-repeat of *RELN* have also supported its contribution to the genetic risk of autism [112, 113, 115]. Others have also reported significant differences in the transmission of the reelin alleles of exon 22 and intron 59 SNPs to autistic subjects [114]. However, results have not been uniformly positive. Krebs *et al* performed a transmission disequilibrium test (TDT) analysis of the CGG-repeat polymorphism in 167 Caucasian families and found no evidence of linkage or association [119]. Similarly, another two groups failed to find a significant association of *RELN* CGG repeat polymorphisms with liability to autism [116, 117].

The association between *RELN* and ASD were also found in other ethnic groups besides Caucasian populations. Recently, a significant genetic association between the *RELN* SNP2 (located in intron 59) and ASD was reported in a Chinese Han population, and the combination of *RELN* SNP1/SNP2/SNP3/SNP4, all in strong linkage disequilibrium, were reported to have a significant association with ASD [111].

ii. Human serotonin transporter gene (SLC6A4)

The human serotonin transporter, encoded by *SLC6A4,* localizes to chromosome 17q11.1-q12 and consists of 15 exons [214]. *SLC6A4* was considered as a candidate gene for autism primarily based on the elevated blood serotonin levels found in a number of autistic probands, as well as the efficacy of potent serotonin transporter inhibitors in reducing rituals and routines [215, 216]. Using the TDT, positive associations of a 5-HTTLPR polymorphism found in the promoter region of the *SLC6A4* gene with autism have been identified by 4 family-based studies and 2 case-control studies [121, 123, 125-127]. Other groups have performed both family-based and case-control analysis and found significant associations of the *SLC6A4* polymorphism with autism [122, 124]. In contrast to these positive reports, 9 family-based studies failed to find evidence for associations of the *SLC6A4* polymorphism with autism [130, 132-134, 136-140], as well as a case-control study [128]. An Indian group performed a series of studies but found no persuasive evidence of the association of the *SLC6A4* polymorphisms with autism [129, 135, 217]. In addition, a systematic review and meta-analysis failed to find a significant overall association of the serotonin polymorphisms examined and autism [131].

iii. Gamma-aminobutyric acid receptor gene (GABR)

Gamma-aminobutyric acid (GABA) is the chief inhibitory neurotransmitter in the brain, acting by binding to a GABA receptor. The receptor is a multimeric transmembrane receptor that consists of five subunits arranged around a central pore. The GABA receptor subunits are homologous, but are both structurally and functionally diverse [144]. Three of the GABA receptor subunit genes (*GABRB3, GABRA5* and *GABRG3*) are localized to chromosome 15q11-q13, one of the most complex regions in the genome involved with genome instability, gene expression, imprinting and recombination [156].

The region 15q11-q13 was originally associated with ASD based on several studies which reported a common duplication of this region in ASD subjects [147, 148, 152, 154]. A chromosome-engineered mouse model for human 15q11-13 duplication was developed with autistic features [141, 143, 153]. Cook *et al* examined markers across this region for linkage disequilibrium in 140 families with ASD, detecting significant linkage disequilibrium between *GABRB3* and ASD [218]. This finding was confirmed by others as well [145, 146, 151]. Also, two SNPs located within the *GABRG3* gene were associated with ASD using the Pedigree Disequilibrium Test (PDT) [144]. An independent study demonstrated nominally significant associations between six markers across the *GABRB3* and *GABRA5* genes [142]. Moreover, using ordered-subset analysis (OSA) another group provided evidence of increased linkage at the *GABRB3* locus [149]. Other research has also identified significant association and gene-gene interactions of GABA receptor subunit genes in autism [150].

Nonetheless, conflicting evidence has also been reported. Other groups have reported limited or no association between GABA receptor polymorphisms and autism [155, 156]. Similarly, another group conducted a full genome search for autism susceptibility loci including seven microsatellite markers from 15q11-q13, and found no significant evidence of association or linkage [157]. Thus the linkage results are at best inconclusive.

iv. Neuroligin genes (NLGN)

The marked difference in sex ratio for ASD justifies the exploration of genes on the sex chromosome, among which the neuroligin genes (*NLGN*) are perhaps the most widely studied. Five *NLGN* have been identified in the human genome, which are localized at 3q26(*NLGN1*), 17p13 (*NLGN2*), Xq13 (*NLGN3*), Xp22.3 (*NLGN4*), and Yq11.2 (*NLGN4Y*) respectively. They encode a family of cell-adhesion molecules, the neuroligans, essential for the formation of functional neural synapses [163, 169].

The earliest report regarding the potential association of *NLGN* genes and ASD came from the study of multiple Swedish families [163]. The authors screened for *NLGN3* mutations in 36 affected sib-pairs and 122 trios with ASD. They found one *de novo* mutation in *NLGN4* in one family. This mutation creates a stop codon leading to premature termination of the protein. In another family, a C to T transition in *NLGN3* was identified that changed a highly conserved arginine residue into cysteine (R451C) within the esterase domain. It was inherited from the mother. Following this report, several other groups studied this gene but found little support for common mutations of the gene. Limited support came from a Portuguese group, who found missense changes in *NLGN4* as well as the protein-truncating mutations in ASD [162]. A Finnish group conducted a molecular genetic analysis of *NLGN1, NLGN3, NLGN4*, and *NLNG4Y*. Their results suggested neuroligin mutations most probably represent rare causes of autism and concluded that it was unlikely that the allelic variants in these genes would be major risk factors for autism [166]. Others have also failed to obtain positive results, casting doubt on the earlier conclusion [164, 165, 167-169].

Other reports about mutations of *NLGN3* or *NLGN4* have identified splice variants in both genes [161]. Three groups recently reported one missense variant and two single substitutions in independent autistic samples, indicating that a defect of synaptogenesis may predispose to autism [158-160].

v. Human oxytocin receptor gene (OXTR)

Oxytocin is a nine-amino-acid peptide synthesized in the hypothalamus. Apart from regulating lactation and uterine contraction, oxytocin acts as a neuromodulator in the central nervous system [219, 220]. Both animal experiments and clinical research have confirmed the role oxytocin plays in social and repetitive behaviors [221]. Therefore the oxytocin system might be potentially involved in the pathogenesis of ASD, and the human oxytocin receptor gene (*OXTR*) has been regarded as a most promising candidate gene to study.

Indeed, research pertaining to the potential association between *OXTR* and autism has come to positive conclusions. Using family-based and population-based association tests, SNPs and haplotypes in the *OXTR* have been reported to confer risk for ASD in different ethnic groups [170, 172-174]. They have also been associated with IQ and adaptive behavior scale scores [172]. Furthermore, a recent study identified significant increases in the DNA methylation status of OXTR in peripheral blood cells and temporal cortex, as well as decreased expression of *OXTR* mRNA in the temporal cortex of autism cases, suggesting that epigenetic dysregulation may be involved in the pathogenesis of ASD [171].

vi. MET

The human *MET* gene encodes a transmembrane receptor tyrosine kinase of the hepatocyte growth factor/scatter factor (HGF/SF) [222]. Though primarily identified as an oncogene, MET plays crucial roles in neuronal development [222-224]. Moreover, impaired MET signaling causes abnormal interneuron migration and neural growth in the cortex, as well as decreased proliferation of granule cells, which matches many of the features found in autistic brains [223, 225].

Campbell and colleagues have done a series of studies regarding the association between MET signaling and autism. They first reported the genetic association of a common C allele in the promoter region of *MET*, which results in significant decrease in *MET* promoter activity and altered binding of specific transcription factor complexes [179]. Then they found significantly decreased MET protein levels and increased mRNA expression for proteins involved in regulating MET signaling activity [226]. Furthermore, they screened the exons and 5′ promoter regions for variants in the five genes encoding the proteins that regulate *MET* expression, finding that genetic susceptibility impacting multiple components of the MET signaling pathway contributes to ASD risk [178]. Most recently, they found that the *MET* C allele influences two of the behavioral domains of the autism triad [175]. Other groups have also provided supportive evidence that *MET* gene variations may play a role in autism susceptibility [176, 177].

vii. SLC25A12

SLC25A12 locates in the chromosome 2q31 region, encoding the mitochondrial aspartate/glutamate carrier (AGC1), a key protein involved in mitochondrial function and ATP synthesis. Since the physiological function of neurons greatly depends on energy supply, any alteration in mitochondrial function or ATP synthesis could lead to corresponding changes in neurons [227]. Recently mitochondrial hyperproliferation and partial respiratory chain block were found in two autistic patients, suggesting *SLC25A12* could be a promising candidate gene [228].

Following this report, several studies for genetic variants of the gene were performed. Three different ethnic groups reported linkage and association between ASD and two SNPs (i.e. rs2056202 and rs2292813) in *SLC25A12* [180, 182, 183], while another three independent groups failed to reveal significant association [184-186]. Another group associated one SNP (rs2056202) with ASD but not the other [181]. Thus, the findings so far are inconclusive.

viii. Other candidate genes

The glutamate receptor 6 gene (*GRIK2* or *GluR6*) is located at chromosome 6q21. Given that glutamate is the principal excitatory neurotransmitter in the brain and it is involved in cognitive functions such as memory and learning, *GRIK2* was proposed as a gene candidate for ASD [229]. Unfortunately, the limited reports have very different results. Genetic studies in a Caucasian population, Chinese Han and Korean trios provided positive evidence, but using different SNPs [187-189]. Another report failed to find any association of *GRIK2* with autism in an Indian population [189].

Contactin associated protein-2 (*CNTNAP2*) belongs to the neurexin family, within which several members have been identified as being related to autism [230]. A recent research report identified a homozygous mutation of *CNTNAP2* in Amish children with pervasive developmental disorders, seizures, and language regression [196]. Five other studies have supported this finding that *CNTNAP2* may be a genetic susceptibility factor in autism [191-195]. Another group found that *CNTNAP2* provided a strong male affection bias in ASD [193].

Glyoxalase 1 is a cytosolic, ubiquitously expressed, zinc metalloenzyme enzyme involved in scavenging toxic α-oxoaldehydes formed during cellular metabolic reactions. Proteomics analysis found glyoxalase 1 increased in autism brains, and subsequent sequencing of its gene (*GLO1*) identified that homozygosity for a polymorphism of the gene, A419 *GLO1*, resulted in decreased enzyme activity and association with autism [198], although this conclusion was not confirmed by other studies [199, 200]. In addition, one group found a protective effect of the A419 allele of *GLO1* [197].

TPH1 and *TPH2* encode rate-limiting enzymes that control serotonin biosynthesis. TPH1 is primarily expressed peripherally, while TPH2 is found exclusively in brain tissue. However, despite evidence for the potential involvement of the serotonin system in the etiology of autism, only one of three reports to date conservatively has supported the notion that *TPH2* plays a role in autism susceptibility [197, 201, 202].

4. Environmental factors

4.1 Prenatal factors

The association between prenatal insults and the pathogenesis of autism has been reported recent decades. Early in 2005, Beversdorf *et al.* conducted surveys regarding incidence and timing of prenatal stressors. They found a higher incidence of prenatal stressors in autism at 21-32 weeks gestation, which peaks at 25-28 weeks. Their finding supported the hypothesis of prenatal stressors as a potential contributor to autism, and the timing was consistent with the embryological age suggested by neuroanatomical findings seen in the cerebellum in autism [231]. More specifically, Meyer *et al* demonstrate that the effects of maternal immune challenge between middle and late gestation periods in mice are dissociable in terms of several neuropsychiatric disorders including autism [232]. However, this conclusion was challenged by another group of scientists. Ploeger *et al.* proposed pleiotropic effects during a very early and specific stage of embryonic development, namely early organogenesis (day 20 to day 40 after fertilization) in order to explain the effect of uterine disturbances to the development of autism [233]. They provided ample evidence from literature for the association between autism and many different kinds of physical anomalies such as limb deformities, craniofacial malformations, brain pathology, and anomalies in other organs, which agrees with the hypothesis that pleiotropic effects are involved in the development of autism.

Drugs are the most important prenatal factors affecting embryo and fetal development. Cumulating data support the relationships between maternal medication and fetogeneous diseases including autism. The obnoxious drug thalidomide turned out not only to relate to fetal abnormality but also to autism. Stromland group retrospectively investigated 100 Swedish thalidomide embryopathy cases and found possible association of thalidomide embryopathy with autism [234]. Another example of drug relating to autism is valproate. Williams *et al* reported six cases whose clinical phenotype was compatible with both fetal valproate syndrome (FVS) and autism. Although the sample size is small, the authors claimed the association between this known teratogen and autism had both clinical and research implications [235]. Similarly, Rasalam group provided another line of evidence that prenatal exposure to sodium valproate is a risk factor for the development of an ASD [236].

Another prenatal factor is intrauterine inflammation. Kannan *et al* conducted an animal study to demonstrate intrauterine inflammation results in alterations in cortical serotonin and disruption of serotonin-regulated thalamocortical development in the newborn brain therefore resulting in impairment of the somatosensory system, such as autism [237]. More persuasive evidence comes from Girard's report. According to their results, end of gestation exposure of pregnant rats to systemic microbial product such as lipopolysacharide (LPS) is an independent risk factor for neurodevelopmental diseases such as cerebral palsy, mental deficiency, and autism. And coadministration of IL-1 receptor antagonist with LPS alleviated the detrimental effects caused by LPS [238].

In addition, maternal complications of pregnancies are proved to be associated with autism. One group performed a discriminant analysis to explore perinatal complications as predictors for autism. They found three maternal medical conditions including urinary infection, high temperatures, and depression to be highly significant and contribute to the separation between the autistic and normal subjects [239].

4.2 Postnatal factors

Heavy metals have also been generally considered to contribute to the pathogenesis of autism. Mercury is one of the most widely studied heavy metals. Palmer *et al* studied the association between environmentally released mercury, special education and autism rates in Texas using data from the Texas Education Department and the United States Environmental Protection Agency, and found there was a significant increase in the rates of special education students and autism rates associated with increases in environmentally released mercury. They reported a 43% increase in the rate of special education services and a 61% increase in the rate of autism [240]. Windham group included 284 children with ASD and 657 controls from the San Francisco Bay area in order to explore possible associations between autism spectrum disorders (ASD) and environmental exposures. Their results suggested a potential association between autism and estimated metal concentrations including mercury, cadmium, nickel [241]. Consistent with previous results, Geier *et al* conducted a prospective study which provided biochemical/genomic evidence for mercury susceptibility/toxicity in ASDs indicating a causal role for mercury [242, 243], and they further explored the threshold effect of mercury in a recent publication [244]. In spite of these different pieces of evidence, disagreement exists. IP *et al* performed a cross-sectional cohort study to compare the hair and blood mercury levels of autistic children and a group of normal children. There was no difference in the mean mercury levels. Thus, they concluded that there is no causal relationship between mercury as an environmental neurotoxin and autism [245].

In addition of mercury, lead is also associated with autism. Very early evidence came from a case report, which explored the interaction and possible casual relationship of an elevated blood-lead and autism, as well as treatment of the behavioral symptoms [246]. Later, Canfield *et al* concluded that blood lead concentrations, even those below 10 microgram per deciliter, were inversely associated with children's IQ scores at three and five years of age, and associated declines in IQ were greater at these concentrations than at higher concentrations [247]. Supporting these results, Yorbik group reported that autism could be associated with significant decrease in excretion rate of lead [248].

Hazardous air pollutants have long been related to the development of autism and more evidences have begun to emerge in recent years. Kalkbrenner *et al* conducted a case-control study to screen perinatal exposure to 35 hazardous air pollutants using 383 children with autism spectrum disorders and, as controls, 2,829 children with speech and language impairment. Although the results were biased by exposure misclassification of air pollutants and the use of an alternate developmental disorder as the control group, they provided evidence based on their analysis that methylene chloride, quinoline, and styrene were the plausible candidate exposures for autism spectrum disorders [249]. In another study conducted by Windham group, trichloroethylene, and vinyl chloride have also been related to autism [241].

However, one should notice that the currently available data are mainly derived from epidemiological studies. Considering the limited sample sizes and the different populations, the previous results are hardly conclusive. Further research is needed to explore the possible mechanisms underlying these results.

5. Mouse models for autism research

Mouse models provide a powerful strategy to explore experimentally candidate genes for autism susceptibility, and to use environmental challenges to induce gene mutations and cell pathology early in development. Mouse models have also been used to investigate the effects of alterations in signaling pathways on neuronal migration, neurotransmission and brain anatomy, which are relevant to findings in autistic subjects [250]. These models have elucidated neuropathology that might underlie the autism phenotype.

There are currently several mouse models for autism research, most of which are primarily developed by knocking out different candidate genes for other neuropsychiatric diseases such as fragile X syndrome [250, 251], Rett syndrome [252], but now are used as autistic models because of their autistic-like behaviors. Other examples include *Engrailed 1&2* and *PTEN* genetic mice [253, 254]. In addition, there is another group of models constructed by surgical or toxic treatments of candidate regions in the brain, in general during development [255]. Some other reports regarding autistic-like behaviors in BALB/c and A/J mice have also been seen [250, 256-258].

Here the author would like to stress an inbred mouse strain for autistic research. BTBR T(+)*tf/J* mouse, also named as BTBR mouse, is an inbred strain with black top coat and blond undercoat. Anatomically BTBR mice get total absence of the corpus callosum, and severely reduced hippocampal commissure, which are also attributed to their phenotypes [259-262]. Although primarily used as type 2 diabetes model [263-268] and phenylketonuria (PKU) model [269-274], BTBR mice were recently found to be a promising mice model for autism research because they exhibited the three core symptoms for diagnosing autism [275-282]. Using this strain, several groups have begun to explore the pathogenesis of autism. It was well documented that circulating corticosterone is higher in the BTBR than in B6. And higher basal glucocorticoid receptor mRNA and higher oxytocin peptide levels were detected in the brains of BTBR as compared to B6, although their relationship to autism remain disputable [283, 284]. In the meanwhile, potential treatments for autism have been proposed based on the experimental results using BTBR mice. Two independent groups confirm the efficacy of the SERT blocker, fluoxetine for enhancement of social interactions [285, 286]. Another experiment reported repetitive self-grooming behavior in the BTBR mouse model of autism was blocked by the mGluR5 antagonist Methyl-6-phenylethynyl-pyridine (MPEP) [287]. Behavioral therapies offer another option for autism treatment, Young group reported social peers rescued autism-relevant sociability deficits in adolescent BTBR mice, but not cross-fostering [288, 289].

However, the tools to analyze these animals are not yet standardized, and an important effort needs to be made. Crawley *et al* proposed three standards to evaluate animal model, namely face validity (i.e. resemblance to the human symptoms), construct validity (i.e. similarity to the underlying causes of the disease) and predictive validity (i.e. expected responses to treatments that are effective in the human disease) [290]. Using these standards, newly developed tests are used to screen more animal models for autism research.

6. Summary and conclusions

Autism spectrum disorders (ASD) is a common neurodevelopment disorder. Diagnosed before three years old, autistic children present significant language delays, social and communication challenges, as well as abnormal repetitive and restrictive behaviors. It is reported that ASD occur in all racial, ethnic and socioeconomic groups, yet are about four times more likely to occur in boys than in girls probably due to the extremes of typical male neuroanatomy of autism.

The relationship between immune disorders and ASD has been proposed based on series of evidences.Secondly, genetic predisposition is considered to be involved in the etiology of ASD. Cumulative evidences indicated ASD had a strong genetic background, both gene-gene and gene-environment interactions attribute to the etiology of autism. Also, it's now generally accepted that ASD is a group of multi-genetic diseases, in which environmental factors play an important part. Given the early onset of the symptoms, prenatal exposures to environmental challenges are considered the major risk factors leading to subsequent mortality of ASD. Various factors have been proven to be potentially detrimental to early neurosystem development, including maternal use of pharmaceutical agents with neurotoxic effects, intrauterine exposure to viral infections or maternal stress , as well as exposure to high levels of environmental pollutants such as heavy metals . Similarly, neonatal exposure to such risk factors may also lead to mortality of ASD, which has been proven in animal studies as well as clinical reports.

At last, ASD animal models provide a feasible and relatively easy way to morphologically and functionally study the etiology of ASD in different levels, and to testify the effectiveness of the potential interventions. Recent advances in this field provide both inbred strains such as BTBR *T+ tf/J* mice and mutant lines. Other mice models for fragile X syndrome, Rett syndrome have also been used for autism related studies due to the autistic-like behaviors exhibited in these patients.

In conclusion, data remain inconclusive for the majority of candidate genes tested so far. Still, we have good reason to be optimistic regarding gene discovery in ASD now and in the future. Cytogenetic, linkage, association studies and array analysis have provided promising results. Emerging genetic technologies and analysis tools offer even more powerful approaches for developing insights into the etiology of ASD. In addition, genetic studies facilitate other autism research such as biochemical and neuroimaging studies, which will, in turn, provide evidence and valuable clues to direct future genetic studies.

7. References

Lord, C., M. Rutter and A. Le Couteur, *Autism Diagnostic Interview-Revised: a revised version of a diagnostic interview for caregivers of individuals with possible pervasive developmental disorders.* J Autism Dev Disord, 1994. 24(5): p. 659-85.

Lord, C., et al., *Autism diagnostic observation schedule: a standardized observation of communicative and social behavior.* J Autism Dev Disord, 1989. 19(2): p. 185-212.

Van Naarden, B.K., et al., *Evaluation of a methodology for a collaborative multiple source surveillance network for autism spectrum disorders--Autism and Developmental Disabilities Monitoring Network, 14 sites, United States,* 2002. MMWR Surveill Summ, 2007. 56(1): p. 29-40.

Nonkin, A.R., et al., *Evaluation of a Records-Review Surveillance System Used to Determine the Prevalence of Autism Spectrum Disorders.* J Autism Dev Disord, 2010.

Krause, I., et al., *Brief report: immune factors in autism: a critical review.* J Autism Dev Disord, 2002. 32(4): p. 337-45.

Lintas, C. and A.M. Persico, *Autistic phenotypes and genetic testing: state-of-the-art for the clinical geneticist.* J Med Genet, 2009. 46(1): p. 1-8.

Baron-Cohen, S., R.C. Knickmeyer and M.K. Belmonte, *Sex differences in the brain: implications for explaining autism.* Science, 2005. 310(5749): p. 819-23.

Williams, J.G., J.P. Higgins and C.E. Brayne, *Systematic review of prevalence studies of autism spectrum disorders.* Arch Dis Child, 2006. 91(1): p. 8-15.

Prevalence of autism spectrum disorders - *Autism and Developmental Disabilities Monitoring Network, United States, 2006.* MMWR Surveill Summ, 2009. 58(10): p. 1-20.

Prevalence of autism spectrum disorders--autism and developmental disabilities monitoring network, six sites, United States, 2000. MMWR Surveill Summ, 2007. 56(1): p. 1-11.

Prevalence of autism spectrum disorders--autism and developmental disabilities monitoring network, 14 sites, United States, 2002. MMWR Surveill Summ, 2007. 56(1): p. 12-28.

King, M. and P. Bearman, *Diagnostic change and the increased prevalence of autism.* Int J Epidemiol, 2009. 38(5): p. 1224-34.

Nonkin, A.R., et al., *Evaluation of a Records-Review Surveillance System Used to Determine the Prevalence of Autism Spectrum Disorders.* J Autism Dev Disord, 2010.

Comi, A.M., et al., *Familial clustering of autoimmune disorders and evaluation of medical risk factors in autism.* J Child Neurol, 1999. 14(6): p. 388-94.

Molloy, C.A., et al., *Familial autoimmune thyroid disease as a risk factor for regression in children with Autism Spectrum Disorder:* a CPEA Study. J Autism Dev Disord, 2006. 36(3): p. 317-24.

Mouridsen, S.E., et al., *Autoimmune diseases in parents of children with infantile autism: a case-control study.* Dev Med Child Neurol, 2007. 49(6): p. 429-32.

Sweeten, T.L., et al., *Increased prevalence of familial autoimmunity in probands with pervasive developmental disorders.* Pediatrics, 2003. 112(5): p. e420.

Careaga, M., J. Van de Water and P. Ashwood, *Immune dysfunction in autism: a pathway to treatment.* Neurotherapeutics, 2010. 7(3): p. 283-92.

Cabanlit, M., et al., *Brain-specific autoantibodies in the plasma of subjects with autistic spectrum disorder.* Ann N Y Acad Sci, 2007. 1107: p. 92-103.

Wills, S., et al., *Detection of autoantibodies to neural cells of the cerebellum in the plasma of subjects with autism spectrum disorders.* Brain Behav Immun, 2009. 23(1): p. 64-74.

Ashwood, P., S. Wills and J. Van de Water, *The immune response in autism: a new frontier for autism research.* J Leukoc Biol, 2006. 80(1): p. 1-15.

Enstrom, A., et al., *Increased IgG4 levels in children with autism disorder.* Brain Behav Immun, 2009. 23(3): p. 389-95.

Heuer, L., et al., Reduced levels of immunoglobulin in children with autism correlates with behavioral symptoms. Autism Res, 2008. 1(5): p. 275-83.

Trajkovski, V., L. Ajdinski and M. Spiroski, *Plasma concentration of immunoglobulin classes and subclasses in children with autism in the Republic of Macedonia: retrospective study.* Croat Med J, 2004. 45(6): p. 746-9.

Ashwood, P., et al., *Altered T cell responses in children with autism.* Brain Behav Immun, 2010.

Comi, A.M., et al., *Familial clustering of autoimmune disorders and evaluation of medical risk factors in autism.* J Child Neurol, 1999. 14(6): p. 388-94.

Sweeten, T.L., et al., *Increased prevalence of familial autoimmunity in probands with pervasive developmental disorders.* Pediatrics, 2003. 112(5): p. e420.
Molloy, C.A., et al., *Familial autoimmune thyroid disease as a risk factor for regression in children with Autism Spectrum Disorder: a CPEA Study.* J Autism Dev Disord, 2006. 36(3): p. 317-24.
Jyonouchi, H., S. Sun and ". H", *Proinflammatory and regulatory cytokine production associated with innate and adaptive immune responses in children with autism spectrum disorders and developmental regression.* J Neuroimmunol, 2001. 120(1-2): p. 170-9.
Molloy, C.A., et al., *Elevated cytokine levels in children with autism spectrum disorder.* J Neuroimmunol, 2006. 172(1-2): p. 198-205.
Li, X., et al., *Elevated immune response in the brain of autistic patients.* J Neuroimmunol, 2009. 207(1-2): p. 111-6.
Ashwood, P., et al., *Elevated plasma cytokines in autism spectrum disorders provide evidence of immune dysfunction and are associated with impaired behavioral outcome.* Brain Behav Immun, 2010.
Singer, H.S., et al., *Antibodies against fetal brain in sera of mothers with autistic children.* J Neuroimmunol, 2008. 194(1-2): p. 165-72.
Braunschweig, D., et al., *Autism: maternally derived antibodies specific for fetal brain proteins.* Neurotoxicology, 2008. 29(2): p. 226-31.
Zimmerman, A.W., et al., *Maternal antibrain antibodies in autism.* Brain Behav Immun, 2007. 21(3): p. 351-7.
Croen, L.A., et al., *Maternal mid-pregnancy autoantibodies to fetal brain protein: the early markers for autism study.* Biol Psychiatry, 2008. 64(7): p. 583-8.
Braunschweig, D., et al., *Autism: maternally derived antibodies specific for fetal brain proteins.* Neurotoxicology, 2008. 29(2): p. 226-31.
Singh, V.K. and W.H. Rivas, *Prevalence of serum antibodies to caudate nucleus in autistic children.* Neurosci Lett, 2004. 355(1-2): p. 53-6.
Trajkovski, V., L. Ajdinski and M. Spiroski, *Plasma concentration of immunoglobulin classes and subclasses in children with autism in the Republic of Macedonia: retrospective study.* Croat Med J, 2004. 45(6): p. 746-9.
Enstrom, A., et al., *Increased IgG4 levels in children with autism disorder.* Brain Behav Immun, 2009. 23(3): p. 389-95.
Morris, C.M., A.W. Zimmerman and H.S. Singer, *Childhood serum anti-fetal brain antibodies do not predict autism.* Pediatr Neurol, 2009. 41(4): p. 288-90.
Stern, L., et al., *Immune function in autistic children.* Ann Allergy Asthma Immunol, 2005. 95(6): p. 558-65.
Goodwin, M.S., M.A. Cowen and T.C. Goodwin, *Malabsorption and cerebral dysfunction: a multivariate and comparative study of autistic children.* J Autism Child Schizophr, 1971. 1(1): p. 48-62.
Horvath, K. and J.A. Perman, *Autism and gastrointestinal symptoms.* Curr Gastroenterol Rep, 2002. 4(3): p. 251-8.
Kuddo, T. and K.B. Nelson, *How common are gastrointestinal disorders in children with autism?.* Curr Opin Pediatr, 2003. 15(3): p. 339-43.
Molloy, C.A. and P. Manning-Courtney, *Prevalence of chronic gastrointestinal symptoms in children with autism and autistic spectrum disorders.* Autism, 2003. 7(2): p. 165-71.

Fernell, E., U.L. Fagerberg and P.M. Hellstrom, *No evidence for a clear link between active intestinal inflammation and autism based on analyses of faecal calprotectin and rectal nitric oxide.* Acta Paediatr, 2007. 96(7): p. 1076-9.

Wakefield, A.J., et al., *Enterocolitis in children with developmental disorders.* Am J Gastroenterol, 2000. 95(9): p. 2285-95.

Horvath, K., et al., *Gastrointestinal abnormalities in children with autistic disorder.* J Pediatr, 1999. 135(5): p. 559-63.

Ashwood, P., et al., *Spontaneous mucosal lymphocyte cytokine profiles in children with autism and gastrointestinal symptoms: mucosal immune activation and reduced counter regulatory interleukin-10.* J Clin Immunol, 2004. 24(6): p. 664-73.

Ashwood, P. and A.J. Wakefield, *Immune activation of peripheral blood and mucosal CD3+ lymphocyte cytokine profiles in children with autism and gastrointestinal symptoms.* J Neuroimmunol, 2006. 173(1-2): p. 126-34.

Jyonouchi, H., et al., *Dysregulated innate immune responses in young children with autism spectrum disorders: their relationship to gastrointestinal symptoms and dietary intervention.* Neuropsychobiology, 2005. 51(2): p. 77-85.

DeFelice, M.L., et al., *Intestinal cytokines in children with pervasive developmental disorders.* Am J Gastroenterol, 2003. 98(8): p. 1777-82.

D'Eufemia, P., et al., *Abnormal intestinal permeability in children with autism.* Acta Paediatr, 1996. 85(9): p. 1076-9.

Caglayan, A.O., *Genetic causes of syndromic and non-syndromic autism.* Dev Med Child Neurol, 2010. 52(2): p. 130-8.

Abrahams, B.S. and D.H. Geschwind, *Advances in autism genetics: on the threshold of a new neurobiology.* Nat Rev Genet, 2008. 9(5): p. 341-55.

Bailey, A., et al., *Autism as a strongly genetic disorder: evidence from a British twin study.* Psychol Med, 1995. 25(1): p. 63-77.

Steffenburg, S., et al., *A twin study of autism in Denmark, Finland, Iceland, Norway and Sweden.* J Child Psychol Psychiatry, 1989. 30(3): p. 405-16.

Liu, K., N. Zerubavel and P. Bearman, *Social demographic change and autism.* Demography, 2010. 47(2): p. 327-43.

Hoffman, E.J. and M.W. State, *Progress in cytogenetics: implications for child psychopathology.* J Am Acad Child Adolesc Psychiatry, 2010. 49(8): p. 736-51; quiz 856-7.

Piggot, J., et al., *Neural systems approaches to the neurogenetics of autism spectrum disorders.* Neuroscience, 2009. 164(1): p. 247-56.

Levitt, P. and D.B. Campbell, *The genetic and neurobiologic compass points toward common signaling dysfunctions in autism spectrum disorders.* J Clin Invest, 2009. 119(4): p. 747- 54.

Kumar, R.A. and S.L. Christian, *Genetics of autism spectrum disorders.* Curr Neurol Neurosci Rep, 2009. 9(3): p. 188-97.

Betancur, C., T. Sakurai and J.D. Buxbaum, *The emerging role of synaptic cell-adhesion pathways in the pathogenesis of autism spectrum disorders.* Trends Neurosci, 2009. 32(7): p. 402-12.

Vissers, L.E., et al., *A de novo paradigm for mental retardation.* Nat Genet, 2010. 42(12): p. 1109-12.

Choi, M., et al., *Genetic diagnosis by whole exome capture and massively parallel DNA sequencing*. Proc Natl Acad Sci U S A, 2009. 106(45): p. 19096-101.
Robinson, P.N., *Whole-exome sequencing for finding de novo mutations in sporadic mental retardation*. Genome Biol, 2010. 11(12): p. 144.
Bilguvar, K., et al., *Whole-exome sequencing identifies recessive WDR62 mutations in severe brain malformations*. Nature, 2010. 467(7312): p. 207-10.
Sanders, S., *Whole-exome sequencing: a powerful technique for identifying novel genes of complex disorders*. Clin Genet, 2011. 79(2): p. 132-3.
Betancur, C., *Etiological heterogeneity in autism spectrum disorders: More than 100 genetic and genomic disorders and still counting*. Brain Res, 2010.
Buxbaum, J.D., et al., *Evidence for a susceptibility gene for autism on chromosome 2 and for genetic heterogeneity*. Am J Hum Genet, 2001. 68(6): p. 1514-20.
Shao, Y., et al., *Phenotypic homogeneity provides increased support for linkage on chromosome 2 in autistic disorder*. Am J Hum Genet, 2002. 70(4): p. 1058-61.
Rabionet, R., et al., *Analysis of the autism chromosome 2 linkage region: GAD1 and other candidate genes*. Neurosci Lett, 2004. 372(3): p. 209-14.
Wu, S., et al., *Association of the neuropilin-2 (NRP2) gene polymorphisms with autism in Chinese Han population*. Am J Med Genet B Neuropsychiatr Genet, 2007. 144B(4): p. 492-5.
Blasi, F., et al., *SLC25A12 and CMYA3 gene variants are not associated with autism in the IMGSAC multiplex family sample*. Eur J Hum Genet, 2006. 14(1): p. 123-6.
Szatmari, P., et al., *Mapping autism risk loci using genetic linkage and chromosomal rearrangements*. Nat Genet, 2007. 39(3): p. 319-28.
Ramoz, N., et al., *An analysis of candidate autism loci on chromosome 2q24-q33: evidence for association to the STK39 gene*. Am J Med Genet B Neuropsychiatr Genet, 2008. 147B(7): p. 1152-8.
Philippi, A., et al., *Association of autism with polymorphisms in the paired-like homeodomain transcription factor 1 (PITX1) on chromosome 5q31: a candidate gene analysis*. BMC Med Genet, 2007. 8: p. 74.
Ma, D., et al., *A genome-wide association study of autism reveals a common novel risk locus at 5p14.1*. Ann Hum Genet, 2009. 73(Pt 3): p. 263-73.
Weiss, L.A., et al., *A genome-wide linkage and association scan reveals novel loci for autism*. Nature, 2009. 461(7265): p. 802-8.
Shinawi, M., et al., *Recurrent reciprocal 16p11.2 rearrangements associated with global developmental delay, behavioural problems, dysmorphism, epilepsy, and abnormal head size*. J Med Genet, 2010. 47(5): p. 332-41.
Kumar, R.A., et al., *Recurrent 16p11.2 microdeletions in autism*. Hum Mol Genet, 2008. 17(4): p. 628-38.
Kim, S.J., et al., *Transmission disequilibrium testing of the chromosome 15q11-q13 region in autism*. Am J Med Genet B Neuropsychiatr Genet, 2008. 147B(7): p. 1116-25.
Sutcliffe, J.S., et al., *Partial duplication of the APBA2 gene in chromosome 15q13 corresponds to duplicon structures*. BMC Genomics, 2003. 4(1): p. 15.
Nurmi, E.L., et al., *Linkage disequilibrium at the Angelman syndrome gene UBE3A in autism families*. Genomics, 2001. 77(1-2): p. 105-13.
Shen, Y., et al., *Clinical genetic testing for patients with autism spectrum disorders*. Pediatrics, 2010. 125(4): p. e727-35.

Ma, D.Q., et al., *Dissecting the locus heterogeneity of autism: significant linkage to chromosome 12q14.* Mol Psychiatry, 2007. 12(4): p. 376-84.

Alvarez, R.A., et al., *Association of common variants in the Joubert syndrome gene (AHI1) with autism.* Hum Mol Genet, 2008. 17(24): p. 3887-96.

Qin, J., et al., *Association study of SHANK3 gene polymorphisms with autism in Chinese Han population.* BMC Med Genet, 2009. 10: p. 61.

Kumar, R.A., et al., *A de novo 1p34.2 microdeletion identifies the synaptic vesicle gene RIMS3 as a novel candidate for autism.* J Med Genet, 2010. 47(2): p. 81-90.

Noor, A., et al., *Disruption at the PTCHD1 Locus on Xp22.11 in Autism Spectrum Disorder and Intellectual Disability.* Sci Transl Med, 2010. 2(49): p. 49ra68.

Segurado, R., et al., *Confirmation of association between autism and the mitochondrial aspartate/glutamate carrier SLC25A12 gene on chromosome 2q31.* Am J Psychiatry, 2005. 162(11): p. 2182-4.

Cukier, H.N., et al., *Identification of chromosome 7 inversion breakpoints in an autistic family narrows candidate region for autism susceptibility.* Autism Res, 2009. 2(5): p. 258-66.

Sakurai, T., et al., *Association analysis of the NrCAM gene in autism and in subsets of families with severe obsessive-compulsive or self-stimulatory behaviors.* Psychiatr Genet, 2006. 16(6): p. 251-7.

Hutcheson, H.B., et al., *Examination of NRCAM, LRRN3, KIAA0716, and LAMB1 as autism candidate genes.* BMC Med Genet, 2004. 5: p. 12.

Marui, T., et al., *Association of the neuronal cell adhesion molecule (NRCAM) gene variants with autism.* Int J Neuropsychopharmacol, 2009. 12(1): p. 1-10.

Marui, T., et al., *Association between autism and variants in the wingless-type MMTV integration site family member 2 (WNT2) gene.* Int J Neuropsychopharmacol, 2010. 13(4): p. 443-9.

Barnby, G., et al., *Candidate-gene screening and association analysis at the autism-susceptibility locus on chromosome 16p: evidence of association at GRIN2A and ABAT.* Am J Hum Genet, 2005. 76(6): p. 950-66.

McCauley, J.L., et al., *Genome-wide and Ordered-Subset linkage analyses provide support for autism loci on 17q and 19p with evidence of phenotypic and interlocus genetic correlates.* BMC Med Genet, 2005. 6: p. 1.

Christian, S.L., et al., *Novel submicroscopic chromosomal abnormalities detected in autism spectrum disorder.* Biol Psychiatry, 2008. 63(12): p. 1111-7.

Marshall, C.R., et al., *Structural variation of chromosomes in autism spectrum disorder.* Am J Hum Genet, 2008. 82(2): p. 477-88.

Sebat, J., et al., *Strong association of de novo copy number mutations with autism.* Science, 2007. 316(5823): p. 445-9.

Cho, S.C., et al., *Copy number variations associated with idiopathic autism identified by whole-genome microarray-based comparative genomic hybridization.* Psychiatr Genet, 2009. 19(4): p. 177-85.

Qiao, Y., et al., *Phenomic determinants of genomic variation in autism spectrum disorders.* J Med Genet, 2009. 46(10): p. 680-8.

Cusco, I., et al., *Autism-specific copy number variants further implicate the phosphatidylinositol signaling pathway and the glutamatergic synapse in the etiology of the disorder.* Hum Mol Genet, 2009. 18(10): p. 1795-804.

Babatz, T.D., et al., *Copy number and sequence variants implicate APBA2 as an autism candidate gene.* Autism Res, 2009. 2(6): p. 359-64.
Wang, K., et al., *Common genetic variants on 5p14.1 associate with autism spectrum disorders.* Nature, 2009. 459(7246): p. 528-33.
Pinto, D., et al., *Functional impact of global rare copy number variation in autism spectrum disorders.* Nature, 2010. 466(7304): p. 368-72.
Glessner, J.T., et al., *Autism genome-wide copy number variation reveals ubiquitin and neuronal genes.* Nature, 2009. 459(7246): p. 569-73.
Geschwind, D.H. and P. Levitt, *Autism spectrum disorders: developmental disconnection syndromes.* Curr Opin Neurobiol, 2007. 17(1): p. 103-11.
Li, H., et al., *The association analysis of RELN and GRM8 genes with autistic spectrum disorder in Chinese Han population.* Am J Med Genet B Neuropsychiatr Genet, 2008. 147B(2): p. 194-200.
Ashley-Koch, A.E., et al., *Investigation of potential gene-gene interactions between APOE and RELN contributing to autism risk.* Psychiatr Genet, 2007. 17(4): p. 221-6.
Dutta, S., et al., *Reelin gene polymorphisms in the Indian population: a possible paternal 5'UTR-CGG-repeat-allele effect on autism.* Am J Med Genet B Neuropsychiatr Genet, 2007. 144B(1): p. 106-12.
Serajee, F.J., H. Zhong and H.A. Mahbubul, *Association of Reelin gene polymorphisms with autism.* Genomics, 2006. 87(1): p. 75-83.
Skaar, D.A., et al., *Analysis of the RELN gene as a genetic risk factor for autism.* Mol Psychiatry, 2005. 10(6): p. 563-71.
Devlin, B., et al., *Alleles of a reelin CGG repeat do not convey liability to autism in a sample from the CPEA network.* Am J Med Genet B Neuropsychiatr Genet, 2004. 126B(1): p. 46-50.
Li, J., et al., *Lack of evidence for an association between WNT2 and RELN polymorphisms and autism.* Am J Med Genet B Neuropsychiatr Genet, 2004. 126B(1): p. 51-7.
Zhang, H., et al., *Reelin gene alleles and susceptibility to autism spectrum disorders.* Mol Psychiatry, 2002. 7(9): p. 1012-7.
Krebs, M.O., et al., *Absence of association between a polymorphic GGC repeat in the 5' untranslated region of the reelin gene and autism.* Mol Psychiatry, 2002. 7(7): p. 801-4.
Persico, A.M., et al., *Reelin gene alleles and haplotypes as a factor predisposing to autistic disorder.* Mol Psychiatry, 2001. 6(2): p. 150-9.
Sutcliffe, J.S., et al., *Allelic heterogeneity at the serotonin transporter locus (SLC6A4) confers susceptibility to autism and rigid-compulsive behaviors.* Am J Hum Genet, 2005. 77(2): p. 265-79.
Coutinho, A.M., et al., *Evidence for epistasis between SLC6A4 and ITGB3 in autism etiology and in the determination of platelet serotonin levels.* Hum Genet, 2007. 121(2): p. 243-56.
Jr Cook, E., et al., *Evidence of linkage between the serotonin transporter and autistic disorder.* Mol Psychiatry, 1997. 2(3): p. 247-50.
Anderson, B.M., et al., *Examination of association of genes in the serotonin system to autism.* Neurogenetics, 2009. 10(3): p. 209-16.
Cho, I.H., et al., *Family-based association study of 5-HTTLPR and the 5-HT2A receptor gene polymorphisms with autism spectrum disorder in Korean trios.* Brain Res, 2007. 1139: p. 34-41.

McCauley, J.L., et al., *Linkage and association analysis at the serotonin transporter (SLC6A4) locus in a rigid-compulsive subset of autism.* Am J Med Genet B Neuropsychiatr Genet, 2004. 127B(1): p. 104-12.

Coutinho, A.M., et al., *Variants of the serotonin transporter gene (SLC6A4) significantly contribute to hyperserotonemia in autism.* Mol Psychiatry, 2004. 9(3): p. 264-71.

Zhong, N., et al., *5-HTTLPR variants not associated with autistic spectrum disorders.* Neurogenetics, 1999. 2(2): p. 129-31.

Guhathakurta, S., et al., *Analysis of serotonin receptor 2A gene (HTR2A): association study with autism spectrum disorder in the Indian population and investigation of the gene expression in peripheral blood leukocytes.* Neurochem Int, 2009. 55(8): p. 754-9.

Ma, D.Q., et al., *Association and gene-gene interaction of SLC6A4 and ITGB3 in autism.* Am J Med Genet B Neuropsychiatr Genet, 2010. 153B(2): p. 477-83.

Huang, C.H. and S.L. Santangelo, *Autism and serotonin transporter gene polymorphisms: a systematic review and meta-analysis.* Am J Med Genet B Neuropsychiatr Genet, 2008. 147B(6): p. 903-13.

Persico, A.M., et al., *Lack of association between serotonin transporter gene promoter variants and autistic disorder in two ethnically distinct samples.* Am J Med Genet, 2000. 96(1): p. 123-7.

Wu, S., et al., *Lack of evidence for association between the serotonin transporter gene (SLC6A4) polymorphisms and autism in the Chinese trios.* Neurosci Lett, 2005. 381(1-2): p. 1-5.

Ramoz, N., et al., *Lack of evidence for association of the serotonin transporter gene SLC6A4 with autism.* Biol Psychiatry, 2006. 60(2): p. 186-91.

Guhathakurta, S., et al., *Population-based association study and contrasting linkage disequilibrium pattern reveal genetic association of SLC6A4 with autism in the Indian population from West Bengal.* Brain Res, 2008. 1240: p. 12-21.

Tordjman, S., et al., *Role of the serotonin transporter gene in the behavioral expression of autism.* Mol Psychiatry, 2001. 6(4): p. 434-9.

Maestrini, E., et al., *Serotonin transporter (5-HTT) and gamma-aminobutyric acid receptor subunit beta3 (GABRB3) gene polymorphisms are not associated with autism in the IMGSA families. The International Molecular Genetic Study of Autism Consortium.* Am J Med Genet, 1999. 88(5): p. 492-6.

Klauck, S.M., et al., *Serotonin transporter (5-HTT) gene variants associated with autism?.* Hum Mol Genet, 1997. 6(13): p. 2233-8.

Betancur, C., et al., *Serotonin transporter gene polymorphisms and hyperserotonemia in autistic disorder.* Mol Psychiatry, 2002. 7(1): p. 67-71.

Koishi, S., et al., *Serotonin transporter gene promoter polymorphism and autism: a family-based genetic association study in Japanese population.* Brain Dev, 2006. 28(4): p. 257-60.

Takumi, T., *A humanoid mouse model of autism.* Brain Dev, 2010.

McCauley, J.L., et al., *A linkage disequilibrium map of the 1-Mb 15q12 GABA(A) receptor subunit cluster and association to autism.* Am J Med Genet B Neuropsychiatr Genet, 2004. 131B(1): p. 51-9.

Nakatani, J., et al., *Abnormal behavior in a chromosome-engineered mouse model for human 15q11-13 duplication seen in autism.* Cell, 2009. 137(7): p. 1235-46.

Menold, M.M., et al., *Association analysis of chromosome 15 gabaa receptor subunit genes in autistic disorder.* J Neurogenet, 2001. 15(3-4): p. 245-59.

Buxbaum, J.D., et al., *Association between a GABRB3 polymorphism and autism.* Mol Psychiatry, 2002. 7(3): p. 311-6.

Kim, S.A., et al., *Association of GABRB3 polymorphisms with autism spectrum disorders in Korean trios.* Neuropsychobiology, 2006. 54(3): p. 160-5.

Kwasnicka-Crawford, D.A., W. Roberts and S.W. Scherer, *Characterization of an autism-associated segmental maternal heterodisomy of the chromosome 15q11-13 region.* J Autism Dev Disord, 2007. 37(4): p. 694-702.

Bolton, P.F., et al., *Chromosome 15q11-13 abnormalities and other medical conditions in individuals with autism spectrum disorders.* Psychiatr Genet, 2004. 14(3): p. 131-7.

Shao, Y., et al., *Fine mapping of autistic disorder to chromosome 15q11-q13 by use of phenotypic subtypes.* Am J Hum Genet, 2003. 72(3): p. 539-48.

Ma, D.Q., et al., *Identification of significant association and gene-gene interaction of GABA receptor subunit genes in autism.* Am J Hum Genet, 2005. 77(3): p. 377-88.

Yoo, H.K., et al., *Microsatellite marker in gamma - aminobutyric acid - a receptor beta 3 subunit gene and autism spectrum disorders in Korean trios.* Yonsei Med J, 2009. 50(2): p. 304-6.

Cai, G., et al., *Multiplex ligation-dependent probe amplification for genetic screening in autism spectrum disorders: efficient identification of known microduplications and identification of a novel microduplication in ASMT.* BMC Med Genomics, 2008. 1: p. 50.

Aldinger, K.A. and S. Qiu, *New mouse genetic model duplicates human 15q11-13 autistic phenotypes, or does it?.* Dis Model Mech, 2010. 3(1-2): p. 3-4.

Depienne, C., et al., *Screening for genomic rearrangements and methylation abnormalities of the 15q11-q13 region in autism spectrum disorders.* Biol Psychiatry, 2009. 66(4): p. 349- 59.

Curran, S., et al., *An association analysis of microsatellite markers across the Prader- Willi/ Angelman critical region on chromosome 15 (q11-13) and autism spectrum disorder.* Am J Med Genet B Neuropsychiatr Genet, 2005. 137B(1): p. 25-8.

Martin, E.R., et al., *Analysis of linkage disequilibrium in gamma-aminobutyric acid receptor subunit genes in autistic disorder.* Am J Med Genet, 2000. 96(1): p. 43-8.

Maestrini, E., et al., *Serotonin transporter (5-HTT) and gamma-aminobutyric acid receptor subunit beta3 (GABRB3) gene polymorphisms are not associated with autism in the IMGSA families. The International Molecular Genetic Study of Autism Consortium.* Am J Med Genet, 1999. 88(5): p. 492-6.

Zhang, C., et al., *A neuroligin-4 missense mutation associated with autism impairs neuroligin-4 folding and endoplasmic reticulum export.* J Neurosci, 2009. 29(35): p. 10843-54.

Pampanos, A., et al., *A substitution involving the NLGN4 gene associated with autistic behavior in the Greek population.* Genet Test Mol Biomarkers, 2009. 13(5): p. 611-5.

Yan, J., et al., *Analysis of the neuroligin 4Y gene in patients with autism.* Psychiatr Genet, 2008. 18(4): p. 204-7.

Talebizadeh, Z., et al., *Novel splice isoforms for NLGN3 and NLGN4 with possible implications in autism.* J Med Genet, 2006. 43(5): p. e21.

Yan, J., et al., *Analysis of the neuroligin 3 and 4 genes in autism and other neuropsychiatric patients.* Mol Psychiatry, 2005. 10(4): p. 329-32.

Jamain, S., et al., *Mutations of the X-linked genes encoding neuroligins NLGN3 and NLGN4 are associated with autism.* Nat Genet, 2003. 34(1): p. 27-9.

Wermter, A.K., et al., *No evidence for involvement of genetic variants in the X-linked neuroligin genes NLGN3 and NLGN4X in probands with autism spectrum disorder on high functioning level.* Am J Med Genet B Neuropsychiatr Genet, 2008. 147B(4): p. 535-7.

Blasi, F., et al., *Absence of coding mutations in the X-linked genes neuroligin 3 and neuroligin 4 in individuals with autism from the IMGSAC collection.* Am J Med Genet B Neuropsychiatr Genet, 2006. 141B(3): p. 220-1.

Ylisaukko-oja, T., et al., *Analysis of four neuroligin genes as candidates for autism.* Eur J Hum Genet, 2005. 13(12): p. 1285-92.

Gauthier, J., et al., *NLGN3/NLGN4 gene mutations are not responsible for autism in the Quebec population.* Am J Med Genet B Neuropsychiatr Genet, 2005. 132B(1): p. 74-5.

Vincent, J.B., et al., *Mutation screening of X-chromosomal neuroligin genes: no mutations in 196 autism probands.* Am J Med Genet B Neuropsychiatr Genet, 2004. 129B(1): p. 82- 4.

Talebizadeh, Z., et al., *Do known mutations in neuroligin genes (NLGN3 and NLGN4) cause autism?.* J Autism Dev Disord, 2004. 34(6): p. 735-6.

Liu, X., et al., *Association of the oxytocin receptor (OXTR) gene polymorphisms with autism spectrum disorder (ASD) in the Japanese population.* J Hum Genet, 2010. 55(3): p. 137- 41.

Gregory, S.G., et al., *Genomic and epigenetic evidence for oxytocin receptor deficiency in autism.* BMC Med, 2009. 7: p. 62.

Lerer, E., et al., *Association between the oxytocin receptor (OXTR) gene and autism: relationship to Vineland Adaptive Behavior Scales and cognition.* Mol Psychiatry, 2008. 13(10): p. 980-8.

Jacob, S., et al., *Association of the oxytocin receptor gene (OXTR) in Caucasian children and adolescents with autism.* Neurosci Lett, 2007. 417(1): p. 6-9.

Wu, S., et al., *Positive association of the oxytocin receptor gene (OXTR) with autism in the Chinese Han population.* Biol Psychiatry, 2005. 58(1): p. 74-7.

Campbell, D.B., et al., *Association of MET with social and communication phenotypes in individuals with autism spectrum disorder.* Am J Med Genet B Neuropsychiatr Genet, 2010. 153B(2): p. 438-46.

Jackson, P.B., et al., *Further evidence that the rs1858830 C variant in the promoter region of the MET gene is associated with autistic disorder.* Autism Res, 2009. 2(4): p. 232-6.

Sousa, I., et al., *MET and autism susceptibility: family and case-control studies.* Eur J Hum Genet, 2009. 17(6): p. 749-58.

Campbell, D.B., et al., *Genetic evidence implicating multiple genes in the MET receptor tyrosine kinase pathway in autism spectrum disorder.* Autism Res, 2008. 1(3): p. 159-68.

Campbell, D.B., et al., *A genetic variant that disrupts MET transcription is associated with autism.* Proc Natl Acad Sci U S A, 2006. 103(45): p. 16834-9.

Turunen, J.A., et al., *Mitochondrial aspartate/glutamate carrier SLC25A12 gene is associated with autism.* Autism Res, 2008. 1(3): p. 189-92.

Silverman, J.M., et al., *Autism-related routines and rituals associated with a mitochondrial aspartate/glutamate carrier SLC25A12 polymorphism.* Am J Med Genet B Neuropsychiatr Genet, 2008. 147(3): p. 408-10.

Segurado, R., et al., *Confirmation of association between autism and the mitochondrial aspartate/glutamate carrier SLC25A12 gene on chromosome 2q31.* Am J Psychiatry, 2005. 162(11): p. 2182-4.

Ramoz, N., et al., *Linkage and association of the mitochondrial aspartate/glutamate carrier SLC25A12 gene with autism.* Am J Psychiatry, 2004. 161(4): p. 662-9.
Chien, W.H., et al., *Association study of the SLC25A12 gene and autism in Han Chinese in Taiwan.* Prog Neuropsychopharmacol Biol Psychiatry, 2010. 34(1): p. 189-92.
Rabionet, R., et al., *Lack of association between autism and SLC25A12.* Am J Psychiatry, 2006. 163(5): p. 929-31.
Blasi, F., et al., *SLC25A12 and CMYA3 gene variants are not associated with autism in the IMGSAC multiplex family sample.* Eur J Hum Genet, 2006. 14(1): p. 123-6.
Kim, S.A., et al., *Family-based association study between GRIK2 polymorphisms and autism spectrum disorders in the Korean trios.* Neurosci Res, 2007. 58(3): p. 332-5.
Shuang, M., et al., *Family-based association study between autism and glutamate receptor 6 gene in Chinese Han trios.* Am J Med Genet B Neuropsychiatr Genet, 2004. 131B(1): p. 48-50.
Jamain, S., et al., *Linkage and association of the glutamate receptor 6 gene with autism.* Mol Psychiatry, 2002. 7(3): p. 302-10.
Dutta, S., et al., *Glutamate receptor 6 gene (GluR6 or GRIK2) polymorphisms in the Indian population: a genetic association study on autism spectrum disorder.* Cell Mol Neurobiol, 2007. 27(8): p. 1035-47.
Poot, M., et al., *Disruption of CNTNAP2 and additional structural genome changes in a boy with speech delay and autism spectrum disorder.* Neurogenetics, 2010. 11(1): p. 81-9.
Arking, D.E., et al., *A common genetic variant in the neurexin superfamily member CNTNAP2 increases familial risk of autism.* Am J Hum Genet, 2008. 82(1): p. 160-4.
Alarcon, M., et al., *Linkage, association, and gene-expression analyses identify CNTNAP2 as an autism-susceptibility gene.* Am J Hum Genet, 2008. 82(1): p. 150-9.
Bakkaloglu, B., et al., *Molecular cytogenetic analysis and resequencing of contactin associated protein-like 2 in autism spectrum disorders.* Am J Hum Genet, 2008. 82(1): p. 165-73.
Rossi, E., et al., *A 12Mb deletion at 7q33-q35 associated with autism spectrum disorders and primary amenorrhea.* Eur J Med Genet, 2008. 51(6): p. 631-8.
Strauss, K.A., et al., *Recessive symptomatic focal epilepsy and mutant contactin-associated protein-like 2.* N Engl J Med, 2006. 354(13): p. 1370-7.
Sacco, R., et al., *Case-control and family-based association studies of candidate genes in autistic disorder and its endophenotypes: TPH2 and GLO1.* BMC Med Genet, 2007. 8: p. 11.
Junaid, M.A., et al., *Proteomic studies identified a single nucleotide polymorphism in glyoxalase I as autism susceptibility factor.* Am J Med Genet A, 2004. 131(1): p. 11-7.
Wu, Y.Y., et al., *Lack of evidence to support the glyoxalase 1 gene (GLO1) as a risk gene of autism in Han Chinese patients from Taiwan.* Prog Neuropsychopharmacol Biol Psychiatry, 2008. 32(7): p. 1740-4.
Rehnstrom, K., et al., *No association between common variants in glyoxalase 1 and autism spectrum disorders.* Am J Med Genet B Neuropsychiatr Genet, 2008. 147B(1): p. 124-7.
Coon, H., et al., *Possible association between autism and variants in the brain-expressed tryptophan hydroxylase gene (TPH2).* Am J Med Genet B Neuropsychiatr Genet, 2005. 135B(1): p. 42-6.
Ramoz, N., et al., *Family-based association study of TPH1 and TPH2 polymorphisms in autism.* Am J Med Genet B Neuropsychiatr Genet, 2006. 141B(8): p. 861-7.
Goffinet, A.M., *Events governing organization of postmigratory neurons: studies on brain development in normal and reeler mice.* Brain Res, 1984. 319(3): p. 261-96.

Goffinet, A.M., *The embryonic development of the cerebellum in normal and reeler mutant mice.* Anat Embryol (Berl), 1983. 168(1): p. 73-86.
Goffinet, A.M., *The embryonic development of the inferior olivary complex in normal and reeler (rlORL) mutant mice.* J Comp Neurol, 1983. 219(1): p. 10-24.
D'Arcangelo, G., et al., *A protein related to extracellular matrix proteins deleted in the mouse mutant reeler.* Nature, 1995. 374(6524): p. 719-23.
Del, R.J., et al., *A role for Cajal-Retzius cells and reelin in the development of hippocampal connections.* Nature, 1997. 385(6611): p. 70-4.
Curran, T. and G. D'Arcangelo, *Role of reelin in the control of brain development.* Brain Res Brain Res Rev, 1998. 26(2-3): p. 285-94.
Bailey, A., et al., *A clinicopathological study of autism.* Brain, 1998. 121 (Pt 5): p. 889-905. Fatemi, S.H., et al., *Dysregulation of Reelin and Bcl-2 proteins in autistic cerebellum.* J Autism Dev Disord, 2001. 31(6): p. 529-35.
Fatemi, S.H., J.M. Stary and E.A. Egan, *Reduced blood levels of reelin as a vulnerability factor in pathophysiology of autistic disorder.* Cell Mol Neurobiol, 2002. 22(2): p. 139-52.
Fatemi, S.H., et al., *Reelin signaling is impaired in autism.* Biol Psychiatry, 2005. 57(7): p. 777-87.
Scherer, S.W., et al., *Human chromosome 7: DNA sequence and biology.* Science, 2003. 300(5620): p. 767-72.
Ramamoorthy, S., et al., *Antidepressant- and cocaine-sensitive human serotonin transporter: molecular cloning, expression, and chromosomal localization.* Proc Natl Acad Sci U S A, 1993. 90(6): p. 2542-6.
Kim, S.J., et al., *Transmission disequilibrium mapping at the serotonin transporter gene (SLC6A4) region in autistic disorder.* Mol Psychiatry, 2002. 7(3): p. 278-88.
McDougle, C.J., et al., *A double-blind, placebo-controlled study of fluvoxamine in adults with autistic disorder.* Arch Gen Psychiatry, 1996. 53(11): p. 1001-8.
Guhathakurta, S., et al., *Serotonin transporter promoter variants: Analysis in Indian autistic and control population.* Brain Res, 2006. 1092(1): p. 28-35.
Jr Cook, E., et al., *Linkage-disequilibrium mapping of autistic disorder, with 15q11-13 markers.* Am J Hum Genet, 1998. 62(5): p. 1077-83.
Lucht, M.J., et al., *Associations between the oxytocin receptor gene (OXTR) and affect, loneliness and intelligence in normal subjects.* Prog Neuropsychopharmacol Biol Psychiatry, 2009. 33(5): p. 860-6.
Yamasue, H., et al., *Oxytocin, sexually dimorphic features of the social brain, and autism.* Psychiatry Clin Neurosci, 2009. 63(2): p. 129-40.
Green, J.J. and E. Hollander, *Autism and oxytocin: new developments in translational approaches to therapeutics.* Neurotherapeutics, 2010. 7(3): p. 250-7.
Powell, E.M., W.M. Mars and P. Levitt, *Hepatocyte growth factor/scatter factor is a motogen for interneurons migrating from the ventral to dorsal telencephalon.* Neuron, 2001. 30(1): p. 79-89.
Streit, A.C. and C.D. Stern, *Competence for neural induction: HGF/SF, HGF1/MSP and the c-Met receptor.* Ciba Found Symp, 1997. 212: p. 155-65; discussion 165-8.
Park, M., et al., *Mechanism of met oncogene activation.* Cell, 1986. 45(6): p. 895-904. Levitt, P., K.L. Eagleson and E.M. Powell, *Regulation of neocortical interneuron development and the implications for neurodevelopmental disorders.* Trends Neurosci, 2004. 27(7): p. 400-6.
Campbell, D.B., et al., *Disruption of cerebral cortex MET signaling in autism spectrum disorder.* Ann Neurol, 2007. 62(3): p. 243-50.
Del, A.A. and J. Satrustegui, *Molecular cloning of Aralar, a new member of the mitochondrial*

carrier superfamily that binds calcium and is present in human muscle and brain. J Biol Chem, 1998. 273(36): p. 23327-34.

Filipek, P.A., et al., *Mitochondrial dysfunction in autistic patients with 15q inverted duplication.* Ann Neurol, 2003. 53(6): p. 801-4.

Shimizu, E., et al., *NMDA receptor-dependent synaptic reinforcement as a crucial process for memory consolidation.* Science, 2000. 290(5494): p. 1170-4.

Burbach, J.P. and B. van der Zwaag, *Contact in the genetics of autism and schizophrenia.* Trends Neurosci, 2009. 32(2): p. 69-72.

Beversdorf, D.Q., et al., *Timing of prenatal stressors and autism.* J Autism Dev Disord, 2005. 35(4): p. 471-8.

Meyer, U., et al., *The time of prenatal immune challenge determines the specificity of inflammation-mediated brain and behavioral pathology.* J Neurosci, 2006. 26(18): p. 4752- 62.

Ploeger, A., et al., *The association between autism and errors in early embryogenesis: what is the causal mechanism?.* Biol Psychiatry, 2010. 67(7): p. 602-7.

Stromland, K., et al., *Autism in thalidomide embryopathy: a population study.* Dev Med Child Neurol, 1994. 36(4): p. 351-6.

Williams, G., et al., *Fetal valproate syndrome and autism: additional evidence of an association.* Dev Med Child Neurol, 2001. 43(3): p. 202-6.

Rasalam, A.D., et al., *Characteristics of fetal anticonvulsant syndrome associated autistic disorder.* Dev Med Child Neurol, 2005. 47(8): p. 551-5.

Kannan, S., et al., *Decreased cortical serotonin in neonatal rabbits exposed to endotoxin in utero.* J Cereb Blood Flow Metab, 2010.

Girard, S., et al., *IL-1 receptor antagonist protects against placental and neurodevelopmental defects induced by maternal inflammation.* J Immunol, 2010. 184(7): p. 3997-4005.

Wilkerson, D.S., et al., *Perinatal complications as predictors of infantile autism.* Int J Neurosci, 2002. 112(9): p. 1085-98.

Palmer, R.F., et al., *Environmental mercury release, special education rates, and autism disorder: an ecological study of Texas.* Health Place, 2006. 12(2): p. 203-9.

Windham, G.C., et al., *Autism spectrum disorders in relation to distribution of hazardous air pollutants in the san francisco bay area.* Environ Health Perspect, 2006. 114(9): p. 1438- 44.

Geier, D.A. and M.R. Geier, *A prospective study of mercury toxicity biomarkers in autistic spectrum disorders.* J Toxicol Environ Health A, 2007. 70(20): p. 1723-30.

Geier, D.A., et al., *A comprehensive review of mercury provoked autism.* Indian J Med Res, 2008. 128(4): p. 383-411.

Geier, D.A., et al., *Blood mercury levels in autism spectrum disorder: Is there a threshold level?.* Acta Neurobiol Exp (Wars), 2010. 70(2): p. 177-86.

Ip, P., et al., *Mercury exposure in children with autistic spectrum disorder: case-control study.* J Child Neurol, 2004. 19(6): p. 431-4.

Eppright, T.D., J.A. Sanfacon and E.A. Horwitz, *Attention deficit hyperactivity disorder, infantile autism, and elevated blood-lead: a possible relationship.* Mo Med, 1996. 93(3): p. 136-8.

Canfield, R.L., et al., *Intellectual impairment in children with blood lead concentrations below 10 microg per deciliter.* N Engl J Med, 2003. 348(16): p. 1517-26.

Yorbik, O., et al., *Chromium, cadmium, and lead levels in urine of children with autism and typically developing controls.* Biol Trace Elem Res, 2010. 135(1-3): p. 10-5.

Kalkbrenner, A.E., et al., *Perinatal exposure to hazardous air pollutants and autism spectrum disorders at age 8.* Epidemiology, 2010. 21(5): p. 631-41.

Moy, S.S. and J.J. Nadler, *Advances in behavioral genetics: mouse models of autism.* Mol Psychiatry, 2008. 13(1): p. 4-26.

Mineur, Y.S., L.X. Huynh and W.E. Crusio, *Social behavior deficits in the Fmr1 mutant mouse.* Behav Brain Res, 2006. 168(1): p. 172-5.

Zoghbi, H.Y., *MeCP2 dysfunction in humans and mice.* J Child Neurol, 2005. 20(9): p. 736-40.

Kuemerle, B., et al., *The mouse Engrailed genes: a window into autism.* Behav Brain Res, 2007. 176(1): p. 121-32.

Cheh, M.A., et al., *En2 knockout mice display neurobehavioral and neurochemical alterations relevant to autism spectrum disorder.* Brain Res, 2006. 1116(1): p. 166-76.

Andres, C., *Molecular genetics and animal models in autistic disorder.* Brain Res Bull, 2002. 57(1): p. 109-19.

Brodkin, E.S., *BALB/c mice: low sociability and other phenotypes that may be relevant to autism.* Behav Brain Res, 2007. 176(1): p. 53-65.

Brodkin, E.S., et al., *Social approach-avoidance behavior of inbred mouse strains towards DBA/2 mice.* Brain Res, 2004. 1002(1-2): p. 151-7.

Moy, S.S., et al., *Sociability and preference for social novelty in five inbred strains: an approach to assess autistic-like behavior in mice.* Genes Brain Behav, 2004. 3(5): p. 287- 302.

Yang, M., A.M. Clarke and J.N. Crawley, *Postnatal lesion evidence against a primary role for the corpus callosum in mouse sociability.* Eur J Neurosci, 2009. 29(8): p. 1663-77.

Wahlsten, D., P. Metten and J.C. Crabbe, *Survey of 21 inbred mouse strains in two laboratories reveals that BTBR T/+ tf/tf has severely reduced hippocampal commissure and absent corpus callosum.* Brain Res, 2003. 971(1): p. 47-54.

Kusek, G.K., et al., *Localization of two new X-linked quantitative trait loci controlling corpus callosum size in the mouse.* Genes Brain Behav, 2007. 6(4): p. 359-63.

MacPherson, P., et al., *Impaired fear memory, altered object memory and modified hippocampal synaptic plasticity in split-brain mice.* Brain Res, 2008. 1210: p. 179-88.

Hudkins, K.L., et al., *BTBR Ob/Ob mutant mice model progressive diabetic nephropathy.* J Am Soc Nephrol, 2010. 21(9): p. 1533-42.

Flowers, J.B., et al., *Abdominal obesity in BTBR male mice is associated with peripheral but not hepatic insulin resistance.* Am J Physiol Endocrinol Metab, 2007. 292(3): p. E936- 45.

Lan, H., et al., *Distinguishing covariation from causation in diabetes: a lesson from the protein disulfide isomerase mRNA abundance trait.* Diabetes, 2004. 53(1): p. 240-4.

Nadler, S.T., et al., *Normal Akt/PKB with reduced PI3K activation in insulin-resistant mice.* Am J Physiol Endocrinol Metab, 2001. 281(6): p. E1249-54.

Stoehr, J.P., et al., *Genetic obesity unmasks nonlinear interactions between murine type 2 diabetes susceptibility loci.* Diabetes, 2000. 49(11): p. 1946-54.

Ranheim, T., et al., *Interaction between BTBR and C57BL/6J genomes produces an insulin resistance syndrome in (BTBR x C57BL/6J) F1 mice.* Arterioscler Thromb Vasc Biol, 1997. 17(11): p. 3286-93.

Gersting, S.W., et al., *Pahenu1 is a mouse model for tetrahydrobiopterin-responsive phenylalanine hydroxylase deficiency and promotes analysis of the pharmacological chaperone mechanism in vivo.* Hum Mol Genet, 2010. 19(10): p. 2039-49.

Martynyuk, A.E., et al., *Epilepsy in phenylketonuria: a complex dependence on serum phenylalanine levels.* Epilepsia, 2007. 48(6): p. 1143-50.

Ercal, N., et al., *Oxidative stress in a phenylketonuria animal model.* Free Radic Biol Med, 2002. 32(9): p. 906-11.

McDonald, J.D., *Postnatal growth in a mouse genetic model of classical phenylketonuria.* Contemp Top Lab Anim Sci, 2000. 39(6): p. 54-6.

Sarkissian, C.N., et al., *A heteroallelic mutant mouse model: A new orthologue for human hyperphenylalaninemia.* Mol Genet Metab, 2000. 69(3): p. 188-94.

Zagreda, L., et al., *Cognitive deficits in a genetic mouse model of the most common biochemical cause of human mental retardation.* J Neurosci, 1999. 19(14): p. 6175-82.

Pobbe, R.L., et al., *General and social anxiety in the BTBR T+ tf/J mouse strain.* Behav Brain Res, 2010.

Pobbe, R.L., et al., *Expression of social behaviors of C57BL/6J versus BTBR inbred mouse strains in the visible burrow system.* Behav Brain Res, 2010. 214(2): p. 443-9.

Wohr, M., F.I. Roullet and J.N. Crawley, *Reduced scent marking and ultrasonic vocalizations in the BTBR T+tf/J mouse model of autism.* Genes Brain Behav, 2010.

Roullet, F.I., M. Wohr and J.N. Crawley, *Female urine-induced male mice ultrasonic vocalizations, but not scent-marking, is modulated by social experience.* Behav Brain Res, 2010.

Scattoni, M.L., L. Ricceri and J.N. Crawley, *Unusual repertoire of vocalizations in adult BTBR T+tf/J mice during three types of social encounters.* Genes Brain Behav, 2010.

Pearson, B.L., et al., *Motor and cognitive stereotypies in the BTBR T+tf/J mouse model of autism.* Genes Brain Behav, 2010.

McFarlane, H.G., et al., *Autism-like behavioral phenotypes in BTBR T+tf/J mice.* Genes Brain Behav, 2008. 7(2): p. 152-63.

Moy, S.S., et al., *Mouse behavioral tasks relevant to autism: phenotypes of 10 inbred strains.* Behav Brain Res, 2007. 176(1): p. 4-20.

Silverman, J.L., et al., *Low stress reactivity and neuroendocrine factors in the BTBR T(+)tf/J mouse model of autism.* Neuroscience, 2010.

Frye, C.A. and D.C. Llaneza, *Corticosteroid and neurosteroid dysregulation in an animal model of autism, BTBR mice.* Physiol Behav, 2010. 100(3): p. 264-7.

Chadman, K.K., *Fluoxetine but not risperidone increases sociability in the BTBR mouse model of autism.* Pharmacol Biochem Behav, 2010.

Gould, G.G., et al., *Density and Function of Central Serotonin (5-HT) Transporters, 5-HT(1A) and 5-HT(2A) Receptors, and Effects of their Targeting on BTBR T+tf/J Mouse Social Behavior.* J Neurochem, 2010.

Silverman, J.L., et al., *Repetitive self-grooming behavior in the BTBR mouse model of autism is blocked by the mGluR5 antagonist MPEP.* Neuropsychopharmacology, 2010. 35(4): p. 976-89.

Yang, M., et al., *Social peers rescue autism-relevant sociability deficits in adolescent mice.* Autism Res, 2010.

Yang, M., V. Zhodzishsky and J.N. Crawley, *Social deficits in BTBR T+tf/J mice are unchanged by cross-fostering with C57BL/6J mothers.* Int J Dev Neurosci, 2007. 25(8): p. 515-21.

Crawley, J.N., *Designing mouse behavioral tasks relevant to autistic-like behaviors.* Ment Retard Dev Disabil Res Rev, 2004. 10(4): p. 248-58.

Permissions

All chapters in this book were first published by InTech Open; hereby published with permission under the Creative Commons Attribution License or equivalent. Every chapter published in this book has been scrutinized by our experts. Their significance has been extensively debated. The topics covered herein carry significant findings which will fuel the growth of the discipline. They may even be implemented as practical applications or may be referred to as a beginning point for another development.

The contributors of this book come from diverse backgrounds, making this book a truly international effort. This book will bring forth new frontiers with its revolutionizing research information and detailed analysis of the nascent developments around the world.

We would like to thank all the contributing authors for lending their expertise to make the book truly unique. They have played a crucial role in the development of this book. Without their invaluable contributions this book wouldn't have been possible. They have made vital efforts to compile up to date information on the varied aspects of this subject to make this book a valuable addition to the collection of many professionals and students.

This book was conceptualized with the vision of imparting up-to-date information and advanced data in this field. To ensure the same, a matchless editorial board was set up. Every individual on the board went through rigorous rounds of assessment to prove their worth. After which they invested a large part of their time researching and compiling the most relevant data for our readers.

The editorial board has been involved in producing this book since its inception. They have spent rigorous hours researching and exploring the diverse topics which have resulted in the successful publishing of this book. They have passed on their knowledge of decades through this book. To expedite this challenging task, the publisher supported the team at every step. A small team of assistant editors was also appointed to further simplify the editing procedure and attain best results for the readers.

Apart from the editorial board, the designing team has also invested a significant amount of their time in understanding the subject and creating the most relevant covers. They scrutinized every image to scout for the most suitable representation of the subject and create an appropriate cover for the book.

The publishing team has been an ardent support to the editorial, designing and production team. Their endless efforts to recruit the best for this project, has resulted in the accomplishment of this book. They are a veteran in the field of academics and their pool of knowledge is as vast as their experience in printing. Their expertise and guidance has proved useful at every step. Their uncompromising quality standards have made this book an exceptional effort. Their encouragement from time to time has been an inspiration for everyone.

The publisher and the editorial board hope that this book will prove to be a valuable piece of knowledge for researchers, students, practitioners and scholars across the globe.

List of Contributors

Hiroshi Tanaka
Department of School Health Science, Faculty of Education Hirosaki University, Japan
Department of Pediatrics, Hirosaki University Hospital, Japan

Tadaatsu Imaizumi
Department of Vascular Biology, Hirosaki University Graduate School of Medicine, Japan

Konstantina G. Yiannopoulou
Neurological Department, Laiko General Hospital of Athens, Greece

Jagat R. Kanwar, Bhasker Sriramoju and Rupinder K. Kanwar
Laboratory of Immunology and Molecular Biomedical Research (LIMBR), Centre for Biotechnology and Interdisciplinary Biosciences (BioDeakin), Institute for Technology in Nanomedicine & Research Innovation, Deakin University Waurn Ponds, Geelong, Australia

James Crooks and Bruno Gran
University of Nottingham, United Kingdom

Ewa Robak and Tadeusz Robak
Medical University of Lodz, Poland

Soyoung Lee, Satoshi Serada, Minoru Fujimoto and Tetsuji Naka
National Institute of Biomedical Innovation, Laboratory of Immune Signal, Japan

Adrienn Angyal and Gabriella Sarmay
Dept. of Immunology, Eotvos Lorand University, Budapest, Hungary

Jozsef Prechl
Immunology Research Group of the Hungarian Academy of Sciences, at Eotvos Lorand University, Budapest, Hungary

Gyorgy Nagy
Buda Hospital of Hospitaller Brothers of St. John, Budapest, Hungary

Elisabetta L. Romeo, Giuseppina T. Russo, Annalisa Giandalia, Provvidenza Villari, Angela A. Mirto, Giuseppa Perdichizzi and Domenico Cucinotta
Department of Internal Medicine, University of Messina, Messina, Italy

Mariapaola Cucinotta
Section of Nuclear Medicine, Department of Radiology, University of Messina, Messina, Italy

Guang-Xian Zhang
Thomas Jefferson University, Philadelphia, USA

Elena Puertollano, María A. Puertollano, Gerardo Álvarez de Cienfuegos and Manuel A. de Pablo
University of Jaén, Faculty of Experimental Sciences, Div. of Microbiology Jaén, Spain

David I. Stott and Donna McIntyre
Institute of Infection, Immunity & Inflammation, University of Glasgow, Glasgow, Scotland, U.K.

Xiaohong Li and Hua Zou
New York State Institute for Basic Research in Developmental Disabilities, USA

Index

Printed in the USA
CPSIA information can be obtained
at www.ICGtesting.com
JSHW061339150424
61201JS00005B/74

9 781639 279067